T0214393

Advances in Prevention Science

The emergent field of prevention science focuses on the application of theories derived from epidemiologic studies, human development, human behavior, genetics, and neuroscience to develop and evaluate cognitive and behavioral interventions. Research over the past two decades has dramatically changed the impact that preventive interventions have had on a number of problem behaviors including substance use and abuse, sexually transmitted infections including HIV and AIDS, violence and injuries, juvenile delinquency, academic failure, obesity, and even lifestyle-related diseases such as hypertension and cardiovascular disorders, cancer, and diabetes.

This book series was conceived to summarize our accumulated knowledge to date and its application to practice. In addition, the series provides suggestions for both short- and long-term research. Having moved forward knowledge about these social and health areas and how to prevent them with various degrees of success, the editors and authors of the series wish to make these findings available to researchers, practitioners, policy makers, social science students, and the public.

More information about this series at http://www.springer.com/series/8822

Kris Bosworth
Editor

Prevention Science in School Settings

Complex Relationships and Processes

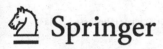 Springer

Editor
Kris Bosworth
College of Education
University of Arizona
Tucson
Arizona
USA

Advances in Prevention Science
ISBN 978-1-4939-4995-3   ISBN 978-1-4939-3155-2 (eBook)
DOI 10.1007/978-1-4939-3155-2

Springer Science+Business Media LLC New York is part of Springer Science+Business Media
(www.springer.com)

Foreword

My entire academic career has focused on adolescent health, and for much of that time, my research has addressed one central question: "Why do young people raised in the most adverse conditions do well?" It was never a mystery to me why they did poorly, but what protects so many who grow up in violent homes and communities?

As a pediatrician, I was always convinced that family was central; however, many who live with adversity, do not have parents, perhaps as a consequence of death, divorce, incarceration, or addiction. What about them? What protects them?

In the mid-1990s, we began to get a glimpse of the answer. Through the National Longitudinal Study of Adolescent Health (or Add Health for short), we saw that, second only to parents, school was the single most protective force in the lives of young people. The protective effect of school was not solely through expanding educational horizons and long-term options (though they certainly make a difference), but in addition, the effects were on the short-term health and risk behaviors as well, and the protective factors were not reserved just for educational achievers.

Simply stated, we saw that adult connections in school were associated with better outcomes for every health risk behavior we studied. There was a strong inverse correlation between alcohol, tobacco, and marijuana use and school connectedness. So too, the same inverse relationship was seen between emotional distress (depression, suicidal thoughts, and attempts) and interpersonal violence, deviant behavior (i.e., shoplifting), and pregnancy. For example, where school connectedness was at the lowest level, about 19% of 11th and 12th grade girls reported ever having been pregnant. When it was at its highest level, it was 0.1%. It was clear that young people who were in school environments where they felt connected, they were also less likely than peers to participate in a range of health-compromising behaviors, and central to school connectedness was teacher support (and while we did not measure it, I suspect this would be true for other adults as well). When young people felt that teacher support was high, not only were they less likely to participate in health-compromising behaviors but they were less likely than peers to initiate such behaviors over time as well.

Let me give a few examples. When school connectedness was reported to be high, 3.2% of students surveyed transitioned to getting drunk regularly over a 1 year period of time; where it was low, it was nearly twice that figure, at 6.2%. The same was seen with marijuana: transition to regular use over a year period of time was 4.8%, but it was 2.6% when connectedness was high. Suicide attempts were half as likely among connected than nonconnected teens, and teacher support was associated with significantly less involvement with violence as well.

These findings are not about pregnancy or drug abuse or violence prevention programs per se. Where high-quality programs exist, they are unquestionably valuable. But these findings are about creating a school climate where expectations for achievement are as high as the supports provided to students.

But how do we take these data to implementation? The present volume takes us down that path. It takes us beyond health education in schools to health-promoting schools. It takes a wide-angle lens to schools as a critical forum that can improve the health and well-being of all children and youth. As Sect. 4 of the book underscores, there are strong connections between education and prevention science. So too, health and education are inexorably linked.

Because the effects of school are multidimensional, the needs are for multidisciplinary engagement and collaboration. As such, this volume is as valuable for the health educator as it is for the prevention scientist. It provides the prevention scientist the tools and perspectives to develop effective collaborations with schools, and it provides the educator the understanding of where education and prevention science goals overlap. It is as critical a read for child health providers as it is for educators, for it provides each the understandings into each other's worlds. We talk about breaking down silos but few actually do it. This book is about children, not professional domains. It provides critically important lessons and perspectives for all who are interested in the health and well-being of America's children.

Schools are the cornerstone of our children's health and well-being. As we must provide families what they need to support their children, we must provide America's schools the tools and resources to excel. This book significantly contributes to that toolbox. Our children deserve nothing less. As I noted previously, second only to parents, schools have the potential for the protection of young people from health-compromising behaviors while concurrently expanding horizons and improving life options.

August, 2014   Robert W. Blum, MD, MPH, PhD
                                                            William H. Gates
                                                          Sr. Professor and Chair
                                                       Johns Hopkins University

Preface

> *If schools are to succeed in their educational mission, the threat of drug use and abuse must be recognized and effective preventive interventions implemented. (Bukoski, 1986, p. 112)*

Prevention science refers to programming to deter adolescents from engaging in a variety of risk behaviors, from use of alcohol, tobacco, and other drugs (ATOD) to suicide, dropping out of school, and violence. Prevention researchers have hailed from a variety of fields—primarily medicine, public health, social work, and psychology—almost any field but education. Yet, the most efficient venue to reach the target audience of adolescents, who may be engaging in risky behavior, is and always has been in schools.

Historically, prevention programs have been separate curricula designed to be delivered outside the "regular" curricula in a school. These curricula are written by researchers with little or no experience in the day-to-day operations of elementary or secondary schools. These interventions are intended for delivery by teachers who have little knowledge of the principles of prevention. The result is a long-standing disconnect that has curtailed the potential success of prevention programming and has diminished opportunities for thousands of adolescents to have the prevention information and skills they need to make healthy lifestyles choices.

Prevention Science in School Settings takes a unique perspective on the history and current practice of prevention science. This volume is designed to provide both prevention researchers and educators with perspectives on the role of schools and educators in the practice of prevention. Additionally, educators can learn more about the principles of prevention science to have a deeper understanding of how the integration of prevention science into existing school structures can meet educators' goals for academic success and a positive culture. This volume has several unique features. First, authors in this volume are respected researchers and practitioners from both education and prevention research. Another feature is that in each chapter, research is supplemented with anecdotes and case studies, illustrating the practice and pitfalls of prevention, putting a practical, real-world spin on the theory that is presented. Third, the majority of seasoned prevention professionals usually focus on one target field or issue—such as curbing drug abuse, bullying, suicide, or dropping out—the present volume encompasses all of these concerns and how they can be addressed within a school setting. Nowhere else can both educators and prevention professionals, with an interest in school-based interventions, and education professionals, with interest in prevention, find such a comprehensive overview of the history and current practice of the prevention field, along with opportunities for cross-disciplinary collaboration.

The major aim of this volume is to build capacity in both prevention specialists and researcher and educators at the intersection of their interests. An underlying theme in the chapters is the opportunities to improve effectiveness of prevention programming through integrating prevention with educational goals and resources and opportunities to improve educational outcomes by engaging with prevention research and practice. The contributing authors explore both educational policy and prevention practices from 1970 to the present and offer some predictions for how prevention science might position itself in the next decades. The four sections address:

1. Setting the context for school-based prevention
2. Prevention science: Origins and evolution of practice
3. Research in and with schools: Toward productive prevention partnerships
4. School-based prevention: Protective schools at work

In Chap. 1, Bosworth discusses the parallel tracks of prevention and education and addresses some opportunities for a deepening relationship between the two disciplines. In the first chapter of the section on setting the context, Sugimoto and Carter outline the history, the stresses, and the accomplishments in the American education system from 1970 to the present. They frame their discussion in terms of the various discourses that are present and the challenges that educators are facing within the school context. In Chap. 3, Bosworth, Pena, and Judkins describe the various levels of leadership within American schools, ranging from the role of the school board and setting policy to the leadership standards for superintendents and principals. Nitza, Fineran, and Dobias, in Chap. 4, describe the impact of school counselors in schools and the opportunities for counselors to be key actors in prevention programming and activities. Dana and Hooser, in Chap. 5, use a case study of a hypothetical teacher to outline the responsibilities and stresses that typical teachers face in the twenty-first-century classroom. The chapter identifies opportunities for engaging teachers in prevention activities as well as a description of how teachers, in their daily interaction with students, become the "frontline" prevention workers. In Chap. 6, the final chapter in this section, Diane Allensworth describes the role of health education and health services, including nurses, school clinic in the schools, and where the interface is with the work of prevention.

The second section focuses on the origin and evolution of prevention science. In Chap. 7, Bosworth and Sloboda describe the history of activities built on expertise, theories, and strategies from diverse theoretical and disciplinary perspectives, such as social work, medicine, and psychology, melded together into a body of knowledge and theories that can be called prevention science. A discussion of curriculum development, which is the main approach that traditionally has been used in schools, is documented by Hecht and Pettigrew in Chap. 8. In Chap. 9, Rohrbach and Dyal describe dilemmas and challenges of scaling up evidence-based prevention programming.

Research that documents the epidemiology of various risk-taking behaviors and evaluation research form the heart of prevention science. The majority of these studies are conducted in schools, so this section outlines various approaches to conducting research in schools. In Chap. 10, Sullivan and colleagues discuss schools as the venues for prevention programming and offer numerous case examples providing strategies for improving data collection within a school setting via partnerships. Kendziora, Dymnicki, Faria, Windham, and Osher discuss evaluating and researching school-based prevention in Chap. 11. In Chap. 12, Debnam, Bradshaw, Pas, and Johnson examine schools as the unit of analysis and provide many case examples of strategies to enhance relationships with schools during all phases of the research process.

In the final section, some current issues are discussed to illustrate how prevention science and education partner to enhance protective factors and reduce risky behaviors. Fletcher, in Chap. 13, focuses on projects and studies that have examined school climate and culture as the main prevention intervention in contrast to implementing a specific curriculum. This chapter provides detail on three environmental change projects in Great Britain, Australia, and the United States. In Chap. 14, Newman and Dusenbury focus on a set of programs and processes that are concerned with social emotional learning (SEL). They describe the basic principles of SEL, and they highlight specific programs, curricula, and activities that support student learning in this area. Eklund, Bosworth, and Bauman, in Chap. 15, explore various aspects of school safety, including issues of discipline, bullying, and dating violence. In Chap. 16, LaFromboise and Husain identify risk factors for youth suicide and describe the relationship of other risk factors to suicide. Elaine Allensworth, in Chap. 17, describes how dropping out of high school is a public health issue because of the relationship between lower educational attainment and negative health outcomes. Thus, dropout prevention is a critical issue in schools and is possibly the area where principles of prevention and academics are most closely aligned.

Taken together, these chapters provide the background for both aspiring and seasoned prevention scientists and educators to work more effectively together in reducing risk factors and enhancing protective factors in students. Each field has its own theoretical underpinnings, political pressures, and mission. Although, at times, it may seem like they move in parallel tracks, closer examination of the themes in this volume can help identify the common ground essential to promote positive youth development and support resiliency.

Reference

Bukoski, W. J. (1986). School-based substance abuse prevention: A review of program research. *Journal of Children in Contemporary Society, 18*(1–2), 95–115. doi:10.1300/J274v18n01_06.

Acknowledgements

This volume would not be possible without the careful review and critical feedback from reviewers Raphel Garcia, Dr. Jason Hurwitz, Dr. Maryann Judkins, Nancy Kaufman, Dr. Mark Saliba, and Kathy Spicer. Editors Kirsteen Anderson and Betsy Bounds provided hours of copy editing. Sally Showalter and Jenni Schultz supported with the numerous tasks inherent in preparing a volume such as this. The support from the series editors, Dr. Zili Sloboda and Dr. Hanno Petras, and the editor at Springer, Khristina Queja, was essential.

As a young educator, I was introduced to the concept of prevention through a *Health Related Behavior Project* that the University of Wisconsin–Madison conducted under the leadership of Dr. David H. Gustafson, who became an important mentor. Since then, many professionals from both the fields of education and prevention provided invaluable guidance, vision, and support throughout my journey of linking education and prevention. These generous professionals include Jean Ajamie at the Arizona Department of Education, Dr. Joyce Epstein at Johns Hopkins, Dr. Phyllis Gingiss at the University of Houston, Dr. Robert Hawkins and Dr. D. Paul Moberg at the University of Wisconsin–Madison, Dean Ron Marx at the University of Arizona, Dr. Bill Bukoski at N.I.D.A., and Dr. Anna Ochoa-Becker at Indiana University. Arizona superintendents Calvin Baker, Dr. J. Robert Hendricks, Dr. John Pedicone, and Dr. Maria Menconi have embraced prevention as an integral part of the education within their districts and have actively explored opportunities for full partnerships between education and prevention science. The generosity of Lester and Roberta Smith to provide an endowment that has provided support for this project.

Finally, this volume could never have been completed without the support and encouragement of my family, especially my husband and partner, LaMont Schultz.

Contents

Part III   Research in and with Schools

**Part IV   Relationships Between Education and Prevention
           Science—Parallel Tracks**

Contributors

Elaine Allensworth University of Chicago Consortium on Chicago School Research, Chicago, IL, USA

Sheri Bauman School Counseling Program, University of Arizona, Tucson, AZ, USA

Kris Bosworth Department of Educational Policy and Practice, University of Arizona, Tucson, AZ, USA

Catherine P. Bradshaw Curry School of Education, University of Virginia, Charlottesville, VA, USA

Kathy Carter Teaching, Learning, and Sociocultural Studies, University of Arizona College of Education, Tucson, AZ, USA

Nancy Fichtman Dana School of Teaching and Learning, University of Florida, Gainesville, FL, USA

Katrina J. Debnam Johns Hopkins Bloomberg School of Public Health, Baltimore, MD, USA

Diane DeMuth Allensworth Kent State University, Snellville, GA, USA

Brian Dobias Indiana University–Purdue University Fort Wayne, Fort Wayne, USA

Linda Dusenbury Collaborative for Academic, Social, and Emotional Learning, Southern Pines, NC, USA

Stephanie R. Dyal Department of Preventive Medicine, University of Southern California, Los Angeles, CA, USA

Allison Dymnicki American Institutes for Research, Washington, DC, USA

Katie Eklund School Psychology Program, University of Arizona, Tucson, AZ, USA

Ann-Marie Faria American Institutes for Research, Washington, DC, USA

Albert D. Farrell Department of Psychology, Virginia Commonwealth University, Richmond, VA, USA

Kerrie R. Fineran Indiana University–Purdue University Fort Wayne, Fort Wayne, USA

Adam Fletcher DECIPHer, School of Social Sciences, Cardiff University, Cardiff, UK

Michael L. Hecht The Pennsylvania State University, State College, PA, USA

REAL Prevention, Gillette, NJ, USA

Angela Hooser Department of Teaching and Learning, University of South Florida, Tampa, FL, USA

Shadab Hussain Graduate School of Education, Standford University, Stanford, CA, USA

Sarah Lindstrom Johnson Arizona State University, Tempe, USA

Maryann Judkins Department of Educational Policy and Practice, University of Arizona, Tucson, AZ, USA

Kimberly Kendziora American Institutes for Research, Washington, DC, USA

Teresa D. LaFromboise Graduate School of Education, Standford University, Stanford, CA, USA

Jessica Newman American Institutes for Research (AIR), Chicago, IL, USA

Amy Nitza Indiana University–Purdue University Fort Wayne, Fort Wayne, USA

David Osher American Institutes for Research, Washington, DC, USA

Elise T. Pas Johns Hopkins Bloomberg School of Public Health, Baltimore, MD, USA

Tricia Pena E.C.H.O. 360 Education Consulting, Vail, AZ, USA

Jonathan Pettigrew University of Tennessee, Knoxville, TN, USA

Hugh Downs School of Human Communication, Tempe, AZ, USA

Louise A. Rohrbach Department of Preventive Medicine, University of Southern California, Los Angeles, CA, USA

Zili Sloboda Applied Prevention Science, Inc., Akron, USA

Amanda T Sugimoto Teaching, Learning, and Sociocultural Studies, University of Arizona College of Education, Tucson, AZ, USA

Terri N. Sullivan Department of Psychology, Virginia Commonwealth University, Richmond, VA, USA

Kevin S. Sutherland Special Education and Disability Policy, School of Education, Virginia Commonwealth University, Richmond, VA, USA

Katherine A. Taylor Department of Psychology, Virginia Commonwealth University, Richmond, VA, USA

Amy Windham American Institutes for Research, Washington, DC, USA

Chapter 1
Exploring the Intersection of Schooling and Prevention Science

Kris Bosworth

Over time, prevention scientists have come to recognize the value of working jointly with the education system to have a positive impact on young people's lives. Since risky behavior such as alcohol and other drug use, aggressive and disruptive behavior, poor nutrition, or premature sexual activity can disrupt the learning process, academic outcomes can be improved through attention to prevention programs or processes. This is particularly important during middle and high school.

The second decade of children's lives is critical to their development and is second only to the rapid growth in the first 2 years of their life. Simultaneously, there is sporadic and significant growth in skeletal, psychological, and cognitive systems as well as sexual maturation. Although teens generally are resistant to diseases, this rapid period of physical growth is not without its risks. These are the years when young people experiment with adult activities and roles. Often they run into difficulties because of their immature cognitive control system in their developing brain (Steinberg 2007).

Working backward from many problems and diseases in adulthood such as alcohol or drug addiction, depression, heart disease, and lung disease, many scientists have identified the habits that may lead to these conditions such as binge drinking, tobacco use, fat and sugar intake, etc. that are developed in adolescence as preventable causes of these costly adult maladies (Troumbourou et al. 2007). Assuming it is better to prevent something from happening rather than a more costly response to crises, medical professionals, scientists, and educators approach adolescence as an opportunity to divert young people from risk-taking behavior that could lead to either premature death or morbidity, or lead to the habits that are precursors of later adult onset diseases and problems.

K. Bosworth (✉)
Educational Policy and Practice, University of Arizona, 1430 E 2nd Street,
Tucson, AZ 85721, USA
e-mail: bosworthk@email.arizona.edu

© Springer Science+Business Media New York 2015   1
K. Bosworth (ed.), *Prevention Science in School Settings,*
Advances in Prevention Science, DOI 10.1007/978-1-4939-3155-2_1

Adolescents come in contact with three major social institutions during the second decade of life: family, community, and school. Each may serve as venues for addressing prevention of risky behavior. In this decade, family who have been the primary socializing entity for children take on a different role, as adolescents break away from their family to form their own personal identity.

The community always has offered options for young people such as clubs, organizations, recreational facilities, and religious organizations. Community practices such as vigilantly enforcing laws about the sale of alcohol, curfews, and expanding access to mental-health services provide clear messages to teens about unacceptable behavior and offer a more protective environment. Additionally, these community structures and the people who organize and staff them are critical role models for young people as they move into adulthood.

Next to families, schools are the most powerful protective entity for young people (Blum et al. 2002). The public school system, like no other institution in America, is charged with taking in any and all children within the community and providing them with a high-quality educational experience that will prepare them for adult citizenship. Some young people entering school come from supportive and caring homes with enormous resources, while others are born into abusive and neglectful environments. Regardless of the background, educators are charged with preparing all students to be college and career ready. The role of schools will be explored in the next section.

1.1 Educational Environment

Although schools have a major role in providing the academic skills that young people will need to pursue careers, and be informed citizens in a democracy, schools in reality provide many more opportunities to either enhance or deter the developmental process of this transition from adolescence to adulthood. Although schools as institutions are not responsible for the nation's problems with alcohol, tobacco and other drugs, depression and suicide, and violence, it is within the school that these risk-taking behaviors present themselves and become clear detractors from the primary academic mission of the public schools.

In today's educational environment of decreasing resources and increasing accountability based on a limited number of metrics (e.g., standardized test scores), schools are faced with a complex set of challenges that essentially ask the question, "How can we balance the needs of the individual student for growth and development while maintaining our integrity and role as an educational institution?"

The role that schools play in socializing students is often referred to as the *hidden curriculum*. The hidden curriculum is a term that was coined by Philip W. Jackson in 1968 in his book, *Life in Classrooms*. The hidden curriculum often results in the unintended consequences of education that are not openly taught within the school day. This includes expressions of values, norms, and beliefs that are modeled (for better or worse) in everyday interactions in classrooms and throughout the school environment. The hidden curriculum exemplifies the role that schools play in the socialization of young people. Without conscious planning, the everyday interactions in a school subtly impact students' psychosocial growth and development (Jackson, 1968).

Educators' behavior can have a negative impact on students. A coach, who bullies players regularly, not only provides a role model for inappropriate behavior, but sends the message that such behavior is acceptable in the entire school. Additionally, a student may feel that adults cannot be trusted to deal with other bullying situations between students (Cornbleth 1984). How educators react to harassment and bullying in schools is an example of how the hidden curriculum can impact adolescent development. Until the past 20 years, bullying behaviors were not recognized as a serious problem. Students were told, "Boys will be boys" when such harassing activity occurred, and for girls social exclusion was considered part of the female teen culture. As research discovered increasing numbers of detrimental effects from bullying behaviors, the values, norms, and beliefs within a school needed to change so that they were not supportive of that kind of behavior. Without the change in this hidden curriculum on bullying behavior and the reaction to it, evidence-based bullying prevention programs would be less successful. The norms, values, and belief systems of both the adults and students that supported bullying would counteract any prevention or intervention (Wang et al. 2013).

For many students, the values, norms, and beliefs expressed in the hidden curriculum are supportive of positive development. For other students, that same environment might be toxic and impede normal development. The more the students' own values and beliefs systems mirrored that of the school's, the more they felt connected to that school, and the less likely they were to experiment in risk-taking behavior (McNeely et al. 2002). This sense of connectedness has been explored in a major national study *(The Adolescent Health Study: Add Health)* which surveyed over 90,000 adolescents, following them for several years. What the researchers discovered was that students who felt connected to their school also exhibited far less negative and risk-taking behavior in all different domains, including alcohol, tobacco and other drug abuse, depression, violence, suicide, disruptive behavior, and unplanned pregnancy (Blum et al. 2002).

With the proliferation of new drugs being used by teens and increases in teen pregnancy in the 1980s and 1990s, prevention scientists developed interventions, primarily curricular, to help students make better decisions about risk-taking behavior (see Chap. 8). Schools, where the vast majority of adolescents spent a good proportion of their day, were seen as an obvious place to introduce prevention concepts into the school's educational curriculum. Not only did most teens attend school, but the educational mission of schools is a good match for use of a prevention curricula. Over time, prevention researchers and program developers sought cooperation and buy-in from educators asking them to survey students and evaluate prevention interventions. However, prevention professionals faced multifaceted challenges working in the educational environment.

1.2 Educational Priorities

Schools are complex organizations. They are funded by a mix of sources from local, state, and federal governments, as well as commercial enterprises such as sales from vending machines. Educators function at the will of local elected officials as a policy-making school board, as well as regulations from state and federal government. Many different systems within the school organization need to be understood to be able impact change. An example of a guide of the systems that directly impacts the success of a prevention intervention is the *Protective Schools Model* (Bosworth 2000). The following factors that are included in the Protective Schools Model can guide educators and preventionists in their thinking about what systems need to be considered when planning for a prevention intervention or change: Vision, school climate, leadership, academic program, research-based prevention, continuum of services, professional development, home and community relationships, funding, and resources and data to guide decision-making.

Although the primary responsibility of educators is academic success of their students, many educators identify their responsibility as developing the "whole child." Developing academic skills are only one consideration in the development of the whole child. Social-emotional learning is also essential and must be integrated and aligned with academics in every aspect of schooling including funding priorities, curriculum development, safety policies, parent and community relationships, staff professional development, and discipline policies. (Liew 2012)

Most educators especially in the middle school or high school years identify that alcohol, illegal drugs, and aggression present barriers to learning. However, educators rarely reach out to prevention scientists for assistance in dealing with behavioral issues that affect learning (Zins et al. 2007). The more pressing issues of assessment, providing services for an increasing number of special education students, technology integration, and basic teaching methods are generally the topics of professional development and topics that are presented at conferences for public school educators. In a recent survey of over 1700 teachers in seven urban and rural districts in the southwest, about 15 % identified a high need for training in health issues such as obesity and depression. Further, interest in participating in training about alcohol and other drugs was reported by 11 % of the respondents (Bosworth et al. 2011). In another study using focus groups, Finley found that teachers were looking for more training on dealing with school-based violence (2003). However, none of the participants in this study had taken the initiative to talk to administrators at either the site or district level about their concerns. In conclusion, Finley suggests that training "…should include ways to integrate conflict resolution and [teaching] methods to create a healthy school and classroom climate…" (p. 65)

1.3 Prevention Science

The prevention process is also complex. It begins with data that facilitate the understanding of the processes that lead to an adolescent experimenting with drugs or engaging in risky behavior. With a solid grounding in behavior change strategies, the program developers with advanced degrees in a discipline related to changing human behavior design an approach. This approach is tested in a limited number of settings to evaluate it with rigorous methods to determine its effectiveness. Once proven effective, the developers need to brand it, package it, and develop a marketing plan so that schools and communities can use the approach. Schools play a critical role in the gathering of the needs assessment data and in serving as sites for the pilot testing and evaluation.

Prevention scientists develop interventions in a protected greenhouse environment where conditions for randomized control trials were as close to ideal as possible. Once the effectiveness of an intervention was determined, then it needed to move out of the greenhouse into the real world, such as a windowsill in an average home. That transition was bumpy at best. To extend the plant metaphor, it is rare that a plant that is cultured and nurtured in such a protected environment as a greenhouse will survive outside of that environment without an extreme amount of care. Hence, the prevention interventions developed by psychologists, drug addiction personnel, mental health personnel, public health personnel, and others in universities or think tank settings had difficulty transitioning to a real-world public school setting. Rarely was an educator sitting at the table as an equal in the development of prevention materials, prevention curricula, or prevention strategies. Educators have often been approached by prevention researchers or developers about implementing an intervention at their site or about serving as a setting for data collection from their students. Educators may review the finished product, but rarely are involved in the needs assessment of development stages. Although most educators do not have much background in the principles of prevention, some prevention expertise exists outside the research and curriculum development communities.

There is a growing need for professionals with prevention expertise outside of research settings. In the public schools, with funds from the Title IV of the Safe and Drug Free Schools program, state and district level prevention specialists were hired to direct prevention programs in schools and local communities. People hired into these roles came from a variety of disciplines including health education, public health, nursing, counseling, social work, or other human service special training. Often, their training in prevention relied on their employer or on self-initiated knowledge seeking. The prevention science field had not yet developed enough to provide standardized certification for prevention specialists. As a result, the quality of the prevention program that could be established varied considerably across the country.

In summary, just as educators do not have an extensive knowledge of the theoretical underpinnings of prevention science, prevention scientists often approach schools with a naïve understanding or appreciation about school structures and organization or about the public pressures for accountability. The conscious development of partnerships can establish the foundation prevention interventions that are a seamless part of schools' structure.

1.4 Integration Opportunities

For many years, educators and prevention scientists were working on similar concerns about the growth and development of young people, but in parallel universes, and not connecting very effectively with each other. Few examples of partnerships in which joint decisions were made about goals and resources to increase the likelihood of healthy youth development exist.

One example of a partnership between educators and prevention researchers is the Child Development Project. In 1980, prevention researcher, Eric Schaps, formed the Developmental Studies Center. The team of educational and behavioral experts he led concentrated on developing programs and materials that could be integrated into classrooms and after-school venues. These now evidence-based programs focused on the development of community within the classroom through academic materials and processes (Battistich et al. 2000).

Although past connections between educators and prevention scientists have been tenuous, in the past decade, the interests and practices of both of these professional groups are coming together in five areas. These represent opportunities for more focused conversations and a development or uncovering of "like-mindedness." These areas include:

• Evidence-based practice
• Multiple-tiered support systems (MTSS)
• Data-based decision-making
• Health disparities/Achievement gap
• School climate and culture

1.4.1 Evidence-Based Practice

Since the inauguration of the National Institute on Drug Abuse (NIDA) as a lead actor in the prevention campaign against drug abuse, a focus of the drug abuse prevention community has been to identify practices and programs that are effective in preventing early onset or problems related to alcohol, tobacco, and other drugs. Research has focused on evaluations and randomized control trials to design and implement practices that will have assured benefits in this area. The grand plan was to create a number of evidence-based practices that a state, a school, or a community would implement with assurances that these practices would be effective. This focus on evidence-based practice grew out of a field in which many people had approaches to prevention that lacked a theoretical base or had a theoretical base (such as scare tactics) that had shown to be ineffective and in some cases, counterproductive (Bosworth and Sailes 1993).

In the education community, for decades, curriculum and teaching practice had been driven by teacher preference at the classroom level. Another influence on what was taught was relying on texts published by the major textbook publishers. There were few rigorous evaluations or randomized control trials of specific curricula or specific practices that would serve to guide teachers, principals, and curricula specialists in identifying those curricula and practices that would lead to increase levels of learning. At a similar time frame when NIDA was focusing on evaluation of prevention programs in schools, the US Department of Education was investing in more rigorous studies and evaluations of academic-oriented curriculum and practices.

In both the education arena and prevention arena, lists of model programs and effective curricula have been established. In the prevention realm, the Substance Abuse Mental Health Services Administration's (SAMSHA) National Registry for Evidence-Based Programs and Practices (NREPP) (http://www.nrepp.samhsa.gov) list and the University of Colorado Blueprints Project (http://www.colorado.edu/cspv/blueprints/) specifically focus on prevention curricula and programs from all areas. What Works Clearinghouse from the US Department of Education (http://ies.ed.gov/ncee/wwc/) focuses on educational programs and strategies that have research evidence to back their effectiveness. Included in the What Works Clearinghouse, are also several prevention programs that target school climate, discipline, and student behavior. This clearinghouse with its bank of effective interventions in both prevention and academics is an example of a resource for the possible integration of education and prevention. Educators searching for a reading intervention could be exposed to a prevention intervention that may respond to a classroom concern. Prevention scientists can find a way to connect with the most effective academic interventions and find opportunities to connect prevention strategies to academic curricula or schooling processes.

1.4.2   Multitiered Support Systems

In both prevention and education, researchers and practitioners are employing the framework of multitiered support systems (MTSS) to organize both academic and behavioral interventions. Here again, are parallel developments coming from two different disciplines. In the education realm, special education developers and researchers (Robert Horner and George Sugai at the University of Oregon) developed a multitiered system of behavioral support for all students in a school (Sugai and Horner 2002). The system known as Positive Behavior Intervention and Supports (PBIS) identified three levels of supports that were essential to smooth functioning of an education system, by providing specific behavioral supports determined by the needs of individual students. With this system in place, school climate improved and fewer students were tracked into special education. George Sugai is often quoted as saying, "Good instruction is one of our best behavioral tools and good behavior is one of our best instructional tools"(Sugai 2007).

In PBIS, (described in more detail in several chapters of this book) at the *universal level,* all students and faculty agree on three to five positively stated rules such as *Be prepared, Be responsible, Be safe,* and then the behavior manifestations of those rules are taught to all students. Students are acknowledged for following those rules, either verbally or through some token. The consequences for not following the rules are agreed upon by the faculty and administration. A team of teacher leaders and administrators monitor discipline referrals to identify problem areas such as a spike in referrals originating during the first lunch period in the cafeteria. For students who need additional behavioral supports *(targeted),* several strategies such as group work or additional adult supervision of behavior are provided. If these enhanced behavioral supports are not effective, then more individual attention and programming *(indicated)* is presented to the student. Students who reach this particular level of support might be referred to special education or to additional counseling and family work.

At the same time, PBIS was being developed targeting behavior; a similar tiered model was introduced that had a similar goal of reducing the number of students that would be funneled into special education. Response to Intervention (RTI) was also developed by special educators, specifically to provide an alternative method to identify students with learning disabilities (Hughes and Dexter 2011). The system involves *universal* screening that identifies students who require further interventions beyond standard classroom instruction. When more *intensive* interventions are provided, more assessment is needed for students for whom the supplemental interventions are not being effective. These additional assessments help to determine the core nature of the issue and to evaluate whether special education placement is appropriate. Thus it provides the three levels of support as does PBIS. Research since 2000 has demonstrated that there are academic gains in students that are participating in the entire RTI process and some indication that it does deter or circumvent special education placement (Hughes and Dexter 2011).

The early prevention professionals came from the medical and social service fields and had a treatment orientation. Many who were medically trained and actively involved in developing and implementing treatment using complex and expensive protocols saw the need to prevent people from gaining the problem in the first place. They became advocates for a focus on prevention. (Chap. 7 discusses the transition from treatment to prevention science in more detail.)

Ever since the early 1980s, the prevention field has approached prevention as a three-tiered response using similar language as currently popular in education (Coie et al. 1993). *Universal* interventions are those that are for all people, such as putting fluoride in the drinking water to prevent dental cavities. A *targeted* intervention provides support to those people with identified risk factors, but who have not yet displayed the problem behavior. To continue the dental example, children whose parents have had a lot of dental work would be checked more frequently. Finally, in *indicated* prevention intervention, low-level behavior has occurred and steps are taken to reduce the odds that either the negative or risky behavior will continue. In the dental example, filling a cavity would be an example of an indicated intervention.

Thus, both the education community and the prevention science community have as a core organizational framework a multitiered approach. Prevention scientists and practitioners can partner with schools that are interested in solving behavioral situations using the multitiered support services approach. For example, in searching for an approach to academic or organization issues, such as bullying, truancy, or disrespect, educators use prevention curriculum and materials whether or not they are evidence-based or were a good match for the problem confronting educators.

1.4.3 Data-Based Decision-Making

With the landmark educational legislation (No Child Left Behind [NCLB], 2002) educators were forced to become more data literate and to justify the educational decisions based on data. A primary source of data has been standardized testing, although many schools now use the benchmark testing from RTI, grades, and other academic indicators to identify student skill deficits and improve instruction.

Prevention scientists have been using data for decision-making as a staple in the program development and program planning process. Nationally collected data on behavior from Monitoring the Future (MTF; http://www.monitoringthefuture. org) study and from the Centers for Disease Control and Prevention (CDC) Youth Risk Behavior Surveillance System (YRBSS; http://www.cdc.gov/HealthyYouth/ yrbs/index.htm) have provided prevention researchers, as well as national, state, and local policy-makers, data for making decisions in allocation of funds, program development priorities, and other prevention-related activities. These national data sets offer the opportunity to evaluate trends and gauge program and policy success.

Although educators at all levels have become much more facile in using data for decision-making about academics, most have not developed yet the same skills in using data to deal with behavioral or safety-prevention issues. However, one of the tenants of MTSS that are gaining popularity nationwide is basing decisions based on behavioral data.

Thus, both educators and prevention scientists are becoming more skilled at collecting and evaluating data that eventually will be the source of the need for program implementation. Data about behavior can become a common language for educators and prevention professionals to facilitate partnerships for improving student lifestyles.

1.4.4 Health Disparities/Achievement Gap

In both education and prevention, it is acknowledged universally that there are different rates of risk and success related to race, ethnicity, and poverty. In the public health and prevention field, these are known as health disparities. The rates of diseases, mortality, and morbidity among ethnic minorities and people living in poverty are much higher than the rates among white, middle, and upper class people (CDC 2011). For youth, it is particularly striking in the area of suicide; where as one particular ethnic group (American Indians) have a much higher rate of suicide (Gone and Trimble 2012). It is not universally true, however, that white students are much more likely to experiment with alcohol, tobacco, and other drugs than are students of any other race or ethnicity. Yet, the health problems that lead to premature mortality and morbidity in adults such as smoking, poor diet, lack of exercise, alcohol, and other drug addictions are the preventable causes of things such as heart disease, lung disease, etc. that are costly both in terms of medical care and in terms of quality of life. These risk factors for later health issues are born in the adolescent and young adult years (Sawyer et al. 2012).

In education, the disparity and the achievements of students of color and low-income students becomes apparent quite early in all subjects (Ladson-Billings 2009). Academic achievement gaps are apparent in standardized test scores, as well as in outcomes in adolescence such high school graduation, rates, college admissions and completion, and career opportunities (Hernandez 2011). Additionally, specific preventable health conditions such as obesity are connected to achievement (Stuart et al. 2008)

The links between public health and prevention and student outcomes are informing policy in the public health community. The premier public health organization (American Public Health Association; APHA) adopted a policy identifying high school graduation as a public health issue (APHA 2010). This policy is supported by current evidence that improving graduation rates to reduce health disparities in addition to improving health in general might be a more potent strategy than investing solely in more costly medical interventions.

1.4.5   School Climate and Culture

> When we view [academic and behavioral] problems that come from the struggles of an individual student, it is an impossible problem to solve. When viewed as a problem of the design of schools as systems, they become solvable (Allensworth 2015, in this volume).

Increasingly, researchers from both education and prevention are discovering the power of the climate and culture in schools as foundational to strong academic performance and decreases in risk-taking behavior. Components of the hidden curriculum discussed earlier are found in the constructs of climate and culture. Hoy reviewed decades of research in identifying the organizational characteristics of schools that support achievement for all students regardless of their socioeconomic status (Hoy 2012). He concludes that for both elementary and secondary schools "….efficacy, trust, and academic emphasis (in the school) produce a powerful force that engenders motivation, creates optimism and, channels behavior toward the accomplishment of high academic goals (Hoy 2012, p. 86).

The effects of school climate extend to academic-related behaviors. Lee and Burkham (2003) explored the factors that influence a student's decision to drop out of school before graduation. They found that above and beyond student's individual behaviors or backgrounds, school organizational structures have strong effects on a student's decisions to drop out of school.

As discussed earlier, the Add Health study (McNeely et al. 2002) linked students' feelings of connectedness to schools as a protective factor for a myriad of teen risk-taking including alcohol, tobacco and other drug use, depression, suicide, deviant behavior, and pregnancy. For example, recent research into the dynamics of bullying has expanded to include not only student characteristics and behaviors, but an exploration to social-contextual factors. This line of inquiry has uncovered how features of the environment can mitigate or perpetuate bullying (Espelage et al. 2014). The authors report that, "A healthy school community is not hospitable to bullying behavior and other forms of aggression/violence, but building and maintaining such communities is an evolving, complex process" (p. 236).

School climate and culture offers, perhaps, the best opportunity for like-mindedness between educators and prevention scientists. Research opportunities abound as there is much more to learn about how climate influences both academics and development, as well how climate can be changed. A number of evidence-based programs and strategies, such as PBIS and other MTSS, have been developed to create and maintain positive climates. Many states have infrastructures that support various multitiered interventions. Thus, training, coaching, and support are available to support educators. The intervention and scaling-up process is another area with many unanswered research questions.

1.5 Future Issues

Because of their common interests in the healthy human growth and development, educators and prevention professionals have numerous opportunities for collaboration and partnerships. In a time of diminishing resources, pooling resources and expertise will be value-added for this country's health and future. Rapid advances in technology and neuroscience must be considered in both the future of education and prevention. These burgeoning areas offer numerous opportunities for collaborative exploration.

1.5.1 Technology

Technology offers both opportunity and challenge for education and prevention professionals. Adolescents are electronically connected via Twitter, Snapshot, Instagram, and Yik Yak. Changes in their technology move faster than researchers can learn about the impact of them within social structures. It is not clear how the technology has changed the dynamics of teen risk-taking behavior or of learning. Understanding the dynamics of technology in teen communication will require the best research.

For practitioners and program developers from both fields, the challenge is how to take advantage of the technology to improve the delivery of evidence-based curricula or programs. Additionally, technology can enhance professional development and coaching for teachers and other educators who are implementing these practices (Neiger et al. 2012).

Not only can technology enhance prevention program delivery, but technology increases the capacity for more complex analysis of data that can facilitate the understanding of the dynamics of risk and protective factors. These analytic tools can provide support for both qualitative and quantitative methods and will be essential in understanding the complex nation of the changing dynamics that result from expanding venues for communication through technology.

1.5.2   Neuroscience

Another scientific development that can change both prevention and education is the advances in neuroscience (Paus 2005). Statistics related to issues such as automobile crashes, binge drinking, and delinquency support the claim that adolescents engage in more risk-taking behavior than older people (Steinberg 2007). Advances in neuroscience allow scientists to disentangle the neurological functions that relate to risk-taking. For example, Perry and colleagues (2010) found that engaging the brain's "PFC inhibitory processes ... may reduce risk-related behaviors" (p. 124). The authors suggest that this knowledge could impact the design of effective public service announcements, the development of cognitive exercises, physical activity, or feedback control training.

Neuroscience presents a number of social and organizational opportunities for increased prevention and educational impact. Noted adolescent development researcher, Laurence Steinberg, reports that based on information from neuroimaging technology, risk-taking more often occurs when adolescents are in a group of their peers (2007).

In other neuroscience research, development neuroscientist, B.J. Casey concludes from reviewing recent human imaging and animal work that, " ...rather than trying to eliminate adolescent risk-taking behavior that has not been a successful enterprise to date, a more constructive strategy may be to provide access to risky and exciting activities under controlled settings and limit harmful risk-taking opportunities" (Casey and Jones 2010, p. 16).

A challenge for both educators and prevention scientists is twofold. First, clear communication channels must be developed between neuroscientist and prevention scientists and educators. Second, lessons from neuroscience need to be translated into educational policy and practices and implemented in settings where teens congregate.

1.5.3 Next Steps

Although educators and prevention scientists are grounded in different disciplines and paradigms, both groups of professionals have a common interest in the healthy growth and development of young people. Research and practical experience point to ways in which education and prevention can partner to create powerful research and evidence-based interventions that will support positive development. This volume provides educators an opportunity to learn from prominent prevention researchers about the processes and challenges of helping young people make healthy choices. For prevention scientists, leading educators writing in this volume describe the dynamics of the complex American educational system and provide examples of opportunities for linkages with prevention science. Both seasoned and aspiring educators and prevention scientists have the opportunity to use the information in this volume to cultivate strong partnerships that can lay the foundation for the more positive youth development.

References

American Public Health Association. (2010). Public health and education: working collaboratively across sectors to improve high school graduation as a means to eliminate health disparities. (Policy 20101). https://www.apha.org/policies-and-advocacy/public-health-policy-statements/policy-database/2014/07/09/14/35/public-health-and-education-working-collaboratively-across-sectors-to-improve-high-school-graduation.

Battistich, V., Schaps, E., Watson, M., Solomon, D., & Lewis, C. (2000). Effects of the child development project on students' drug use and other problem behaviors. *Journal of Primary Prevention, 21*(1), 75–99. doi:10.1023/A:1007057414994.

Blum, R. W., McNeely, C., & Rinehart, P. M. (2002). *Improving the odds: the untapped power of schools to improve the health of teens*. Minneapolis: Center for Adolescent Health and Development, University of Minnesota.

Bosworth, K. (2000). Protective schools: linking drug abuse prevention with student success. Tucson: Arizona Board of Regents. www.protectiveschools.org.

Bosworth, K., & Sailes, J. (1993). Content and teaching strategies in 10 selected drug abuse prevention curricula. *Journal of School Health, 63*(6), 247–253. doi:10.1111/j.1746-1561.1993.tb06134.x.

Bosworth, K., Summers, J., & Hernandez, D. (2011). Profiling teacher needs for health and drug prevention information. Report to the Tucson Values Teachers Board, Tucson, AZ.

Casey, B. J., & Jones, R. M. (2010). Neurobiology of the adolescent brain and behavior: implications for substance use disorders. *Journal of the American Academy of Child & Adolescent Psychiatry, 49*(12), 1189–1201. doi:10.1016/j.jaac.2010.08.017.

Centers for Disease Control and Prevention. (2011). CDC health disparities and inequalities report— United States, 2011. *Morbidity and Mortality Weekly Report, 60*(Suppl), 1–116.

Coie, J. D., Watt, N. E., West, S. G., Hawkins, J. D., Asarnow, J. R., Markman, H. J., Ramey, S. L., Shure, M. B., & Long, B. (1993). The science of prevention: a conceptual framework and some directions for a national research program. *American Psychologist, 48*(10), 1013–1022.

Cornbleth, C. (1984). Beyond hidden curriculum? *Journal of Curriculum Studies, 16*(1), 29–36. doi:10.1080/0022027840160105.

Espelage, D. L., Low, S. K., & Jimerson, S. R. (2014). Understanding school climate, aggression, peer victimization, and bully perpetration: Contemporary science, practice, and policy. *School psychology quarterly 29*(3), 233–237. doi: 10.1037/spq0000090

Finley, L. L. (2003). Teachers' perceptions of school violence issues: a case study. *Journal of School Violence, 2*(2), 51–66. doi: 10.1300/J202v02n02_04.

Gone, J. P., & Trimble, J. E. (2012). American Indian and Alaska Native mental health: Diverse perspectives on enduring disparities. *Annual review of clinical psychology 8*(1), 131–160. doi: 10.1146/annurev-clinpsy-032511-143127

Hernandez, D. J. (2011). How third-grade reading skills and poverty influence high school graduation. Annie E. Casey Foundation.

Hoy, W. (2012). School characteristics that make a difference for the achievement of all students: a 40-year odyssey. *Journal of Educational Administration, 50*(1), 76–97. doi: 10.1108/09578231211196078.

Hughes, C. A., & Dexter, D. D. (2011). Response to intervention: a research-based summary. *Theory Into Practice, 50*(1), 4–11.

Jackson, P.W. (1968). *Life in classrooms*. New York: Holt, Rinehart, and Winston.

Ladson-Billings, G. (2009). *The dreamkeepers*. San Francisco: Jossey-Bass.

Lee, V. E., & Burkam, D. T. (2003). Dropping out of high school: The role of school organization and structure. *American Educational Research Journal, 40*(2), 353–393. doi: 10.3102/00028312040002353.

Liew, J. (2012). Effortful control, executive functions, and education: Bringing self-regulatory and social-emotional competencies to the table. *Child Development Perspectives, 6*(2), 105–111. doi: 10.1111/j.1750-8606.2011.00196.x.

McNeely, C. A., Nonnemaker, J. M., & Blum, R. W. (2002). Promoting school connectedness: Evidence from the national longitudinal study of adolescent health. *Journal of School Health, 72*(4), 138–146.

Neiger, B. L. Thackeray, R. & Van Wagen, S. A. (2012). Use of social media in health promotion: purposes, key performance indicators, and evaluation metrics. *Health promotion practice* 13(2), 159–164. doi: 10.1177/1524839911433467

No Child Left Behind (NCLB) Act of 2001, Pub. L. No. 107–110, § 115, Stat. 1425 (2002).

Paus, T. (2005). Mapping brain maturation and cognitive development during adolescence. *Trends in Cognitive Sciences, 9*(2), 60–68. doi:10.1016/j.tics.2004.12.008.

Perry J. L., Joseph J. E., Jiang Y., Zimmerman R. S., Kelly T. H., Darna M., Huettl P., Dwoskin L. P., & Bardo M. T. (2010). Prefrontal cortex and drug abuse vulnerability: Translation to prevention and treatment interventions. *Brain Research Review, 65*(2), 124–149. doi: 10.1016/j.brainresrev.2010.09.001.

Sawyer, S. M., Afift, R. A., Bearinger, L. H., Blackemore, S. Dick, B., Ezeh, A. C., & Patton, G. C. (2012). Adolescence: A foundation for future health. *Lancet, 379*, 1630–1640. doi:10.1016/S0140-6736(12)60072-5

Steinberg, L. (2007). Risk taking in adolescence new perspectives from brain and behavioral science. *Current Directions in Psychological Science, 16*(2), 55–59. doi: 10.1111/j.1467-8721.2007.00475.x.

Stuart, S., Sachs, M., Lidicker, J., Brett, S., Wright, A., Libonati, J. (2008). Decreased scholastic achievement in overweight middle school students. *Obesity, 16*(7), 1535–1538.

Sugai, G. (2007). *Beyond classroom management: school-based mental health and positive behavior support*. (PowerPoint Slides). Presented at University of Connecticut. https://www.pbis.org/resource/124/beyond-classroom-management-school-based-mental-health-and-positive-behavior-support-inside-schoolhouse-door-conference.

Sugai, G., & Horner, R. (2002). The evolution of discipline practices: School-wide positive behavior supports. *Child & Family Behavior Therapy, 24*(1–2), 23–50.

Toumbourou, J. W., Stockwell, T., Neighbors, C., Marlatt, G. A., Sturge, J., & Rehm, J. (2007). Interventions to reduce harm associated with adolescent substance use. *The Lancet, 369*(9570), 1391–1401. doi: 10.1016/S0140-6736(07)60369-9.

Wang, C., Berry, B., & Swearer, S. M. (2013). The critical role of school climate in effective bullying prevention. *Theory Into Practice, 52*(4), 296–302.

Zins, J. E., Bloodworth, M. R., Weissberg, R. P., & Walberg, H. J. (2007). The scientific base linking social and emotional learning to school success. *Journal of Educational and Psychological Consultation, 17*(2–3), 191–210. doi: 10.1080/10474410701413145.

Part I
How Schools Work

Chapter 2
The Story of Schools, Schooling, and Students from the 1960s to the Present

Amanda T Sugimoto and Kathy Carter

Stories have the power to direct and change our lives.
Nell Noddings (1991, p. 157)

Originally, public education consisted of a highly localized school or set of schools that was governed and shaped by the community it served (Spring 2011). As America grew and expanded, so did the role of public education. Horace Mann envisioned the common school as a means to ensure an equal education for all students in order to transmit common cultural and moral ideals (Spring 2011).

Over time, schools became positioned as the panacea for multiple social ills, for example, poverty, inadequately prepared workers, racial inequality, and global economic shortcomings. Currently, the ideal of the common school has been replaced with the vision of market-based, business models of schools and schooling (Ravitch 2013). Given these historical policy shifts, do the diverse institutional narratives diverge from students' lives or converge with them to effect positive changes in their personal and school-based narratives, particularly with regard to their social, emotional, mental, and physical development?

Every day, students and teachers are creating and changing their individual stories within classrooms and schools throughout the country. Concomitantly, institutional narratives, as defined by national funding mandates, policy directives, and federally commissioned reports, are shaping the lives of the individual and collective inhabitants of schools. Long-term *institutional* narratives are often touted as the remedy for struggling schools and students; however, how have these changing policies intersected with or bypassed the diverse and changing *insider* narratives

A. T. Sugimoto (✉) · K. Carter
Teaching, Learning, and Sociocultural Studies, University of Arizona College of Education, 1430 E. Second St., Tucson, AZ 85721, USA
e-mail: ats@email.arizona.edu

K. Carter
e-mail: kcarter@email.arizona.edu

© Springer Science+Business Media New York 2015
K. Bosworth (ed.), *Prevention Science in School Settings*,
Advances in Prevention Science, DOI 10.1007/978-1-4939-3155-2_2

of students who may be at risk for engaging in risky behaviors? Additionally, how have the larger narratives—institutional, collective, and individual—changed over time, and how have these changes shaped the American vision of schooling? This chapter seeks to elucidate the themes and power of these narratives in relation to the public education system, politics, the social images of schooling, and, most importantly, the students who navigate school spaces on a daily basis in the hopes of leading healthy and fulfilling lives.

As we reviewed the historical and ongoing institutional narratives about education, we asked how can these outsider, institutional narratives be situated within the insider spaces, places, and lives of children and schools? The first section of this chapter describes some of the major themes in public education from the 1960s to the present. The second section examines the currently held belief that untrained outsiders and naive newcomers may be the solution to the failing public school system. Finally, we present counter-narratives from students' perspective in an effort to explore how institutional and national educational narratives have changed and shaped students' individual experiences in schools.

2.1 The Central Narratives of Schools: The 1960s to the Present

Institutional narratives contribute to the school environment and culture that individual students encounter on a daily basis. Our examination of the central narratives of schools begins with a discussion of the historical goals and outcomes of the desegregation movement because it was one of the milestone reforms in the recent history of the American public education system and its effects are still being discussed today. Next, we examine how achievement testing and international comparative assessments have contributed to public alarm about the "failure of America's schools" and eventually led to the creation of "A Nation at Risk" (1983), the influential federal report that has influenced educational policy for the last 30 years. This report was followed by a move toward standardization and assessment-driven practices in schools as a result of policy makers' desire to increase student achievement outcomes by controlling teachers. Then, we turn to an examination of the impact of the No Child Left Behind (NCLB) Act (2001) and conclude with an analysis of topics related to school budgets, incentives, Race to the Top, and the Common Core initiative, all of which represent the current ideology of market-based reforms to incentivize education and educators in order to increase test scores. These policy initiatives were designed to improve students' lives, but we are compelled to ask how these reforms diverge from or converge with the insider narratives of students and their developing emotional, social, mental, and physical health and well-being.

2.1.1   Desegregation and Radicalism

The desegregation and radicalism movements of the 1950s and 1960s were de-signed to redress the inequitable power relationships in schools, and by extension in society, both racial inequality and the inequality perpetuated by the traditional canon of schools, schooling, and student–teacher relationships. Although it was an attempt to rectify racial inequalities, the Supreme Court ruling in the *Brown v. Board of Education of Topeka* (1954) case ushered in a time of great unrest in public schools. The ruling overturned the previous Supreme Court decision in *Plessy v. Ferguson* (1896), which created the national doctrine of "separate but equal" that governed many aspects of American life, ranging from restaurants, movie theaters, and restrooms to schools. *Brown v. Board of Education* was grounded in the argu-ment that for racially marginalized populations, the "separate but equal" doctrine unequivocally violated the equal protection clause of the Fourteenth Amendment of the US Constitution. After this initial ruling, it took the court a year to draft a plan for how desegregation should proceed with "all deliberate speed" (United States Courts 2013). Ultimately, it was decided that busing should be the primary tool for integrating schools, a decision that the American public met with a variety of emo-tions, from wariness to open and sometimes brutal hostility.

In keeping with the desire for equality underlying the desegregation movement, Lyndon B. Johnson attempted to redress civil inequality with a set of sweeping policy initiatives termed the War on Poverty. Numerous social welfare programs (e.g., Head Start, food stamps, and Medicare) were created under Johnson's re-form initiatives (Spring 2011). In 1965, President Johnson signed the Elementary and Secondary Education Act (ESEA) into law. ESEA was designed to reduce the achievement gap through the allocation of federal monies to schools with the high-est need. Furthermore, ESEA mandated that schools utilize accountability measures to track students' academic progress (Standerfer 2006).

Concern for the welfare of students, as defined by measures of equality and ac-cess, was widespread throughout the radical reform movements of the 1960s and 1970s. During this time, the idea of common schools existing to create a common culture was abandoned in favor of movements toward multiculturalism and bilin-gualism (Spring 2011). At the same time, there was also a growing concern about the academic performance of America's children. Concerns over the achievement levels of American children, especially compared to their peers in other countries, signaled a change in public discourse and policy that challenged the historic politi-cal discourse which centered reform around concern for students who were at great-est risk for academic underachievement or educational inequality.

2.1.2 Reification of Student Performance and the Achievement Gap

With the naming of the achievement gap in schools during the 1960s, public attention was acutely attuned to uneven student achievement in schools, as measured by standardized tests. This ideological shift from equity to achievement was grounded in the reformists' call for equality, but ultimately resulted in the positioning of student academic achievement over other measures of positive school outcomes, including the prevention of suicide, bullying, and substance abuse or the promotion of positive civic behaviors and engagement.

In 1965, a federal commission was convened to conduct a survey "concerning the lack of availability of equal education opportunities for individuals for reason of race, color, religion, or national origin in public educational institutions" (Coleman et al. 1966, p. iii). The commission's report, commonly known as the Coleman Report after its primary author, found that a majority of American children attended schools that were segregated, which resulted in minority students having less access to curricular and extracurricular resources. Moreover, the commission attempted to correlate student achievement with individual teacher characteristics (i.e., quality and type of college attended, years of teaching experience, salary, scores on vocabulary tests, and mother's educational attainment). The average Black student was found to attend a school with a larger percentage of teachers who were measured as "less able" in the aforementioned characteristics, which, it was argued, negatively affected student achievement levels.

The Coleman Report was the first to articulate a racial and economic division among students that came to be referred to as the *achievement gap* and has become a part of the national discourse on schools, schooling, and importance of academic achievement. The report claimed that schools were not helping students overcome their "non-school disadvantages," specifically, poverty, community attitudes, or parents' low education level. Additionally, academic achievement was strongly related to socioeconomic status and, as a student progressed through school, the achievement gap continued to widen.

Coleman and his coauthors on the commission (1966) defended standardized tests as the most reliable measure of students' academic gains. They claimed that standardized tests were particularly suited for measuring student performance because they were not mere measures of intelligence nor of student attitudes or qualities of character. Rather, standardized tests measured the skills "which are among the most important in our society. Consequently, a pupil's test results at the end of public school provide a good measure of the range of opportunities open to him as he finishes school" (Coleman et al. 1966, p. 20). The Coleman Report served to position student performance on standardized tests as the ultimate measure of a student's skills and knowledge and, by extension, as a means to measure the widening achievement gap.

The story of the reification of student performance is a narrative grounded in a shift from concern over *equity* for all students to *achievement* for all students. In the end, what happened to the insider narratives of students who were not only at risk of academic underachievement but also in danger of engaging in risky behavior? Students' test scores and achievement gains were to become one of the driving forces behind educational reform, particularly when collective student achievement on international assessments was compared.

2.1.3   Achievement Testing and International Comparisons

The narrative of achievement testing in America has been partially defined by a national preoccupation with international rankings, as defined by students' scores on standardized tests. One potential concern with the high priority of achievement tests in education is that test results may have eclipsed concerns about students' emotional, physical, and mental well-being or their potential for larger risk-taking behaviors.

The 1957 launch of the Soviet-engineered space satellite Sputnik ignited public fears about the competitiveness of American citizens in the global economic and educational arena. These fears were compounded by the release of the results from the First International Mathematics Study in the 1960s. Among both 13-year-olds and high school seniors, American students scored near the bottom (Ravitch 2013). Concurrently, in the First International Science Test, American 10-year-olds ranked second, American 14-year-olds ranked sixth, and American high school seniors ranked last, suggesting declining performance in higher grades (Ravitch 2013). Taken collectively, these defining events in American history were used to denounce the public education system's ability to adequately prepare the next generation of citizens.

Since these original international comparative assessments, American students have been perpetually portrayed as lagging behind their counterparts in other countries (Ravitch 2013). The twenty-first-century international testing and comparison movement focused on results from the Programme for International Student Achievement (PISA) assessment and the Trends in International Mathematics and Science Study (TIMSS). The release of the 2010 PISA scores prompted President Obama to call the results "our nation's Sputnik moment." His statement suggests that American schools are once again in decline; however, the actual results do not completely support this interpretation (Berliner and Glass 2014; Cochran-Smith and Lytle 2009; Ravitch 2013).

Of the 70 nations that took part in the 2009 PISA assessment, China was the top nation in all three tested subjects: reading, science, and mathematics (Ravitch 2013). This came as somewhat of a surprise to the international community and contributed to the news media's growing emphasis on the educational power of China, as exemplified by the *New York Times* article by Sam Dillon titled "Top Test Scores from Shanghai Stun Educators" (2010). What this and other articles did not report was that Shanghai represents an elite enclave in China where parents have extra funds to pay large sums for private tutoring services and extra classes for their children (Loveless 2013). Furthermore, Shanghai was the only province that allowed PISA to report their results, whereas America did not specify regions or populations that could be used for international comparison (Loveless 2013).

In truth, since 2000, American students' mathematics and reading scores on PISA have not dramatically changed, and science scores have actually improved. Additionally, in 2012, US fourth and eighth graders performed at or above the international average on the TIMMS (Ravitch 2013). Although American students have failed to secure top-tier scores on international tests, their performance is decidedly less bleak than the elevated rhetoric in the popular media and research would suggest (Berliner and Glass 2014).

International assessments and comparisons have greatly influenced the national discourse about public education, but one document still continues to influence American classroom more than 30 years after its release. This government report built upon growing fears about America's global competitiveness and positioned America as "a nation at risk." Once again, the larger institutional narrative would focus on academic achievement at the expense of addressing students' overall mental, physical, and emotional well-being.

2.1.4   A Nation at Risk

In 1983, a government commission released a report entitled "A Nation at Risk," which stated "Our nation is at risk. Our once unchallenged preeminence in commerce, industry, science, and technological innovation is being overtaken by competitors throughout the world" (National Commission on Excellence in Education 1983, p. 3). The inflammatory report continued, "If an unfriendly foreign power had attempted to impose on America the mediocre educational performance that exists today, we might well view it as an act of war." To combat this "rising tide of mediocrity," the commission called for reform so that America could "retain the slim competitive edge" that it had managed to maintain in the global market.

This report followed in a long-standing tradition of casting the public education system as either the panacea for or perpetuation of America's ills. The report shifted the blame for the loss of industry from corporate management and placed it firmly on supposedly inadequate schools (Ravitch 2013). Unfortunately, the report also positioned the nation as being at risk for economic collapse while overlooking the very children within the report who could also be at risk for a variety of other potentially harmful behaviors and life outcomes. In order to increase economic competitiveness, *A Nation at Risk* called on local communities and states to increase academic standards, improve teacher quality, and reform curriculum (Spring 2011). Furthermore, the report focused on the quality of teacher preparation programs and textbook materials used in schools while calling for more stringent graduation requirements so that high schools would produce students who were capable of succeeding in college (Ravitch 2013).

In answer to this call for increased standards and resources, US states passed more laws and regulations related to education than had been passed in the previous 20 years, most of them focused solely on increasing student achievement. For these lawmakers, the solution was grounded in the ideology of "more": more time in school, more academic courses, more attention to the basics, more teacher evaluations, and more testing (Tyack and Cuban 1995). It is noteworthy that whereas these state and national mandates were designed to increase student achievement, they conspicuously omitted references to reforms to increase students' overall health and well-being.

In some ways, state laws were ideologically aligned with *A Nation at Risk*, but, as Diane Ravitch (2013) noted, the report itself only briefly mentioned testing and positioned a more rigorous and coherent curriculum as the key to reforming American schools. While *A Nation at Risk* focused on the power of curriculum, several national policies arising from that report focused the discourse of the American public and public education on the idea of standards and assessment, a vision that would eventually rewrite the ongoing institutional narrative.

2.1.5   Standards and Assessments

The current accountability movement has its roots in Leon Lessinger's book, *Every Kid a Winner: Accountability in Education* (1970). In his book, Lessinger laid out a vision for public education modeled on the institutional design of hospitals, but not on their concern for patients' physical and mental health. According to Lessinger's model, teachers should be highly trained before being allowed to participate fully in the professional community. Furthermore, schools should be required to publicly report their results from standardized tests so that the community could judge their effectiveness. Lessinger's book was published at a time when the public education system was embroiled in an accountability movement to raise test scores, partially due to concerns over international competiveness and economic stability, and it became the basis of our current system of accountability-driven reforms (Tyack and Cuban 1995).

The accountability movement in the 1970s focused on a "return to the basics" and emphasized the raising of test scores through rote memorization of discrete skills and facts (Tyack and Cuban 1995). The movement was designed to "teacher-proof" education by standardizing teaching practices to focus on the most basic levels of knowledge representation (Rosenholtz 1991). In this paradigm, instruction, assessment, and accountability were intricately interwoven with the aim to increase student achievement. In reality, the emphasis on accountability decreased teachers' freedom to use their professional judgment and placed more pressure on schools, teachers, and students (Tyack and Cuban 1995).

The teacher education community responded to the accountability movement in the 1980s and 1990s by calling for an increased professionalization of the field (Darling-Hammond 1984; Zeichner 1991). The professionalization of the teaching force was proposed as a means to reform school practices by empowering teachers' judgment and knowledge instead of mandating the memorization of basic skills for ease of assessment. Concurrently, national politics and politicians were leading the reformist agenda for increased accountability. For example, President Ronald Reagan ran on a platform that supported school choice and tuition tax credits as a means of increasing student performance by making schools accountable for their performance (Spring 2011).

In response to demands for increased accountability in public education, in 1994, President Bill Clinton signed Goals 2000 into law (Heise 1994). The Act gave federal monies to states specifically so that they could develop their own state standards, which would be used to standardize school curricula (Ravitch 2013). Ultimately, the standardization, assessment, and accountability reform movements were designed to ensure student achievement gains by controlling teachers and classrooms and ignored larger concerns about students' holistic growth and well-being.

2.1.6   Incompetent Teachers: Controlling Teachers by Controlling Outcomes

To maximize student performance, researchers and policy makers spent decades attempting to mandate or describe universal teaching practices that would result in gains in student achievement. A supporter of the process–product ideology in educational research, Nathaniel Gage (1963) defined research as "activity aimed at increasing our power to understand, predict, and control events of a given kind" (p. 96). The act of teaching was defined as "any interpersonal influence aimed at changing the ways in which other persons can or will behave" (p. 96).

By extension, scholars and reformers who subscribed to the process–product paradigm attempted to uncover ways to control teachers' actions in classrooms so as to maximize student achievement outcomes over other behavioral outcomes, e.g., personal, mental, emotional, and social development (Brophy and Good 1984). Given that the process–product paradigm dominated research on teaching for decades and can still be seen in some of the "research-based" strategies and programs that educational reformists tout today, the idea of controlling student outcomes through controlling teachers has been and continues to be a central narrative theme in education.

Accountability and standardization reform measures were designed to "teacher-proof" education (Rosenholtz 1991). The underlying assumption was that teachers were largely to blame for the failure of American schools and needed guidance from outside sources. According to reformers, the solution to underachievement was to mandate incentives and punishments for teachers based on student performance. Rosenholtz (1991) argued that this standardization mentality framed schools as production lines and teachers as "semi-skilled workers" who needed to be "trained" to work effectively in classrooms. The standardization movement contradicted the professionalism movement that had influenced teacher education during the 1980s and 1990s. Standardization led to increased bureaucratic oversight, which, in turn, undermined teachers' collaboration, autonomy, and even commitment to the profession (Rosenholtz 1991).

These historical standardization mandates were a preview of the upcoming value-added accountability measures of teacher effectiveness that were to become a foundation of current accountability measures. Value-added measures treat the student as an independent and fixed variable, with teachers being the dependent variable (i.e., that students' performance defined the effectiveness and value of teachers). The reasoning goes that by measuring a student's progress from year to year, schools would be able to identify gains and losses in student achievement regardless of socioeconomic status or race (Sanders and Rivers 1996). Furthermore, tracking student achievement for 3 years would be sufficient evidence to identify "effective teachers" (Ravitch 2013). In theory, the designation as an effective or ineffective teacher could then be used to make faster decisions about hiring and firing, as well as being tied to teacher compensation, which would ultimately result in higher student achievement scores.

The value-added model and the standardization movement are based on the idea that teachers are a singular determining factor in student achievement. These reform models incorrectly place student outcomes under the direct and complete control of teachers, overlooking outside social factors, for example, family income level, that affect student performance (Berliner 2006; Berliner and Glass 2014). The idea that teachers are in complete control of student outcomes minimizes the "mutual relations among environmental demands and human responses in natural classroom settings" (Doyle 1977, p. 176). The classroom ecology paradigm argues that there are multiple factors in classrooms that affect student outcomes, including the self-interested student (Doyle 1977).

Placing the onus of student achievement firmly on the backs of teachers oversimplified the complex processes that support or hinder student learning and limited the definition of desired student outcomes to academic achievement on tests, thus narrowing the institution's focus to a single measure of student outcomes. What would happen if the institutional definition of student outcomes were broadened beyond a singular focus on achievement measured by standardized tests to better converge with the lives of children in schools? Would students be better served not only academically but also socially and emotionally? Despite these and other debates, educational reformers in the government and the private sector singled out teachers as primarily responsible for student outcomes and issued sweeping accountability mandates under NCLB (2001).

2.1.7   No Child Left Behind

George W. Bush entered his presidency at a time that was perfectly primed for major educational reform. Unlike the desegregation mandate of the 1960s, the push for accountability measures in schools enjoyed bipartisan support in the late twentieth and early twenty-first century. The NCLB (2001) mandated increased student achievement by imposing severe consequences on schools that were not able to meet strict benchmarks. Although NCLB was heralded as a means to increase test scores of students who were most at risk (e.g., those in urban communities and with low socioeconomic status), in practice, the educational reform left behind or failed even to acknowledge specific student groups, such as lesbian, gay, bisexual, and transgender (LGBTQ) youth or English language learners (Carter et al. 2013a; Sugimoto et al. 2013).

President Bush promoted NCLB as a system of accountability and standards that would ensure America's ability to compete in the global economy by increasing student achievement (Spring 2011). The Act required major reform efforts on the part of schools, school districts, and states. Ultimately, NCLB mandated that all students must be tested as proficient in mathematics and reading by 2014; the logistics of accomplishing this monumental task were, however, largely left to the states. To this end, each state was required to determine what proficient looked like, then design high-stakes assessments according to their individualized proficiency standards.

Starting in the 2002–2003 school year, states were required to submit an annual report card to the national government to show student achievement by school and district. This information was made available to the public and was the basis for major systemic decisions, including teacher evaluations, pay raises, and school closures. Furthermore, students in grades 3–8 were required to be tested in reading and mathematics during the 2005–2006 school year, and in science during the 2007–2008 school year. Test results were reported by students' race, ethnicity, income status, disability status, and English proficiency in an effort to specifically track the progress of minority and marginalized students (Ravitch 2013).

Serious consequences could be imposed on schools that failed to meet the federally mandated Annual Yearly Progress (AYP) on these assessments, hence their designation as high-stakes tests. When a school was initially labeled as failing, it was targeted for improvement. If the failing school did not improve within an allotted time, it would be restructured, a process that involved the firing of administrators, teachers, and staff, as well as the possibility of the school being placed under state or private control.

The underlying ideology of NCLB was based on the concept of market-based reforms that positioned public education as a commodity, students as products, and teachers as workers. Supporters argued that yearly assessments, coupled with public reporting of data and potentially serious consequences for schools, would foster healthy competition between schools, thereby improving public education in general. In fact, NCLB focused solely on incentives and sanctions instead of on ways to improve the actual organization and pedagogical practices of schools, changes that could have been of practical benefit to schools and teachers (Ravitch 2013). As a result, teachers increasingly teach to the test, a practice that was considered unprofessional and pedagogically unsound before NCLB (Ravitch 2013). The professionalism movement of the 1980s and 1990s has been replaced by the standardization movement, in which teachers are increasingly being told what to teach, when to teach it, and, in some cases, how to teach it. In fact, some principals proudly state that on any given day, they know exactly what page of the textbook their teachers should be on (Baines 2013).

The push for universal accountability tied to state standards and high-stakes assessments has resulted in a homogenized curriculum that spelled the demise of the multicultural and bilingual education movement of the 1960s and 1970s (Spring 2011). In fact, Kenneth Zeichner (2009) argued that the accountability movement equated multicultural education and teaching for social justice with an overall lack of concern for academic achievement. Extending this argument, we worry that the push for academic accountability has overtaken concern for children's emotional, physical, and mental health and development in schools.

The accountability and testing demands of NCLB forced states, districts, and schools to divert large amounts of money to the creation and implementation of standards and high-stakes tests. This financial outlay cost districts and schools large portions of their already stretched budgets. Schools were stretched even further during the great recession and budget crisis of the early twenty-first century.

2.1.8 School Budgets: Reductions, Incentives, and Race to the Top

The 2008–2009 recession led states to reduce funding levels to schools and school districts (Johnson et al. 2008). Despite these cuts, the fact was that the expense of schooling rose every year, due in part to increasing student enrollments coupled with increases in special services needed for the growing populations of English Language Learners and students with disabilities, and in part to the increased expenditures for testing materials and test preparation after NCLB (Baines 2013). Growing costs and shrinking state funds forced schools to prioritize their spending; therefore, school libraries closed, class sizes increased, and programs like art and physical education were eliminated (Ravitch 2013). Many schools and districts were left searching for new funding sources to make up for shrinking budgets.

When President Obama designed his federal stimulus plan, the American Recovery and Reinvestment Act (2009), $100 billion was earmarked for education, with most of the federal dollars pledged to make up for the state budget shortfalls that threatened teachers' jobs (Ravitch 2013). President Obama and Congress stipulated that $5 billion would be used to ensure the continual supply of teachers, particularly in high-need districts where teachers may have been less likely to enter or stay, given the pressures for ever-increasing test scores (Baines 2013).

The earmarked $5 billion funded the federal program entitled "Race to the Top" (2009). Race to the Top was ideologically grounded in the market-based reform movement, driving the push for accountability of the twenty-first century (Ravitch 2013). The program created a competition between states and local education agencies to apply for highly competitive grants that represented "innovative reforms" (Race to the Top 2009). Applicants were judged based on their ability to increase student achievement, graduation rates, college enrollment, and kindergarten readiness, as well as to improve teacher effectiveness, thereby maintaining reformers' narrow focus on academic achievement instead of larger concerns about students' social-emotional competence and social justice.

Underlying these criteria were eligibility requirements that states and education agencies had to meet to even apply for a Race to the Top grant. These requirements included a plethora of particularistic mandates, including, but not limited to, directives that states must adopt international standards to promote college and career readiness, increase the number of charter schools, use value-added teacher evaluations, and reform failing schools by firing teachers and closing schools (Race to the Top 2009). These eligibility requirements, to some extent, forced struggling states and school districts to adopt the federal educational reform agenda because it offered much-needed educational funding in exchange for ideological and systemic reforms (Ravitch 2013).

Race to the Top marked a departure from previous formula-based federal funding where a certain percentage of federal monies was specifically directed to schools with the highest percentage of poor children. Instead, the open-market mentality resulted in private foundations backing and funding grant writing for their preferred districts, which greatly increased the likelihood of these favored districts winning Race to the Top monies regardless of their student population (Ravitch 2013).

2.1.9 National Curriculum: The Common Core Initiative

In 2009, representatives from 41 states met with the National Governor's Association (NGA) and the Council of Chief State School Officers (CCSSO) to discuss the development of a set of national curricular standards (Mathis 2010). These standards, named the Common Core State Standards, represented a significant reform in the American education system and were positioned as an attempt to increase academic expectations and student achievement (Gallimore and Hiebert 2014). In President Obama's words, "We must raise the expectations for our students, for our schools, and for ourselves to prevent other nations from out-competing us" (Mathis 2010, p. 2). In reality, the national standards movement was based in historical concern over achievement, as measured by standardized assessments, as well as the belief that standardization of education would lead to equitable student experiences and achievement, or the "one-size-fits-all model" (Mathis 2010).

Aligned with this educational model, the Obama administration, along with private and public accountability-focused groups (e.g., the Gates Foundation), were major proponents and funders of the Common Core initiative. These individuals and groups promoted the standards as a means of closing the achievement gap, while concomitantly increasing America's economic and educational competitiveness internationally (Common Core State Standards Initiative 2010a). The NGA and CCSSO delegated the drafting of a set of English language arts and mathematics standards to the Achieve Corporation by the summer of 2009 (Mathis 2010). Unlike previous efforts to create a national curriculum, which involved educational

scholars and educators, the developers of the Common Core Standards met in relative privacy, and the panel included Achieve employees, American College Test
(ACT) and College Board employees, and members of pro-accountability groups.
Alarmingly for some, there was only one K–12 educator on this initial board of
standards creators (Mathis 2010; Ravitch 2013).

The Common Core standards, released in 2010, outlined what students should
learn at each grade level, but not how educators should actually teach the content
(Porter et al. 2011). The developers of the Common Core claimed that the standards
were (a) research- and evidence-based; (b) clear, understandable, and consistently aligned to college and career readiness expectations; (c) based on higher order
thinking skills and a rigorous foundation for content; and (d) designed to build on
the strengths of states' current standards and the standards of other highly competitive countries (Common Core State Standards Initiative 2010a, b, c). By avoiding
pedagogical prescriptiveness, the writers of the standards claimed to have allowed
states, districts, and schools the freedom to choose how they teach, while rectifying
the "patchwork of academic standards" that dominated the previous system of state-
determined standards (Common Core State Standards Initiative 2010a). However,
given the 500-page standards document and the explicitness of what was deemed as
leading students toward college and career readiness, the freedom espoused by the
Common Core developers may actually represent freedom within restraint.

The English language arts (ELA) standards represented a shift from the narrative-based literacy curriculum that traditionally had been a major component of
the K–12 literacy curriculum. In fact, the ELA standards placed a strong emphasis
on the teaching and use of informational and nonfiction texts in schools. During
elementary school, there was an approximately equal emphasis on the use of informational texts and literature, but after fifth grade, the focus on informational
text significantly increased (Coleman and Pimentel 2012; Common Core State
Standards Initiative 2010b). The ELA standards emphasized the skills needed for
reading "complex texts" in order to gather information and create coherent, well-
supported arguments (Common Core State Standards Initiative 2010b). Ultimately,
the progression of the grade-level standards was designed to scaffold students to
reading complex texts independently so that they would be ready to use different
forms of texts when they entered college or the workforce (Coleman and Pimentel
2012).

The use of complex texts also played a significant role in the Common Core
writing curriculum because students were expected to analyze evidence from text
in order to create informational or argumentative pieces (Bunch et al. 2012). Again,
the standards represented a shift from the historical emphasis on narrative-based
writings to a curriculum that emphasized writing to inform or persuade because persuasive and informational writing skills were judged to be more useful to students
after graduation (Coleman and Pimentel 2012). Interestingly, the Common Core
standards emphasized the acquisition and use of Standard English despite previous
scholarship challenging the hegemony of Standard English in schools (Bunch et al.
2012; Lippi-Green 1997; Wiley and Lukes 1996).

In mathematics, the Common Core standards were touted as a reform from the "mile-wide, inch-deep curriculum" created by many state standards to a focus on a "deep, authentic command of mathematical concepts" (Common Core State Standards Initiative 2010c, p. 1). The mathematics standards were designed to focus on fewer concepts that were meant to build upon one another, thereby reducing the need for review at the start of the school year (Common Core Standards Initiative 2010c). Additionally, the standards centered around three concepts that were deemed as critical for students' college and career readiness: (a) conceptual understanding, (b) procedural skills, and (c) fluency and application of skills both in and out of school (Common Core State Standards Initiative 2010c).

Although the Common Core State Standards enjoyed enthusiastic support from the Obama administration and other large corporations and organizations interested in accountability-based reform measures, state adoption of the Common Core standards remained voluntary. However, the US Department of Education made adoption of Common Core or comparable standards a prerequisite for receiving federal funding in many forms, including grant competitions such as Race to the Top (Mathis 2010; Porter et al. 2011).

The adoption of the standards is just the beginning of the massive reform effort that states need to undertake in order to remain in compliance with previous mandates under NCLB (2001). The Common Core developers did not prescribe specific pedagogical practices for educators or create the assessments that need to be used to determine student attainment of the standards in compliance with NCLB's high-stakes testing mandates, which means that school districts and schools are now charged with many of these implementation concerns. A set of independent consortia, the SMARTER Balanced Assessment Coalition and the Partnership for Assessment of Readiness for College and Careers, have been awarded significant amounts of federal and state monies to develop assessments aligned with the Common Core standards (Porter et al. 2011). At the time of this writing, these assessments were not publicly implemented, but there is much speculation and concern about how schools are going to be able to prepare students for these assessments, particularly given the high-stakes decisions that will be attached to student achievement on end-of-year assessments (Gallimore and Hiebert 2014).

Critics of the Common Core initiative are concerned over the speed with which the standards have been created, adopted, and implemented in schools (Gallimore and Hiebert 2014). The standards represent a major shift in curriculum, content, and pedagogy, which requires schools to adopt new textbooks, find new resources, and provide professional development for teachers who are expected to prepare their students for end-of-year, high-stakes assessments (Gallimore and Hiebert 2014; Mathis 2010). Unfortunately, the speed of implementation has made it difficult for districts still recovering from the massive education cuts of 2008–2009 to allocate all of the resources needed for successful implementation (Gallimore and Hiebert 2014).

These concerns point to larger concerns about the historical success of top-down reforms in education (Tyack and Cuban 1995). Teachers have been left with the task of interpreting the standards, experimenting, and modifying their curriculum and instruction in the absence of systematic implementation guidelines or research demonstrating the effectiveness of the standards themselves. Adding to this urgent need for thoughtful research, some scholars have shown that students in states with relatively rigorous standards score no better or worse than students in states with less rigorous standards on the National Assessment of Educational Progress (NAEP) (Mathis 2010). Additionally, despite proponents' claims that the Common Core standards will help American students stay internationally competitive, there is growing research demonstrating that larger social issues (e.g., poverty) affect student performance, and these larger issues cannot be rectified solely by the creation of a national curriculum (Berliner 2006; Berliner and Glass 2014).

Reform movements that were originally intended to increase equity in education have become dominated by concerns for students' academic achievement. Furthermore, the influence of private companies, foundations, and individuals in public education has increased at an alarming rate over the past two decades, with little concern for the long-term impact of these relatively new groups becoming major shaping agents in the central narratives of public education. One reason for this development is the national rhetoric that teachers and schools have historically failed America's children and that people outside of education have the solutions to our public education crisis (Cann 2013).

2.2   Newcomer Narratives: The Power of the Naïve Voices

We now turn to a different set of narratives, those outside the traditional, institutional groups that have wielded power in the policy and funding arenas of school reform. We argue that these newcomer narratives are naive in the sense that they tend to focus on unsophisticated, quick-fix solutions to complex, multifaceted issues in education. It is difficult to imagine that these outsider voices and their untested simplification strategies are going to change the internal suffering of schoolchildren who may be at risk of mental, social, and emotional issues.

In this section, we position the belief in untrained newcomers' abilities to save failing schools within a larger popular discourse about the power of the outsider that has been fueled by movies and the media. Then, we turn to the development and performance of the Teach for America (TFA) program, which placed minimally trained college graduates in some of the nation's neediest schools. Finally, we describe the evolution of the school choice movement through the promotion of the power of vouchers and charter schools to improve the education system through competition.

2.2.1   Motion Picture and Media Stories

The movie industry has perpetuated the myth of the power of the untrained new-comer through its frequent portrayal of school redemption stories. Within this genre is a subgenre of movies that Cann (2013) refers to as "white teacher savior films." These movies highlight the efforts of a single teacher, typically a newcomer, who is able to turn around a group of troubled, inner-city youth plagued by risky be-haviors like violence, substance abuse, and gang involvement. Interestingly, many of the teachers in these movies are not traditionally credentialed through teacher preparation courses and make nontraditional pedagogical choices to increase stu-dent achievement.

The 1995 movie *Dangerous Minds* featured Michelle Pfeiffer as an ex-marine who was able to win over her classroom full of rebellious and sometimes violent inner-city teens through candy bars and Bob Dylan (Bruckheimer et al. 1995). This movie has become an iconic tale of the power of one caring teacher to change the lives of troubled students. *The Substitute* also featured an ex-marine, but one with a decidedly more confrontational style (Mandel 1996). Tom Berenger, an ex-marine and a former CIA operative, posed as a substitute to seek out and punish the high school students who assaulted his fiancée. Through intimidation tactics and force, Berenger was able to reform an urban school that had been overtaken by violent gang members. While these fictional movies portrayed inexperienced, and some-times unqualified, newcomers as the saviors of students and schools, other films focused on the failures of schools themselves.

David Guggenheim's documentary *Waiting for Superman* uncovered the failure of the American public education system by documenting the educational journeys of five inner-city youth (Chilcott and Guggenheim 2010). In this documentary, the savior is not a specific teacher but the charter school that the students are attempt-ing to enroll in through a lottery system. The charter school is cast as the only hope that these inner-city youth have to secure a quality education and safe future. Docu-mentaries and movies like these fuel the public perception that public schools and teachers are the problem and that the solution to the perceived education crisis lies within people and programs outside of the current public education system, a belief that the private reform Teach for America, TFA, was founded upon (Cann 2013).

2.2.2   Teach for America

The power of the nontraditionally trained outsider was the basis of the well-funded and profitable education reform initiative called TFA, of which Wendy Kopp is the founder and CEO. As a Princeton undergraduate, Kopp wrote her thesis about a proposal to create a Peace Corps-style service program to promote and improve teaching in underserved areas. Today, TFA recruits some of America's "brightest college graduates," many with no formal teacher preparation, to work in high-need rural and urban districts (Decker et al. 2004). Recruits are typically given approximately 5 weeks of "intensive training" before the start of the school year and then are placed in classrooms with some of the nation's highest need students (Ravitch 2013). Despite the ostensibly "intensive training," educational newcomers cannot possibly be adequately prepared to work with students who are at risk of not only academic underachievement but also social, emotional, and behavioral issues. Furthermore, TFA perpetuates the myth of the teacher as savior of marginalized students, particularly teachers who come from positions of power and privilege and enter low-socioeconomic-status (SES) schools to work with students from drastically different backgrounds than their own.

Student gains in classrooms with TFA teachers have not been shown to be drastically better. Students who have novice teachers typically perform at an equivalent level on reading and mathematics achievement tests regardless of whether the teacher is TFA or non-TFA (Heilig and Jez 2010). Students of veteran TFA teachers were comparable to students of non-TFA teachers in reading but performed slightly better on mathematics assessments (Decker et al. 2004; Heilig and Jez 2010). There is no clear evidence that TFA teachers improved grade promotion, summer school attendance, or student behavior (Decker et al. 2004). Without definitive evidence of better student gains and outcomes, the cost of TFA has become a particular concern.

Once a TFA teacher is placed in a classroom, the school or district pays TFA a fee ranging from $2000 to $5000 (Ravitch 2013). It is important to note that one of TFA's self-proclaimed goals is to place teachers in high-need, urban schools, schools that are typically underfunded. In addition to paying TFA's fee, the school is responsible for covering the teacher's salary, which is typically lower than average because the recruit is less credentialed and experienced than a traditionally certified teacher (Cann 2013). In exchange for training and access to a powerful network of future professional contacts, recruits are only required to sign a 2-year contract, and most leave the education profession after 2 or 3 years. These high teacher turnover rates cost school systems significant amounts of money for the recruitment and training of replacement teachers (Heilig and Jez 2010).

In fact, the high turnover rate and brief time spent in the classroom may prevent TFA teachers from gaining the experience necessary to work effectively with these high-need student populations (Heilig and Jez 2010; Ravitch 2010). As one TFA alumna said, "It puts you off teaching. We do not have the background in education and are thrown into schools" (Lee 2012). Despite such misgivings and protests, as well as potentially deleterious effects on students' emotional, social, and mental well-being, TFA continues to place unseasoned recruits in schools that have some of the highest need students in the nation. TFA is not the only reform movement in the improve-student-achievement-through-newcomers narrative genre; some voices have heralded alternatives like vouchers and school choice as the solution to failing schools.

2.2.3   Alternatives, Vouchers, and School Choice

One of the basic tenets of NCLB (2001) was that students in failing schools should be given the option to transfer to a different school, thereby increasing competition among schools. The concept of market-based competition portrayed schools and schooling as a "consumer good" instead of a "common good" (Tyack and Cuban 1995). Within this consumer framework, reformists pushed a "commonsense" agenda to privatize and deregulate schools so as to increase the number and quality of schools available for students and parents, particularly for students who were considered to be at risk of failure, behavioral issues, or both (Zeichner 2009).

The idea of vouchers to promote school choice was pioneered by economist Milton Freidman in 1955 (Ravitch 2013). Originally, Friedman envisioned vouchers as an appeasement for religious parents who complained about not receiving any government support to pay for private Catholic school. In 1990, John Chubb and Terry Moe advanced vouchers as the panacea for the overly burdensome bureaucracy that hampered local school boards, principals, and teachers. The argument was that school choice would open up free-market competition, ultimately leading to gains in student achievement by culling the weaker schools (Ravitch 2013).

Milwaukee, Cleveland, and the District of Columbia have publicly funded voucher systems. Despite high hopes, these districts have failed to show significant student achievement gains for underprivileged youth in their schools. Furthermore, the use of vouchers has funneled monies away from the public school system, thereby exacerbating the schooling conditions for students who remain in their local public school (Ravitch 2013).

Charter schools were advanced as another alternative to supposedly failing public schools. The charter school movement is an extension of the privatization movement because it opens the market for the development of schools by companies, teachers, and parents (Spring 2011). NCLB's identification of charter schools as a solution to America's failing education system, despite the fact that no research or empirical evidence exists to support this claim, was the catalyst for the future federal appropriations and tax breaks made available to charter schools (Ravitch 2013). For example, President Obama signed a law in 2009 that encourages the development of charter schools by mandating their semiautonomous status and eligibility to receive federal funding.

Charter schools are not subject to the same level of regulation as public schools, a fact that has made them attractive to proponents of the privatization and market-based reform movement. As a result of reduced oversight, charter schools enroll fewer students with disabilities and behavior issues, and sometimes use a student's disability status as a reason for refusing admission (US Government Accountability Office 2012). Additionally, the lack of regulation means that charter schools "run the gamut from excellence to awful and are, on average, no more innovative or successful than public schools" (Ravitch 2013, p. 156). The explosion of for-profit charter schools has firmly positioned education as a commodity to be traded in exchange for profit without consistent and universal evidence of student achievement gains (Berliner and Glass 2014; Ravitch 2010, 2013). Within this larger rhetoric about educational reform, the student population is diversifying. Insider student narratives provide a counter-narrative to the federal policy and newcomer narratives of schools and schooling in America.

2.3   Counter-Narratives of Students in Schools

Institutional and newcomer narratives have been dominated by calls for overall increased student achievement regardless of race, class, language, culture, or neighborhood. This goal is admittedly admirable, but how effective have such reforms actually been in increasing students' academic achievement *and* their social, emotional, and physical well-being? In this section, we apply critical perspectives to examine the influence of power, privilege, and voice in schools (Carter et al. 2013a, b; Sugimoto et al. 2013) and how these relationships shape the experiences of racially, culturally, linguistically, sexually, ethnically, and socioeconomically diverse as well as differently abled student populations. All of these diverse student groups have been largely ignored in the institutional and newcomer narratives, but given our ongoing research agenda, we have chosen to focus on two special and instructive student groups, English Language Learners and LGBTQ students. Then, we utilize these critical perspectives on race, immigration, language, sexuality, class, and culture to examine how successful previous and current reforms have been in trying to reduce the achievement gap.

2.3.1   Critical Perspectives

Critical theories challenge schools, teachers, and researchers to examine the inequitable power relationships that shape and change the storied experiences of students in schools (see, e.g., Freire 1970/2000 or Pollock 2004). Furthermore, critical theories in education seek to identify sources of inequity, both overt and covert, in order to transform the systemic injustices for the betterment of all students. Many times, the marginalization of students is neither overt nor intentional; rather, it is the result of systemic inequities that have been rationalized as unchangeable or permanent and can create inequity in school cultures that hampers diverse student populations.

The number of students from diverse linguistic, racial, and socioeconomic backgrounds in classrooms is continually increasing, whereas the teaching force remains predominantly unchanged—specifically, Caucasian and middle class with a monolingual English-speaking background (Guarino et al. 2006; Zumwalt and Craig 2005). The result of this demographic discontinuity is that teachers and educators are working with students whose lives are often drastically different than their own. Lisa Delpit referred to the difficulty of teaching "other people's children" as a "deadly fog formed when the cold mist of bias and ignorance meets the warm vital reality of children of color in many of our schools" (Delpit 2006, p. 23). It is not completely understood how this "cold mist of bias and ignorance" converges with students' own developing insider narratives, particularly in terms of students' emotional, mental, and physical well-being as well as their engagement in schools.

Although Delpit focused on race, critical theories apply to all iterations of diversity by challenging teachers, administrators, and school staff "who look at 'other people's children' and see damaged and dangerous caricatures of the vulnerable and impressionable before them" (Delpit 2006, p. xxiii). Teachers' and administrators' characterizations of diverse student populations have real and potentially harmful consequences for diverse students (see, e.g., Yosso et al's (2009) work on microaggressions). Chester Pierce coined *microaggression* in the 1970s to describe daily interactions that intentionally or unintentionally attack and undermine people from a different racial, cultural, or other background to one's own. The consequences of negative characterizations may be compounded by other external and internal factors, leaving students at an increased propensity for engaging in risky, potentially harmful behaviors.

Despite decades of integration efforts, inequity and segregation still exist in schools today. In his seminal book *Savage Inequalities* (1991, 2012), Jonathan Kozol found that the poorest schools were home to "ninety percent Black and Hispanic students," while the wealthiest schools served a majority of White and Asian students (p. 7). Socioeconomic status has created a bifurcated system where equitable access to a quality education and school is still a dream for many minoritized students. In classrooms, English Language Learners and immigrants navigate the complicated, and often unnoticed, hegemony of English and power-normed cultural practices and ideals (Norton and Toohey 2004; Portes and Rumbaut 2001). Power relations around language, culture, and race create a system of segregation in schools whereby English Language Learners and immigrants struggle to achieve linguistic proficiency, academic excellence, and social acceptance (Fu 1995; Suárez-Orozco et al. 2009).

Critical theories also compel educators to examine their practices with sexually diverse students. Currently, many schools employ both overt and covert strategies to make the LGBTQ student population invisible (Ferfolja 2007). Instead of embracing all students and creating safe and comfortable spaces for dialogue about sexual orientation, as well as the harmful effects of bullying, schools choose to silence these students through pedagogical practices or by completely ignoring their existence. Within the power-normed system of public education, racially, linguistically, ethnically, sexually, culturally, and socioeconomically diverse students may struggle to find voice, acceptance, and equitable access to schools and schooling.

A critical perspective on education requires "a consideration of culture, gender, race, instruction, assessment, and communicative practice by stressing that identities and activities are historically constructed in diverse, dynamic, social, and political contexts and that politics will play a role in who is advantaged and who is disadvantaged with respect to these matters" (Norton and Toohey 2004, p. 15). Therefore, the conditions in which diverse student populations attempt to learn cannot be divorced from existing and evolving power relationships within the education system and larger American society nor from how the dominant institutional narratives diverge from individual students' narratives.

2.3.2   Diversity and the Ever-Widening Achievement Gap

The achievement gap has been a primary concern of educational reformists over the past six decades. Numerous public policies and reform movements have been designed to close the achievement gap between diverse groups of students, but the success of these efforts is questionable. Despite massive desegregation and busing programs, a majority of the nation's struggling schools are still home to racial minorities, and many are located in areas with high crime rates, gang members, violence, and instances of substance abuse (Duncan-Andrade 2011). Currently, the concentration of racial and ethnic minorities in America's inner-city schools has become more a result of economic inequity than racial inequity (Berliner and Glass 2014; Kozol 1991, 2012).

Brown v. Board of Education (1954) focused integration efforts on a Black-or-White student binary. This false binary served to overshadow the lagging achievement of other racial and cultural groups, such as Latinos/as or Native Americans (Lomawaima and McCarty 2006; Nieto 2004). This is not meant to minimize the often unthinkable conditions that many Black students historically and currently experience in schools, rather it is meant to complicate the tendency of dichotomous thinking when conceptualizing the achievement gap.

The achievement gap today is defined not only by racial inequality but also by inequality of wealth. Reardon (2011) argued that the income achievement gap is almost twice as large as the racial achievement gap. Kozol's (1991, 2012) book supported this perspective, showing that the poorest schools had the most deteriorated facilities, a marked lack of textbooks and curricular materials, and the highest turnover in teachers and staff, potentially communicating to the students enrolled there that they are not as valued as students in more prosperous neighborhoods. The inequitable distribution of resources creates an achievement gap that exists even before a child enters school and remains relatively stable throughout his or her schooling trajectory (Reardon 2011). Moreover, economic disparities contribute to and are significantly seen in American students' uneven achievement on national and international assessments (Berliner and Glass 2014).

The desegregation movement, NCLB, TFA, and other policies and programs have all been designed to increase student achievement and decrease the achievement gap, but how effective have they been? Barton and Coley (2010) found that the most significant reduction in the achievement gap occurred in the 1970s and 1980s due to the desegregation movement, early childhood education programs, more economic opportunities for minoritized families, and increased federal support for schools serving very large percentages of poor students. From 2004 to 2008, despite numerous reform initiatives and the federal mandate for increased test scores, the achievement gap has stabilized with very little change in student achievement (Barton and Coley 2010).

2.4 Conclusion: What We Know and Where We Need to Go

The complexity of teaching diverse student populations within a system shaped by narratives of power and privilege has been and continues to be a challenge for public schools (Carter 1993; Carter et al. 2012; Carter et al. 2013b; Sugimoto et al. 2013). Despite the efforts of the federal government as well as private corporations, foundations, and individuals, the American public education system is still not reaching and teaching "all students, all the time." Individual, collective, and institutional narratives are being forged, shaped, and changed within this inequitable and complex system of schooling on a daily basis. Institutional narratives of the 1950s and 1960s that focused on increasing equity and access to schools have become dominated by rhetoric over increasing students' academic achievement as measured by high-stakes tests. Concomitantly, the student population has become increasingly diverse and still remains at risk for engaging in potentially dangerous and deleterious behaviors. How can these two divergent sets of narratives converge so that students will be taken care of not only academically but also socially, emotionally, mentally, and physically?

Instead of blaming individuals, programs, or mandates for the failure of American schools, perhaps it is time to revisit the guiding vision of schools and schooling. Horace Mann envisioned schools as designed to ensure the transmission of a common knowledge base, culture, and moral system based on democratic ideals (Spring 2011). The various policies reifying student achievement present the primary purpose of schooling as to increase test scores through standardizing teaching practices and curriculum, incentivizing student performance, and imposing value-added models of teacher evaluation. Privatization and school choice movements have positioned untrained outsiders as the solution to failing schools. Meanwhile, Greenberg et al. (2003) state the purpose of schools is "to educate students to be knowledgeable, responsible, socially skilled, healthy, caring, and contributing citizens" (p. 466).

Undoubtedly, the narrative of American public education has been shaped by all of these visions of the purpose of schooling; perhaps, however, it is time to rethink these visions in relation to their impact on students' own developing lives and stories. Perhaps, it is time to place children's developing humanity ahead of tables of test scores and concerns for equity ahead of one-dimensional definitions of achievement. A focus on social-emotional development, in addition to academic development, is a primary preventative role schools can play in child and youth development. Instead of reducing student outcomes to scores on standardized tests, perhaps, we should move toward a "pedagogy of hope" that fosters students' agency and sense of control over their own destinies (Duncan-Andrade 2011). Within this pedagogy of hope, teachers, administrators, legislators, media representatives, and society in general would be compelled to examine the ongoing narrative of schools as well as the true vision of schooling in America. Instead of "triaging" (Sugimoto et al. 2013) student populations based on test scores and achievement results, the US public education system would be forced to triage around the larger emotional, social, academic, and physical needs of diverse students who are attempting to survive and thrive in schools today. Perhaps, it is time to converge the divergent institutional and individual student narratives so that we will be able to imagine the best kinds of stories to guide and enhance students' lives.

References

American Recovery and Reinvestment Act. (2009). 123 Stat. 115.

Baines, L. (2013, September 6). A bullet for the teacher. (Commentary). *Teachers College Record* ID 17241. http://www.tcrecord.org/Content.asp?ContentId=17241. Accessed 9 September 2013.

Barton, P., & Coley, R. (2010). *The Black–White achievement gap: When progress stopped.* Princeton: Educational Testing Service.

Berliner, D. (2006). Our impoverished view of educational reform. *Teachers College Record, 108*(6), 949–995.

Berliner, D., & Glass, G. (2014). *Myths and lies that threaten America's public schools.* New York: Teachers College Press.

Brophy, J. E., & Good, T. L. (1984). Teacher behavior and student achievement (Occasional Paper No. 73). Institute for Research on Teaching: Michigan State University. http://education.msu.edu/irt/PDFs/OccasionalPapers/op073.pdf. Accessed 23 May 2013.

Brown v. Board of Education. (1954). 347 U.S. 483.

Bruckheimer, J., Simpson, D. (Producer), & Smith, J. (Director). (1995). *Dangerous minds* (Motion picture). United States: Hollywood Pictures.

Bunch, G., Kibler, A., & Pimentel, S. (2012). *Realizing opportunities for English learners in the common core english language arts and disciplinary literacy standards.* Stanford: Understanding Language Initiative.

Cann, C. N. (2013). What school movies and TFA teach us about who should teach urban youth: Dominant narratives as public pedagogy. *Urban Education.* doi:0042085913507458.

Carter, K. (1993). The place of story in the study of teaching and teacher education. *Educational Researcher, 22*(1), 5–12. doi:10.3102/0013189X022001005.

Carter, K., Stoehr, K., & Carter, G. (2012). *Narrating school experience and knowing teaching.* Paper presented at the annual meeting of the American Educational Research Association, Vancouver, Canada.

Carter, K., Stoehr, K., Carter, G., & Sugimoto, A. (2013a). *Gay but not gay: Preservice teachers' narratives of sorrow about LGBTQ students' experiences in K–12 school settings.* Paper presented at the annual meeting of the American Educational Research Association, San Francisco, CA.

Carter, K., Stoehr, K., Carter, G., & Sugimoto, A. (2013b). *Learning to teach out and proud? Preservice teachers' well-remembered narratives of social justice in school and field-based settings.* Paper presented at the annual meeting of the American Educational Research Association, San Francisco, CA.

Chilcott, L. (Producer), & Guggenheim, D. (Director). (2010). *Waiting for Superman.* (Motion picture). United States: Paramount Vantage.

Chubb, J. E., & Moe, T. M. (1990). *Politics, markets, and America's schools.* Washington, DC: Brookings Institution Press.

Cochran-Smith, M., & Lytle, S. L. (2009). *Inquiry as stance: Practitioner research for the next generation.* New York: Teachers College Press.

Coleman, D., & Pimentel, S. (2012). Revised publishers' criteria for the common core state standards in english language arts and literacy, grades 3–12. http://www.corestandards.org/assets/Publishers_Criteria_for_3–12.pdf. Accessed 10 August 2013.

Coleman, J. S., Campbell, E. Q., Hobson, C. J., McPartland, J., Mood, A. M., Weinfield, F. D., & York, R. L. (1966). *Equality of educational opportunity*. Washington, DC: U.S. Government Printing Office.
Common Core State Standards Initiative. (2010a). About the standards. http://www.corestandards. org/about-the-standards/. Accessed 11 August 2013.
Common Core State Standards Initiative. (2010b). Common Core State Standards for english language arts & literacy in history/social studies, science, and technical subjects. http://www. corestandards.org/assets/CCSSI_ELA%20Standards.pdf. Accessed 11 August 2013.
Common Core State Standards Initiative. (2010c). Common Core State Standards for mathematics. http://www.corestandards.org/assets/CCSSI_Math%20Standards.pdf. Accessed 11 August 2013.
Darling-Hammond, L. (1984). *Beyond the commission reports. The coming crisis in teaching*. Santa Monica: Rand Corporation.
Decker, P. T., Mayer, D. P., & Glazerman, S. (2004). *The effects of Teach for America on students: Findings from a national evaluation*. Madison: University of Wisconsin, Institute for Research on Poverty.
Delpit, L. (2006). *Other people's children: Cultural conflict in the classroom*. New York: New Press.
Dillon, S. (7 December 2010). Top test scores from Shanghai stun educators. *New York Times*. http://www.nytimes.com/2010/12/07/education/07education.html?pagewanted=all.
Doyle, W. (1977). Paradigms for research on teacher effectiveness. *Review of Research in Education, 5*(1), 163–198.
Duncan-Andrade, J. (2011). The principal facts: New directions for teacher education. In A. F. Ball & C. A. Tyson (Eds.), *Studying diversity in teacher education* (pp. 309–326). Lanham: Rowman & Littlefield.
Ferfolja, T. (2007). Schooling cultures: Institutionalizing heteronormativity and heterosexism. *International Journal of Inclusive Education, 11*(2), 147–162.
Freire, P. (1970/2000). *Pedagogy of the oppressed*. New York: Continuum International.
Fu, D. (1995). *My trouble is my english: Asian students and the American dream*. Portsmouth: Boynton/Cook.
Gage, N. L. (1963). Paradigms for research on teaching. In N. L. Gage (Ed.), *The handbook of research on teaching* (pp. 94–141). New York: Macmillan.
Gallimore, R., & Hiebert, J. (2014). Red flags on the road to Common Core state standards reform. *Teachers College Record*. ID 17451. http://www.tcrecord.org. Accessed 12 August 2013.
Greenberg, M. T., Weissberg, R. P., O'Brien, M. U., Zins, J. E., Fredericks, L., Resnik, H., & Elias, M. J. (2003). Enhancing school-based prevention and youth development through coordinated social, emotional, and academic learning. *American Psychologist, 58*(6–7), 466–474. doi:10.1037/0003-066X.58.6-7.466.
Guarino, C. M., Santibañez, L., & Daley, G. A. (2006). Teacher recruitment and retention: A review of the recent empirical literature. *Review of Educational Research, 76*(2), 173–208. doi:10.3102/00346543076002173.
Heilig, J. V., & Jez, S. J. (2010). *Teach for America: A review of the evidence*. East Lansing: Great Lakes Center for Education Research & Practice. http://www.greatlakescenter.org/docs/ Policy_Briefs/Heilig_TeachForAmerica.pdf. Accessed 5 May 2013.
Heise, M. (1994). Goals 2000: Educate America Act: The federalization and legalization of educational policy. *Fordham Law Review, 63*, 345–381. http://ir.lawnet.fordham.edu/cgi/viewcontent.cgi?article=3133&context=flr. Accessed 1 May 2013.
Johnson, N., Oliff, P., & Koulish, J. (2008). *Most states are cutting education*. Washington, DC: Center on Budget and Policy Priorities.
Kozol, J. (1991). *Savage inequalities: Children in America's schools*. New York: Crown.
Kozol, J. (2012). *Savage inequalities: Children in America's schools* (1st paperback ed.). New York: Broadway Paperbacks.
Lee, C. (2012). Re: Forbes impact 30: Wendy Kopp (Online forum comment). http://www.forbes. com/impact-30/wendy-kopp.html. Accessed 5 May 2013.

Lessinger, L. M. (1970). *Every kid a winner: Accountability in education.* New York: Simon & Schuster.

Lippi-Green, R. (1997). *English with an accent: Language, ideology, and discrimination in the United States.* New York: Psychology Press.

Lomawaima, K., & McCarty, T. (2006). *To remain an Indian: Lessons in democracy from a century of Native American education.* New York: Teachers College Press.

Loveless, T. (9 October 2013). PISA's China problem (Web log post). http://www.brookings.edu/blogs/brown-center-chalkboard/posts/2013/10/09-pisa-china-problem-loveless. Accessed 20 May 2013.

Mandel, R. (Director). (1996). *The Substitute* (Motion Picture). United States: Orion Pictures.

Mathis, W. J. (2010). *The "Common Core" standards initiative: An effective reform tool?* Boulder: Education and the Public Interest Center & Education Policy Research Unit.

National Commission on Excellence in Education. (1983). *A nation at risk: The imperative for educational reform.* Washington, DC: U.S. Government Printing Office. http://www2.ed.gov/pubs/NatAtRisk/index.html. Accessed 1 May 2013.

Nieto, S. (2004). Black, White, and us: The meaning of *Brown v. Board of Education* for Latinos. *Multicultural Perspectives, 6*(4), 22–25.

No Child Left Behind (NCLB) Act of 2001, 20 U.S.C.A. § 6301 *et seq.*

Noddings, N. (1991). Stories in dialogue: Caring and interpersonal reasoning. In C. Witherell & N. Noddings (Eds.), *Stories lives tell: Narrative and dialogue in education* (pp. 157–170). New York: Teachers College Press.

Norton, B., & Toohey, K. (2004). Critical pedagogies and language learning: An introduction. In B. Norton & K. Toohey (Eds.), *Critical pedagogies and language learning* (pp. 1–17). Cambridge: Cambridge University Press.

Plessy v. Ferguson. (1896). 163 U.S. 537.

Pollock, M. (2004). Race wrestling: Struggling strategically with race in educational practice and research. *American Journal of Education, 111*(1), 25–67.

Portes, A., & Rumbaut, R. G. (2001). Lost in translation. In A. Porter & R. G. Rumbaut (Eds.), *Legacies: The story of the immigrant second generation* (pp. 113–146). Berkeley: University of California Press.

Porter, A., McMaken, J., Hwang, J., & Yang, R. (2011). Common Core standards the new U.S. intended curriculum. *Educational Researcher, 40*(3), 103–116.

Race to the Top Fund. (2009). H.R. 1532 (112th). http://www2.ed.gov/programs/racetothetop/index.html. Accessed 10 May 2013.

Ravitch, D. (2010). *The death and life of the great American school system: How testing and choice are undermining education.* New York: Basic Books.

Ravitch, D. (2013). *Reign of error: The hoax of the privatization movement and the danger to America's public schools.* New York: Alfred A. Knopf.

Reardon, S. F. (2011). The widening academic achievement gap between the rich and the poor: New evidence and possible explanations. In G. J. Duncan & R. J. Murnane (Eds.), *Whither opportunity* (pp. 91–116). New York: Russell Sage Foundation.

Rosenholtz, S. J. (1991). *Teachers' workplace: The social organization of schools.* New York: Teachers College Press.

Sanders, W. L., & Rivers, J. C. (1996). *Cumulative and residual effects of teachers on future student academic achievement.* Knoxville: University of Tennessee Value-Added Research and Assessment Center.

Spring, J. H. (2011). *The American school: A global context from the Puritans to the Obama era.* Boston: McGraw-Hill.

Standerfer, L. (2006). Before NCLB: The history of ESEA. *Principal Leadership, 6*(8), 26–27.

Suárez-Orozco, C., Suárez-Orozco, M. M., & Todorova, I. (2009). The challenge of learning English. In C. Suárez-Orozco, M. M. Suárez-Orozco, & I. Todorova (Eds.), *Learning a new land: Immigrant students in American society* (pp. 146–167). Cambridge: Harvard University Press.

Sugimoto, A., Carter, K., & Stoehr, K. (2013). *A study of preservice teachers' early field-based narratives regarding English learners: Will the plot thicken?* Presented at Southwest Consortium for Innovative Psychology in Education.

Tyack, D. B., & Cuban, L. (1995). *Tinkering toward utopia: A century of public school reform.* Cambridge: Harvard University Press.

United States Courts. (2013). History of Brown v. Board of Education. www.uscourts.gov/educational-resources/get-involved/federal-court-activities/brown-board-education-re-enactment/history.aspx. Accessed 15 May 2013.

U.S. Government Accountability Office. (2012). *Charter schools: Additional federal attention needed to help protect access for students with disabilities* (Publication No. GAO 12-543). Washington, DC: U.S. Government Printing Office.

Wiley, T. G., & Lukes, M. (1996). English-only and standard English ideologies in the U.S. *TESOL Quarterly, 30*(3), 511–535.

Yosso, T. J., Smith, W. A., Ceja, M., & Solorzano, D. G. (2009). Critical race theory, racial microaggressions, and campus racial climate for Latina/o undergraduates. *Harvard Educational Review, 79*(4), 659–691.

Zeichner, K. M. (1991). Contradictions and tensions in the professionalization of teaching and the democratization of schools. *Teachers College Record, 92*(3), 363–379.

Zeichner, K. M. (2009). *Teacher education and the struggle for social justice.* New York: Routledge.

Zumwalt, K., & Craig, E. (2005). Teachers' characteristics: Research on the demographic profile. In M. Cochran-Smith & K. Zeichner (Eds.), *Studying teacher education: The report of the AERA panel on research and teacher education* (pp. 111–156). Mahwah: Lawrence Erlbaum.

Chapter 3
Leadership in American Schools

Kris Bosworth, Tricia Pena and Maryann Judkins

Research and experience of educators have clearly demonstrated that engaging school leaders is essential for successful implementation of any prevention programming (Bosworth et al. 1999; Coffey and Horner 2012; Durlak and DuPre 2008; Fagan and Mihalic 2003). Schools and the districts in which they are embedded are complex social structures with leadership positions at several levels (Keshavarz et al. 2010). This presents opportunities to leverage educational leaders for prevention in numerous ways. Whether at the school principal, district superintendent, or school board level, leaders' support for school climate and prevention initiatives can be the critical factor determining the success of prevention activities and policies. Although educational leaders generally are not involved in the day-to-day implementation of prevention programming or activities, their influence is well documented at several levels and involves a variety of activities, including acquiring resources and providing clear expectations and prompt feedback for staff (Kam et al. 2003).

Durlak and DuPre (2008) reviewed more than 500 studies with strong empirical designs to identify factors that affected the implementation of prevention programs. Two critical factors that emerged from their analysis were: (a) leadership for setting priorities and managing the overall process, and (b) managerial support. Similarly, in a survey of 117 schools implementing Positive Behavior Interventions

K. Bosworth (✉) · M. Judkins
Department of Educational Policy and Practice, University of Arizona, 1430 E 2nd Street, Tucson, AZ 85721, USA
e-mail: boswortk@email.arizona.edu

M. Judkins
e-mail: mjudkins@email.arizona.edu

T. Pena
E.C.H.O. 360 Education Consulting, 19930 S. Sonoita Hwy, Vail, AZ 85641, USA
e-mail: tricia@echo360education.com

© Springer Science+Business Media New York 2015
K. Bosworth (ed.), *Prevention Science in School Settings*,
Advances in Prevention Science, DOI 10.1007/978-1-4939-3155-2_3

and Supports (PBIS), Coffey and Horner (2012) found that PBIS was more likely to be implemented and sustained if administrator support is present. In interviews with school clinicians trained in the Cognitive Behavioral Intervention for Trauma in Schools (CBITS) model, the clinicians stated that administrative support for the intervention helped to overcome barriers such as competing responsibilities, logistical barriers, and lack of parent engagement (Langley et al. 2010). On the other hand, lack of support from administrators is seen as a barrier both to implementation and sustainability (Thaker et al. 2008).

As evidenced by the above research, administrative support is essential to engage educators and school leaders in implementing and sustaining prevention interventions. To improve the implementation and impact of prevention programming, prevention scientists must understand the culture in schools and attend to the roles leadership plays. Because prevention scientists may interface with leaders in the US public school system at several levels, this chapter outlines the national standards that guide educational practice at school board, district, and school levels, and discusses opportunities for prevention scientists to influence this practice. The next section focuses on general leadership standards followed by the various leadership roles (school boards, superintendent, and principal) found within school systems.

3.1   The Hierarchy of Educational Leadership

The cornerstone of a successful democracy is an educated citizenship, and the Founding Fathers considered a free, public education to be the foundation of American democracy. The US Constitution assigns responsibility for schooling to state and local authorities, meaning that each state has generally similar, but not identical, structures and approaches to leadership.

Under federal law, public schools are mandated to educate all children from kindergarten to grade 12. For some populations of students with disabilities, this responsibility extends from prekindergarten to the age at which they complete their individual education plan goals which is age 22 in most states. Societal expectations of public education have evolved over time (see Chap. 1), but under current federal guidelines the primary purpose is to produce graduates who are ready for college or a career after graduation from high school (Porter et al. 2011). Quality educational leadership is essential for establishing the curriculum, instruction, and school climate that enable a school to fulfill this mission (Leithwood and Jantzi 2006).

Across the nation, the general hierarchy of educational leadership has multiple layers. Local primary and secondary public schooling is under the control of school districts' governing boards of usually elected, but occasionally appointed officials, who hire a superintendent to manage operations of all schools within the district. Each school is headed by a principal responsible for operating it within the parameters of district policy. These boards are special-purpose government units with similar powers to a city government. Most districts are independent, but some are under the oversight of a state board of education. In some major metropolitan cities (e.g., Baltimore, Chicago, Oakland, Philadelphia), the mayor appoints members to the board of education.

The US public education is a complex mix of politics and pedagogy. Given that school board members are elected or appointed public officials, they operate in the political arena and can be high-profile local targets for public ire when educational issues arise. The leaders below the school board level generally are professional educators who must meet particular standards and certification requirements. Reflecting this division, the following discussion considers each level of leadership, focusing on the historical context, powers and constraints, and suggestions for prevention scientists.

3.1.1   The Political Level of Educational Leadership: School Boards

The Constitution's charge of local control over schooling meant that citizens needed to develop a mechanism to oversee the education of their children. Initially, school governance was haphazard and was under the oversight of either some elected official (e.g., mayor, police chief) or elite citizen (e.g., bank president) in the community. However, as populations grew and the need for more sophisticated education increased, the governance of schools moved from local governments to a committee or group of citizens appointed for the express purpose of overseeing education (Danzberger 1992, 1994; Land 2002).

The modern approach to school governance originated in Massachusetts in 1837 with the creation of the Massachusetts Board of Education, whose members were solely responsible for oversight and operations of public schools. Horace Mann was appointed the first secretary of this newly created board. Although he never had more than 6 years of schooling in his life, this progressive educator's influence shapes the governance of public schools to this day. He became a national spokesman for the new school board movement. Other states followed Massachusetts' lead and developed a similar organizational structure.

Today, there are an estimated 15,000 school districts, officially known as local education agencies, nationwide, with about 100,000 officials on their boards (Alsbury 2008). School districts in all states except Virginia have taxation authority to fund education, and they also have powers such as eminent domain in order to acquire property for schools. The centralized policy-making body for a school district is the school board (in some states called a school corporation or school committee). The board members' role is to represent the local citizenry by providing lay oversight and policy direction to the schools under their purview. Within their role of leading district policy, board members are responsible for securing and allocating adequate funding, as well as recruiting and maintaining talented staff. They provide the link between the "public values and the professional expertise" of education (Resnick 1999, p. 16). The vast majority of school board members are not professional educators. Instead, to oversee the day-to-day operations of the district, the board hires a professional educator as superintendent.

Over time, school boards have evolved to become patterned along the lines of corporation boards with a chief executive officer (superintendent). Unlike a corporate board, however, a hallmark of school boards has been democratic participation of all members, who have equal voting rights. Consequently, most boards are structured with an uneven number of members to avoid tie votes. In most school districts, school board members are elected freely by all voting-eligible citizens within the district boundaries. Although school board members usually are elected (or occasionally appointed by other local elected officials), the position commonly is unpaid. This situation leads citizens to seek election to a local school board for a variety of reasons other than financial compensation, and occasionally their motivations may cause disharmony on the board. Although school boards usually govern fairly harmoniously and seek to serve the interests of local schoolchildren, there are three situations that may lead to conflict. These could impact the adoption and implementation of a variety of programs including those associated with prevention (Land 2002).

First, some individuals see election to the local school board as a political training ground, where they can gain name recognition and experience working within the political system. For these board members, political considerations may override the best interests of children in their decision-making. Second, some individuals may join a school board in order to champion a single issue, such as eliminating sex education from the curriculum. Such members may not understand nor choose to become well informed about the myriad of other educational policy issues presented to the board. Finally, a board member who represents an identified constituency—such as teachers, residents of a specific neighborhood, or members of a particular racial/ethnic group—often has a specific agenda that is not always compatible with the best interests of all schoolchildren. If the board member champions that constituency to the exclusion of others, conflict with other board members is almost certain to result.

3.1.1.1   The Application of School District Policies to Prevention

Prevention practitioners and scientists can take advantage of the school board's position in the educational hierarchy to advocate for sound prevention policies and practice. The role of school boards is to set policies that guide the operation of the school district despite regular turnover in the composition of the board. Since most school board members are elected officials, they are responsive to public pressure. Public pressure for an issue can initiate policy changes.

Generally, one of the areas where the school board enacts policy is on issues of interest to preventionists, including those that address prevention of alcohol, tobacco, and other drugs use; sex education; weapons; bullying; and truancy. Prevention scientists need to study local school district wellness and related policies prior to approaching a district about implementing a program or doing research to ensure that the policies are compatible with the proposed activity. Some school districts have very broad wellness policies, as exemplified by Charlottesville City Schools Policies and Regulations (2014), where the board-adopted wellness policy includes guidelines "to provide all students and staff…with opportunities, knowledge, and skills necessary to make healthy choices for a lifetime…" (Charlottesville City Schools 2011). Other districts have specific policies around a specific topic or curriculum, which may suggest a history of controversy around that issue. For example, in one southwestern city, sex education was a hotly debated concern in the local community and on the school board. In an era when strong political forces were pushing for the adoption of abstinence-only sex education curricula, this district—which had the highest rate of teen pregnancy in the state—chose after weeks of debate to adopt state guidelines defining "sexuality education as part of public school health curriculum and mandate comprehensive discussions of contraception beginning in middle school" (www.siecus.org 2014. Washington DC).

Board policies can make a difference in student behavior. For example in Boston in 2004, the district passed a policy restricting the sale of sugar-sweetened beverages in the schools. Two years later, researchers found statistically significant declines in student consumption of soda and other sweetened beverages (Cradock et al. 2011). Prevention scientists can gain insights on how to approach a school board with a prevention strategy by becoming familiar with local board policies prior to contacting district or campus-level administrators. For example, before promoting implementing or studying an alternative to suspension program for students referred with drugs on campus, the prevention scientist needs to know what the district policy on possession of drug paraphernalia is. If their policy required mandatory suspension, the disconnect between the policy and the aim of the prevention program would need to be addressed. Researchers may also find it advantageous to be able to quote the language in school district policies when presenting a prevention proposal to school personnel, and to demonstrate how the proposal aligns with those policies. As a prevention project progresses in a district, it is helpful to keep the school board informed with data about how well the project is meeting goals. When appropriate, students who have been involved in the prevention activities can become powerful spokespersons for continuation or additional funding by having students present directly to the board.

Another area where prevention scientists can contribute actively is by giving input to school boards about revising outdated policies or setting new policies to address recently developing issues such as cyberbullying or e-cigarettes. Policy discussions are complex and must take into consideration a variety of contingencies from multiple perspectives, while ideally also aligning with research and best practice. For example, the California School Boards Association (2007) identified the following list of considerations that new or newly revised school district policies regarding cyberbullying should address:

1. Legal issues regarding off-campus activity
2. Education of students, parents, and staff
3. Acceptable use of the district's technological resources

4. Use of filters to block Internet sites
5. Supervision and monitoring of students' online activity
6. Mechanisms for reporting cyberbullying
7. Assessment of imminent threat
8. Investigation of reported incidents
9. Appropriate response to incidents of cyberbullying

Complex policy decisions offer prevention scientists the opportunity to engage school district leadership in policy discussions that can impact many students through organizational change. The school board represents the political level of leadership with accountability from voters. While school board members have power to make policy decisions that can provide essential support to prevention programming or activities, other school leaders (i.e., superintendents and principals) are tasked with the daily implementation and oversight of policies. The next section focuses on positional leadership roles: superintendent and principal and the leadership standards that guide their practice.

3.1.2 The Professional Educator Level of Leadership

In contrast to the public officials at the school board level who govern the school district, the superintendent and site-level administrators are typically professional educators with specific preparation and certification requirements. Overall, these professional educators are responsible for optimizing conditions for learning and for recognizing barriers to learning and implementing strategies to remove them. Although specific certification requirements differ by state, they generally include some combination of course work and internship or practicum.

3.1.2.1 Interstate School Leaders Licensure Consortium (ISLLC) Standards for Educational Leadership

The preparation and work of school leaders nationally is guided by a set of standards developed by the National Policy Board for Educational Administration (NPBEA), of which all major national educational preparation and practice organizations are members. Recognizing the critical role that leadership plays in successful schools, NPBEA first developed and adopted the *Interstate School Leaders Licensure Consortium (ISLLC) Standards for School Leaders* in 1996. Responding to the changing policy context of the US education, NPBEA revised the standards in 2008 to set "high-level policy standards for education leadership. [ISLLC 2008] provides guidance to state policy makers as they work to improve education leadership preparation, licensure, evaluation, and professional development" (Council of Chief State School Officers (CCSSO), 2008, p. 1). The ISLLC standards offer the guiding principles for licensure certification courses, for the practice of school leaders at the superintendent and principal level, and for most educational leadership preparation programs. According to the CCSSO (2008), the six ISLLC standards represent broad high-priority themes that educational leaders must address to promote the success of all students.

1. *"Facilitating the development, articulation, implementation, and stewardship of a vision of learning that is shared and supported by all stakeholders"* (p. 14). Having a clear vision that is shared and supported by all members of the school community is the foundation on which school success is built. Under this standard, school leaders are charged with collecting and using data to identify goals and assess organizational effectiveness. They are also charged with creating and implementing plans to achieve these goals and to promote continuous and sustainable improvement by monitoring and evaluating progress and revising plans when indicated.

2. *"Advocating, nurturing, and sustaining a school culture and instructional program conducive to student learning and staff professional growth"* (p. 14). Critical to student success is both the climate and culture of the school and the quality of the instructional program. The school leader has two responsibilities under this standard: (a) to establish and nurture a culture of collaboration, trust, learning, and high expectations among all stakeholders and (b) to create a motivational learning environment for students that focuses on rigorous and relevant high-quality instruction. They are charged to supervise instruction; set up assessment and accountability systems to monitor student progress; develop high-quality professional development that increases the instructional and leadership capacity of staff; and integrate technology into instruction.

3. *"Ensuring management of the organization, operation, and resources for a safe, efficient, and effective learning environment"* (p. 14). No vision can be realized nor any quality climate and instructional programs implemented without a strong, efficient organization and operations. The school leader is responsible for monitoring and evaluating management and operational systems, as well as obtaining, allocating, aligning, and effectively using human, fiscal, and technological resources. Another function is to provide the structures to ensure that teacher organizational time is focused efficiently on supporting quality instruction and student learning. The standard also places an emphasis on distributive leadership, a philosophy of engaging all members of the school community in contributing to and taking responsibility for the organizational structure. Finally, guarding the welfare and safety of students at all times is of utmost importance. A safe environment powerfully affects student learning and is becoming a critical link with prevention.

4. *"Collaborating with faculty and community members, responding to diverse community interests and needs, and mobilizing community resources"* (p. 15). This standard includes collecting and analyzing data that are relevant to the larger educational environment as well as promoting understanding and use of diverse cultural, social, and intellectual resources in the community. A school leader must build and sustain positive relationships not only with families and

caregivers but also with community partners, public service interests, and the business community.

5. *"Acting with integrity, fairness, and in an ethical manner"* (p. 15). One aspect of performing leadership duties to the highest standard of integrity and fairness is to be aware of and evaluate potential moral and legal consequences of all decisions. Students must be central to the accountability systems and leaders must ensure every student's academic and social success. Finally, in preparing future citizens, school leaders have a responsibility for safeguarding the civic values of democracy, equity, and diversity.

6. *"Understanding, responding to, and influencing the political, social, economic, legal, and cultural context"* (p. 15). At its heart, this standard requires educational leaders to advocate for students and their education. School leaders must understand the complexity of the US society to be able to advocate for children, families, and caregivers in all the aforementioned contexts. They have a responsibility to bring their influence to bear on local, state, district, and national decisions affecting student learning. By assessing, analyzing, and anticipating emerging trends and initiatives, they are able to adapt their leadership strategies accordingly.

The ISLLC standards give educators a common language for discussing the expectations for educational leaders. They provide guidance for leadership preparation programs as well as certification requirements and structures. In addition, they provide important policy guidance for the daily activities of educational leaders and are important tools for performance evaluation and accountability. A particular emphasis in the ISLLC standards is the role educational leaders play as instructional leaders who manage all the various aspects of the school organization that have been shown to promote success for all students.

Reading the ISLLC standards provides a glimpse into the breadth and scope of an educational leader's responsibilities. These standards guide both leadership development and preparation and practice. In the section that follows, the superintendent and principal leadership level is described, and opportunities for prevention scientists to partner with these educational leaders are addressed.

3.1.3   Superintendents

To function efficiently, a school district needs administrators who are professional educators. The district leadership team is led by a superintendent who is hired by the school board. In most districts, the superintendent rises through the ranks of the educational system, typically beginning as a teacher, then moving into some site-level administrative position, such as assistant principal or principal. This generally is followed by a move to the district office in a capacity that oversees policy implementation or technical support districtwide. Some districts have a "grow your own" policy and hire most leaders from their current staff. Other districts seek "fresh eyes" from outside the district or region. Finally, through a combination of university coursework and internships, the individual can earn state certification as a superintendent. Frequent turnover of superintendents is not uncommon, especially in urban districts where the average tenure is about 3 years (Grissom and Andersen 2012; Yee and Cuban 1996). Much of this turnover is related to the labor market as well as to the changes in school board membership following an election (Grissom and Andersen 2012).

The superintendent is the liaison between the administration and the school board. In this position, he or she usually becomes the "face" of the district to many constituencies, such as parents, students, teachers, community members, local and state-elected officials, other school districts, and the business community. Although the superintendent's role varies somewhat by state and district, his or her primary responsibilities are to manage the district efficiently, to implement the vision and policies enacted by the school board, and to comply with the requirements of state and federal laws (Kowalski et al. 2011).

The superintendent has three key leadership roles that need to be carefully balanced and may, at times, conflict with one another. First, the superintendent is the chief executive officer of the school district responsible for managing resources to conduct all necessary operations. As part of this role, superintendents appoint personnel, subject to the approval of the school board. It is the superintendent's responsibility to identify and nurture the other leaders in the district. Second, however, the role of being a liaison with the board requires the superintendent to function as a community leader in the political sphere who can engage the community in a productive dialogue about the needs of the children and influence public perceptions of the district. The end goal of that dialogue is to generate support for the schools in the district, the superintendent, and the board. Finally, the superintendent serves as an instructional leader. In the current era of accountability, instruction is seen as the key determinant of student success, particularly when measured by standardized tests. The superintendent typically assigns accountability for student achievement to an assistant superintendent or director of instruction, who oversees the writing of curriculum and assessments aligned to the state standards, analyzes student achievement data, and proposes to the superintendent any policy changes necessary to keep district policy current and aligned with state law and state board of education requirements (Ziebarth 2002).

As is generally true of any leadership position, a superintendent's responsibilities are shaped by numerous contextual considerations, including district size, community demographics, organizational culture, history, geography, and local political realities. For example, the demographic and geographic characteristics of the local community are relevant in that a rural or relatively isolated community has different sets of needs and priorities than does an urban one. Thus, for some superintendents the most challenging problem may be keeping the district financially stable, whereas for others student achievement or student equity may be at the forefront of their agenda (Bredeson et al. 2011).

As a result, personality types and political strategies that are effective in one environment may not transfer well to a district with a different climate, community relationships, and political situation. For example, as district size increases so do the level of management and bureaucratic complexity. Many tasks that would fall to the superintendent of a large district are delegated to district-level administrators, meaning the superintendent is rarely involved in day-to-day district operations, except when a major issue arises. In smaller districts, a superintendent is more likely to be involved in all day-to-day administrative issues. Either way, a superintendent often must operate in crisis mode with regard to operational issues while maintaining a consistent face in dealings with the school board and community leaders (Grissom and Andersen 2012).

The unique organizational culture of each district also affects the priority assigned to the superintendent's various leadership responsibilities. A school board that values the board liaison and community relations functions of the superintendent would expect him or her to prioritize those activities while delegating managerial and instructional tasks to subordinates in the district office.

A major contextual factor that drives the work of the superintendent is the district's financial situation. The 2008 recession brought numerous school funding challenges at local, state, and federal levels. Decreasing property values and rising home vacancies through foreclosure reduced the revenue, a district could secure through property tax levies. Tightening state budgets have forced cuts in state funding for education, and federal budget cuts have slashed funding for supplemental projects grants. Theories and standards for educational leadership were largely written in better financial times when the main challenge was to expand district programs, not to consolidate or even dismantle them. Thus, they offer minimal guidance to superintendents and school boards facing tough decisions about curtailing spending in the current political and economic situation.

3.1.3.1 Application of the Superintendent's Role to Prevention

Because of their budgetary authority, superintendents have a great deal of power over health and prevention programming in their district through, for example, the number of counselors, health educators, physical education teachers, nutritionists, prevention specialists, and coordinators hired at both district and site levels. In lean fiscal times, a superintendent may also decide to dismantle or curtail the district's health and prevention infrastructure to direct the maximum resources to the classroom and academic preparation. Superintendents with a commitment to health and prevention will seek out additional sources of funding to keep as much of the student wellness infrastructure in place as possible. Because prevention scientists and policy makers often have access to information about funding sources such as federal grants, the relationships they can form with superintendents can facilitate mutually beneficial, jointly funded projects.

In a study of California superintendents, Brown et al. (2001) uncovered an opportunity for prevention scientists to influence a nutrition and activity policy in a district. The researchers interviewed superintendents in California about the factors that guided their decision-making about exercise and nutrition programs. Although the majority expressed support for positive nutrition policies, such as providing healthy food choices in the cafeterias, banning soda machines, and banning fast-food sales in elementary schools, only slightly more than a third (38%) reported having a nutrition policy in their district.

Although the majority of superintendents recognized that district policies endorsing good nutrition on school campuses could "contribute to the reduction of student cancer and heart disease risks in the future...[and] reduction of the number of overweight or obese students," (p. 56) they identified several other factors that influenced their decision-making. These primary factors related to family and community perceptions and political pressure (or lack thereof) placed on the board by constituents. The second powerful consideration was directives from state leaders. In the absence of strong community or parent pressure or state mandates, even superintendents who see the value of heart disease and cancer prevention through nutrition policy and education may not consider it a priority.

An example of how a superintendent can be persuaded to support prevention occurred in one southwestern medium-sized district. When this superintendent, who had 20 years' experience in the district, was approached with the opportunity to partner with a local university to apply for a federal Safe Schools/Healthy Students grant, he was supportive but not particularly enthusiastic. Implementation of the grant-supported prevention programs and activities showed success in reduction of violence on campus and in other risk-taking behavior. During the same time period, the academic performance peaked with all district schools receiving the state's highest rating—excelling. The superintendent now reports that "we were a good district, before the Safe Schools/Healthy Students grant. The programs, such as Positive Behavior Interventions and Support (PBIS) that were implemented during the grant and the training we received in culture and climate with a Safe Schools/ Healthy Students grant have made us a great district. A positive school culture and climate are key." (Baker, personal communication, 2013). What accounts for this change of heart? Data that demonstrated improvement in academic scores and reduction in discipline referrals were key to the superintendent's reevaluation of the importance of the prevention activities.

Four years after the end of that federal funding, the structures and activities initiated during the grant years are still an integral part of district operations. A district-level team with representatives from each school now guides and supports the continuation of PBIS (Sugai and Horner 2006) and the data-based planning process that were the foundation of the grant. Yearly, every faculty member completes a school climate survey (the Protective Schools Assessment (PSA); www.psalinks. org), which is reviewed at each school and at the district to measure progress and set school- and district-level goals.

One superintendent of a medium-sized district reported that one summer, he received over 20 requests for the opportunity to conduct research or implement an innovative program in his district. Some of these requests came from university faculty or graduate students and others from local agencies. He reported that he responded more quickly to requests from people with whom he conversed at some time about district needs. Researchers and professional scientists "should never underestimate the importance of an ongoing relationship: when planning partnerships with schools and districts" (D. Baker, personal communication, 7 July 2014).

In summary, as a professional educator, the superintendent is responsible for the smooth operation of a district, relationships with the community and the board, and the academic success of its students. A person in this position has influence with the school board and with the district organization, including the principals who are responsible at each campus.

3.1.4 Principal

Perhaps the most critical leader for the success of a prevention intervention is the site or building principal (Coffey and Horner 2012). Research shows that if the principal is open to and supportive of a prevention curriculum, the intervention has a better chance of success (See Durlak et al. 2003; Durlak and DuPre 2008).

Although each state has specific mandates about the kind of preparation required to hold a principalship, most states organize the preparation and certification requirements set forth in the ISLLC standards. As with the superintendent, preparation for certification is a combination of course work (e.g., law, finance, curriculum, personnel, supervision of instruction, and leadership theory) and internships and practicum. Generally, principals begin their careers as classroom teachers and are promoted to some school-level leadership position (such as instructional coach, dean of students, or assistant principal) prior to being appointed as principal. Some principals view this position as a step toward a district-level position, whereas others choose to remain in the principal role for the remainder of their career. The principal is the bridge between the superintendent and the school and is the "face" of the school to many constituencies: parents, students, teachers, community members, and the business community.

As the leader on a school campus, the principal is responsible for all the operations of the school, ranging from faulty air conditioning to ensuring academic success for all students to preventing violence. This range of tasks requires both management and leadership skills (e.g., delegating tasks to assistant principals, developing partnerships). The principal's joint role as leader and as manager is complementary in the rapidly changing educational environment, but occasional tension rises between them. In the managerial role, the principal organizes and maintains a safe environment that supports learning, constantly seeking better ways of doing things and inspiring people to be innovative and creative. A well-managed environment is the foundation for leadership organized around a guiding vision and for developing plans and strategies to produce the changes that improve the education of all children in the school (Shriberg and Shriberg 2011). However, management and leadership require different skills, and most principals are more skilled at one than the other. A successful principal will counterbalance his or her strengths by hiring staff that have the opposite strengths. The key is to value and balance both roles, and to understand the processes by which both are accomplished (Shriberg and Shriberg 2011).

Principals typically are evaluated on their contributions to student academic success, as research affirms that the quality of school leadership is second only to the influence of the classroom teacher in student academic success (Leithwood and Jantzi 2006). Student success as measured by achievement tests is often the most influential measure in the evaluation of a principal's performance. Accountability for principals often depends on student test scores. The pressure this implies may lead a principal to place a secondary emphasis on prevention, unless he or she has a deep understanding of the relationship between behavior and academics.

The school culture and climate are most directly under the control of the principal, although the superintendent can play an indirect role through hiring and promotion decisions and mandates passed down to the site level. Numerous studies have demonstrated that a school's culture and climate can serve as an enormous protective factor (see Bosworth 2000). The Adolescent Health (Add Health; Blum et al. 2004) studies show a direct relationship between students' perceived degree of connectedness toward their school and their risk-taking behavior. Blum described positive school culture as the best prevention. Safe, caring, participatory, and responsive school climates tend to foster attachment and bonding to school, and these in turn reduce the incidence of aggressive and other risk-taking behavior (Gregory et al. 2010; Thapa et al. 2013; Wilson 2004). School climate factors along three dimensions have been associated with the level of bullying that occurs: (a) structure and support, (b) relationships, and (c) norms and policies (e.g., McNeely et al. 2002; Thapa et al. 2013). All these dimensions are influenced by the principal and will be considered separately.

3.1.4.1 Application of the Principal's Role to Prevention

Decades of literature in the USA and internationally have highlighted the importance of the leadership support for any successful change including adopting new programs in a school (Fullan 2007; Kallestad and Olweus 2003; Levine and Lezotte 1990; Stoll 1999). Specifically, in a prevention trial of a delinquency prevention program, Kam et al. (2003) found that the two main factors contributing to the success of the intervention were (a) adequate support from school principals and (b) a high degree of classroom implementation. Moreover, significant intervention effects were only found in settings where both principal support and implementation quality were high. Neither factor alone predicted intervention effectiveness. Principal support led to the allocation of sufficient resources, supervision, and professional support to teachers implementing the program. Additionally, they found that principals who are effective leaders promote positive social climates that reinforce norms for safe, positive behavior rather than risk-taking behavior throughout the building (see also Deal 1986; Greenfield 1986; Heck et al. 1990a).

The staff gauges the principal's attitude to determine the relative priority of the multiple activities in any school, so signals of support are crucial. Principals can be very helpful in providing teachers with incentives for implementing prevention programs, which may range from verbal recognition and encouragement to credit hours for meetings and release time for curriculum replication. They also are important liaisons for those who promote the program and rally support for it among parents, students, and the community. A consensus is growing that obtaining principal support for the program is essential because principal leadership partially determines whether teachers' efforts in program implementation are supported.

Forman et al. (2008) surveyed perceptions of prevention curriculum developers about facilitators and barriers to implementation. The majority of developers (79%) identified the principal's leadership style and behavior as an important facilitator of implementation, citing three key characteristics: (a) good management, (b) instructional leadership, and (c) support for the success of the innovation.

Actions that confirm a principal's support for prevention include attending trainings and discussing implementation issues during faculty meetings. Moreover, it is important for the principal to have a positive attitude and belief about the effectiveness of the intervention and to be knowledgeable about how it works. In contrast, more than one third of the developers reported passive resistance from administrators that constituted a barrier to implementation. For example, one developer reported an administrator saying, "I really don't want to know anything about what you're doing but you have my blessing. Go ahead. See you later" (Forman et al. 2008, p. 32).

School and district goals and policies were also important in implementation. More than half of the developers indicated that in instances of successful implementation, the school goals contained an emphasis on mental health and prevention, and that implementation was more successful when it was compatible with school philosophy (Forman et al. 2008).

The culture of a school is a powerful prevention tool the principal controls without having any additional programming or curriculum (Lindstrom et al. 2011; Trickett and Rowe 2012). The following are some examples of how individual principals engage with students and support a positive climate. One high school principal greets students each morning as they enter the school grounds. He shares positive prevention messages in animated and eye-catching ways, one day wearing a hardhat and megaphone while welcoming students and announcing that the school is helping them "build" their futures, another day rolling out a red carpet and calling students the rock stars of the campus. An elementary school principal shares the publicly available discipline data with students each month and rewards good behavior. The principal at the middle school these students feed into also shares discipline data as well as involves groups of students in weekly discussions where they offer suggestions to decrease discipline referrals and increase positive behaviors.

The values and beliefs that a principal has influence their openness to prevention. Bosworth and Earthman (2002) interviewed ten school administrators who had expressed an interest in implementing resiliency-based programs in their schools. Of the ten, five applied to receive extra training and funding in order actually to implement those programs. These five all believed that resiliency was a critical component of the school environment and that it could be promoted at the environmental level. In contrast, the five school administrators who did not pursue additional support viewed resiliency as something that resided in individual students rather than being modifiable through the school-culture and environmental-based intervention.

Raising principal awareness and concern about prevention issues is critical to gaining support. Additionally, understanding the principal's management style and consequently the structure and organization of the school allows prevention experts to gear program implementation to fit with the ebb and flow of the school. Understanding the pressures placed on school leaders can help prevention program developers and researchers demonstrate how a particular program or research study might meet the identified needs of the leader. Many commercially available prevention curricula that can be matched to particular principal and school priorities.

Successfully engaging school leadership in prevention involves building a relationship. A focus group of principals who led their high schools in a strong implementation of PBIS identified approaches to partnerships with prevention scientists that were characterized by mutual trust and respect. These include:

1. Inviting educators to participate in the research.
2. Asking educators what they need to improve their climate and reduce risk-taking behavior and then provide something they requested.
3. Matching the prevention activity or approach with the school vision and needs as well as the state's accountability system.
4. Maintaining contact with educators/leaders after the initial project, research, or funding is over. One research team invited local school leaders to presentations on campus and appropriately included participating leaders as coauthors on papers and academic presentations.

By actively involving and engaging these leaders, the potential for success and sustainability will be maximized.

3.2 Structure and Support

Eliot et al. (2010) cite structure and support as two essential components of climate, reporting that the most effective environment is high in both control and caring. Other important factors are rules that students perceive as fair (Thapa et al. 2013) and unambiguous (Gregory and Cornell 2009; Reinke and Herman 2002). Students perceive disorganized schools to be both unsafe and unsupportive (Unnever and Cornell 2003). A concrete, school-wide discipline plan provides both support and structure for all students, leading to a culture that does not tolerate bullying (Unnever and Cornell 2003).

Positive Relationships Caring, fair, and supportive relationships with both adults and peers are critical components of a climate low in aggression and victimization. Three decades ago, Rutter et al. (1979) found that strong student–teacher relationships predicted higher levels of academic success and lower levels of delinquency. Students who perceive school personnel as "unfriendly, unfair and unsupportive" report being less likely to conform to socially acceptable school rules and norms (Gendron et al. 2011, p. 152).

Norms and Policies Schoolwide policies and norms supporting positive and respectful interactions among everyone in the school community contribute to a bully-resistant climate. Waasdorp et al. (2011) found a positive relationship between feelings of safety and belongingness in schools. But when peers and adults are neutral or nonresponsive to bullying behaviors, the entire student body infers that bullying is tolerated and even accepted (Unnever and Cornell 2003). To reduce bullying incidents and mitigate the harm caused to individuals and the school community, school policy must mandate positive and respectful interactions among adults and students.

Principals have power and authority by virtue of their position, which allows them to influence people in specific ways, control the flow information, direct who does what work and where they do it, and reward or reprimand subordinates. Most principals do not rely on positional power to move their vision and agenda forward, however. The type of power that generally drives success in a school derives from relationships, that is, personal power. Developing relationships with all of the school stakeholders, and harnessing these relationships to increase organizational efficiency to promote student achievement is a critical aspect of a principal's position (Marion and Gonzales 2013).

The principal has considerable discretionary power to shape a culture that reflects his or her vision for the school, but getting the job done requires many "feet on the ground." A number of other building-level administrators are responsible for certain aspects of the educational process. The most prominent of these is the assistant principal (sometimes titled vice principal or dean). Generally, the assistant principal (or one of the assistant principals if there are several) is responsible for student discipline and can contribute to building a positive school culture that will reduce disciplinary incidents.

Teacher leaders are also critical to implementation success. Teachers traditionally have facilitated prevention activities through such leadership behaviors as being open to learning about the intervention, attending training, volunteering to be the primary implementer, and training other teachers. In contrast, teacher-related barriers included teachers being inflexible in their teaching approach, lacking teaching skill, and lacking interest in prevention (Forman et al. 2008).

Teaming is a particularly important strategy in schools. Teams of teachers and other school personnel may be formed to facilitate planning and policy-making, to focus on operations, to lead the school in a new direction, or to improve quality of education. For example, in one district the norm is that all professional staff in the school will serve on a team that deals with some aspect of management. Currently, the school's four operating teams address (a) parent relationships, (b) curriculum development and articulation, (c) school safety, and (d) professional development. Staff members are free to choose one of the teams and work throughout the year to evaluate, monitor, and make suggestions for improvement in their team's focus area. Other schools organize teams by programmatic functions, such as prevention activities, interventions, after-school activities, or athletics. These teams support distributed leadership (Spillane and Diamond 2007), help staff develop leadership skills for administrative positions, and, key to the site climate, provide staff with a voice in the decisions that affect their positions.

3.3 Everyday Activities of Prevention-Minded Educational Leaders

The second author of this chapter had been a high school principal for 13 years in a growing district about 45 minutes drive from the US—Mexican border. During that time, she was a strong advocate for prevention by using the power of her position and the power of her personality. She identified three functions that educational leaders can be encouraged to play in promoting prevention: leading by example, securing funds for prevention programs and curricula, and using the "bully pulpit."

Leading by Example School and district leaders are under a microscope at all times. Their constituents encounter them both in their professional roles and at official functions as well as informally in their activities as members of the community. Their habits and behavior can support or downplay a prevention message. As an example, while a colleague superintendent was out of town for a conference, his teenage son hosted a party that was reported to the police and several arrests were made for underage drinking and curfew violations. The superintendent openly supported the police actions and used this event as an opportunity to lead a community discussion about drinking and partying norms in the community.

Leading by example is also apparent in educational leaders' everyday behaviors in the school. For example, by consistently treating people in a respectful, caring manner models behavior that is antithetical to bullying and aggressive behavior, the leader embeds social skills lessons for both adults and students in everyday interactions. Treating students fairly and equitably during disciplinary actions sends a message of caring and respect for the student as a person while identifying particular behaviors as unacceptable.

Finding Funding Sources The impetus for implementation of prevention activities in a school or schools within a district often comes from outside the district, via either state or federal mandates or participation in curriculum development projects or other research. Funding opportunities are announced at conferences or on web sites. After joining a statewide network of schools implementing PBIS, the principal sought out funding sources including researchers who were interested in collecting data at her school. The initial prevention activities were funded through these grants. Once the local data showed a reduction in risky behavior, the superintendent and the school board became enthusiastic and supported the successful programs after grant funding ended. As a member of a civic organization, the principal has used her contacts with business to solicit funds from local businesses and community groups to provide ongoing prevention materials for students and staff.

Bully Pulpit Educational leaders command respect and so are often given opportunities to speak to a variety of audiences, especially parents and community organizations interested in education. They can use such opportunities to talk about ways to prevent risk-taking behavior as well as to support and encourage prevention activities with families and in the community. After the arrest of three strong students for possession with the intent to sell black tar heroin, the principal organized a community advisory group and partnered with law enforcement, the business community, the medical community, and a local college to offer a series of educational programs for parents.

Principals can use their bully pulpit to educate parents and community members about the issues related to preventing bullying. Dake et al. (2004) encourage principals to educate the public about bullying and intervene consistently when bullying occurs. Recently, this principal focused on a concern about bullying after noticing an increased number of discipline referrals for bullying behaviors.

Social media sites in the school and the district were used to communicate to parents, students, and community members. The school sent out messages and tips to parents encouraging them to have conversations with their children about bullying and cyberbullying as well as verified links to reputable web sites on bullying prevention and intervention. Using social media provides a unique opportunity for communication with busy parents and concerned community members that fills in a possible communication gap between the home and the schoolhouse.

3.4 Conclusion

In sum, school leaders can directly impact prevention through the active support of specific prevention programs, curricula, or activities and creating positive and protective school climate and cultures. Their influence can also be informal and extend outside the school walls to parents and the community.

Educational leaders, whether elected or appointed, are the gatekeepers to implementation of prevention programming in any school or district. Knowing how the district functions and developing relationships with various leaders facilitate successful implementation. Developing those relationships with leaders can have both immediate and long-term benefits (see Chap. 11). If a prevention scientist is housed at a college or university, faculty in the educational leadership department or program can be an important source of information on districts and schools and can offer introductions to innovative leaders who are likely to be interested in prevention activities and research. Ultimately, the success for prevention research or programming in a school or district lies with developing a partnership with school or district leadership.

References

Alsbury, T. L. (2008). *The future of school board governance: Relevancy and revelation.* Blue Ridge Summit: Rowman & Littlefield Education.

Blum, R. W., Libbey, H. P., Bishop, J. H., & Bishop, M. (2004). School connectedness—strengthening health and education outcomes for teenagers. *Journal of School Health, 74*(7), 231–235.

Bosworth, K. (2000). Protective schools: Linking drug abuse prevention with student success. A guide for educators, policy makers, and families.

Bosworth, K., & Earthman, E. (2002). From theory to practice: School leaders' perspectives on resiliency. *Journal of Clinical Psychology, 58*(3), 299–306. doi:10.1002/jclp.10021.

Bosworth, K., Gingiss, P., Potthoff, S., & Roberts-Gray, C. (1999). A Bayesian model to predict the success of the implementation of health and education innovations in school-centered programs. *Evaluation and Program Planning, 22*(1), 1–11. doi:10.1016/S0149-7189(98)00035-4.

Bredeson, P. V., Klar, H. W., & Johansson, O. (2011). Context-responsive leadership: Examining superintendent leadership in context. *Education Policy Analysis Archives, 19*(18). http://epaa.asu.edu/ojs/article/view/739. Accessed 1 April 2014.

Brown, K. M., Akintobi, T. H., & Pitt, S. (2001). *School board member and superintendent survey results: The examination of communication factors affecting policymakers* (Research Report to California Project LEAN of the California Department of Health Services and the Public Health Institute). California Project Lean website: http://www.californiaprojectlean.org/docuserfiles/schoolboardsuperintendentreportfinal2_17_02.pdf. Accessed 14 Jan 2015.

Charlottesville City Schools. (2011). *Wellness policy.* http://www.ccs.k12.va.us/policy/SectionJ/JHCF.pdf. Accessed 14 Jan 2015.

Coffey, J. H., & Horner, R. H. (2012). The sustainability of schoolwide positive behavior interventions and supports. *Exceptional Children, 78*(4), 407–422.

Council of Chief State School Officers (CCSSO). (2008). *Educational leadership policy standards: ISLLC 2008. As adopted by the national policy board for educational administration.* Washington, DC. http://www.ccsso.org/Documents/2008/Educational_Leadership_Policy_Standards_2008.pdf. Accessed 2 Dec 2014.

Cradock, A. L., McHugh, A., Mont-Ferguson, H., Grant, L., Barrett, J. L., Gortmaker, S. L., & Wang, C. (2011). Effect of school district policy change on the consumption of sugar-sweetened beverages among high school students, Boston Massachusetts, 2004–2006. *Preventing Chronic Disease, 8*(4), A74.

Dake, J. A., Price, J. H., Telljohann, S. K., & Funk, J. B. (2004). Principals' perceptions and practices of school bullying prevention activities. *Health Education & Behavior, 31*(3), 372–387. doi:10.1177/1090198104263359.

Danzberger, J. P. (1992). *School boards: A troubled American institution. Facing the challenge: The report of the twentieth century fund task force on school governance.* New York: The Twentieth Century Fund.

Danzberger, J. P. (1994). Governing the nation's schools: The case for restructuring local school boards. *Phi Delta Kappan, 75*(5), 67–73.

Deal, T. E. (1986). New images of organizations and leadership. *Peabody Journal of Education, 63*(3), 1–8. doi:10.1080/01619568609538521.

Durlak, J. A. (2003). Effective prevention and health promotion programming. In *Encyclopedia of primary prevention and health promotion* (pp. 61–69). Springer US. doi:10.1007/978-1-4615-0195-4_6.

Durlak, J. A., & DuPre, E. P. (2008). Implementation matters: A review of research on the influence of implementation on program outcomes and the factors affecting implementation. *American Journal of Community Psychology, 41*(3–4), 327–350. doi:10.1007/s10464-008-9165-0.

Eliot, M., Cornell, D., Gregory, A., & Fan, X. (2010). Supportive school climate and student willingness to seek help for bullying and threats of violence. *Journal of School Psychology, 48*(6), 533–553. doi:10.1016/j.jsp.2010.07.001.

Fagan, A. A., & Mihalic, S. (2003). Strategies for enhancing the adoption of school-based prevention programs: Lessons learned from the Blueprints for violence prevention replications of the life skills training program. *Journal of Community Psychology, 31*(3), 235–253. doi:10.1002/jcop.10045.

Forman, S. G., Olin, S. S., Hoagwood, K. E., Crowe, M., & Saka, N. (2008). Evidence-based interventions in schools: Developers' views of implementation barriers and facilitators. *School Mental Health, 1*(1), 26–36. doi:10.1007/s12310-008-9002-5.

Fullan, M. (2007). The new meaning of educational change. Abingdon: Routledge.

Gendron, B. P., Williams, K. R., & Guerra, N. G. (2011). An analysis of bullying among students within schools: Estimating the effects of individual normative beliefs, self-esteem, and school climate. *Journal of school violence, 10*(2), 150–164 doi:10.1080/15388220.2010.539166.

Greenfield, T. B. (1986). Leaders and schools: Willfulness and nonnatural order in organizations. In T. J. Sergiovanni & J. E. Corbally (eds.), *Leadership and organizational culture: New perspectives on administrative theory and practice* (pp. 142–169). Urbana: University of Chicago Press.

Gregory, A., & Cornell, D. (2009). "Tolerating" adolescent needs: Moving beyond zero tolerance policies in high school. *Theory Into Practice, 48*(2), 106–113. doi:10.1080/00405840902776327.

Gregory, A., Cornell, D., Fan, X., Sheras, P., Shih, T. H., & Huang, F. (2010). Authoritative school discipline: High school practices associated with lower bullying and victimization. *Journal of Educational Psychology, 102*(2), 483–496.doi: 10.1037/a0018562.

Grissom, J. A., & Andersen, S. (2012). Why superintendents turnover. *American Educational Research Journal, 49*(6), 1146–1180. doi:10.3102/0002831212462622.

Heck, R. H., Larsen, T. J., & Marcoulides, G. A. (1990a). Instructional leadership and school achievement: Validation of a causal model. *Educational Administration Quarterly, 26*(2), 94–125. doi:10.1177/0013161X90026002002.

Heck, R., Larsen, T., & Marcoulides, G. (1990b). Principal instructional leadership and school achievement. In annual meeting of the American Educational Research Association, Boston, April.

Kallestad, J. H., & Olweus, D. (2003). Predicting teachers' and schools' implementation of the olweus bullying prevention program: A multilevel study. *Prevention & Treatment, 6*(1), 21. doi:10.1037/1522-3736.6.1.621a.

Kam, C. M., Greenberg, M. T., & Walls, C. T. (2003). Examining the role of implementation quality in school-based prevention using the paths curriculum. *Prevention Science, 4*(1), 55–63. doi:10.1023/A:1021786811186.

Keshavarz, N., Nutbeam, D., Rowling, L., & Khavarpour, F. (2010). Schools as social complex adaptive systems: A new way to understand the challenges of introducing the health promoting schools concept. *Social Science & Medicine, 70*(10), 1467–1474. doi:10.1016/j.socimed.2010.01.34.

Kowalski, T. J., McCord, R. S., Peterson, G. J., Young, P. I., & Ellerson, N. M. (2011). *The American school superintendent: 2010 decennial study*. Plymouth: R & L Education.

Land, D. (2002). Local school boards under review: Their role and effectiveness in relation to students' academic achievement. *Review of Educational Research, 72*(2), 229–278. doi:10.3102/00346543072002229.

Langley, A. K., Nadeem, E., Kataoka, S. H., Stein, B. D., & Jaycox, L. H. (2010). Evidence-based mental health programs in schools: Barriers and facilitators of successful implementation. *School Mental Health, 2*(3), 105–113. doi:10.1007/s12310-010-9038-1.

Leithwood, K., & Jantzi, D. (2006). Transformational school leadership for large-scale reform: Effects on students, teachers, and their classroom practices. *School Effectiveness and School Improvement, 17*(2), 201–227. doi:10.1080/09243450600565829.

Levine, D. U., & Lezotte, L. W. (1990). *Unusually effective schools: A review and analysis of research and practice*. Madison: The National Center for Effective Schools Research and Development.

Lindstrom, S. J., Burke, J. G., & Gielen, A. C. (2014). Urban students' perceptions of the school environment's influence on school violence. *Children & Schools, 34*(2): 92–102. doi:10.1093/cs/cdsO16. Accessed 4 March 2014. (First published online 24 August 2012)

Marion, R., & Gonzales, L. D. (2013). *Leadership in education: Organizational theory for the practitioner.* Long Grove: Waveland Press.

McNeely, C. A., Nonnemaker, J. M., & Blum, R. W. (2002). Promoting school connectedness: Evidence from the national longitudinal study of adolescent health. *Journal of School Health, 72*(4), 138–146. doi:10.1111/j.1746-1561.2002.tb06533.x.

Porter, A., McMaken, J., Hwang, J., & Yang, R. (2011). Common Core Standards: The new U.S. intended curriculum. *Educational Researcher, 40*(3), 103–116. doi:10.3102/0013189X11405038.

Reinke, W. M., & Herman, K. C. (2002). Creating school environments that deter antisocial behaviors in youth. *Psychology in the Schools, 39*(5), 549–559. doi:10.1002/pits.10048.

Resnick, M. A. (1999). Effective school governance: A look at today's practice and tomorrow's promise. http://files.eric.ed.gov/fulltext/ED433611.pdf. Accessed 15 Jan 2015.

Rutter, M., Maughan, B., & Smith, A. (1979). *Fifteen thousand hours: Secondary schools and their impact upon children.* Cambridge: Harvard University Press.

Shriberg D., & Shriberg, A. (2011). *Practicing leadership: Principles and applications* (4th ed.). Hoboken: John Wiley & Sons, Inc.

SIECUS. (2014). SIECUS: Sexuality information and education council of the United States. http://siecus.org/index.cfm. from http://siecus.org/index.cfm. Accessed 11 June 2014.

Spillane, J. P., & Diamond, J. B. (Eds.). (2007). Distributed leadership in practice. New York: Teachers College, Columbia University.

Stoll, L. (1999). Realising our potential: Understanding and developing capacity for lasting improvement. *School effectiveness and school improvement, 10*(4), 503–532. doi:10.1076/sesi.10.4.503.3494.

Sugai, G., & Horner, R. R. (2006). A promising approach for expanding and sustaining schoolwide positive behavior support. *School Psychology Review, 35*(2), 245.

Thaker, S., Steckler, A., Sanchez, V., Khatapoush, S., Rose, J., & Hallfors, D. D. (2008). Program characteristics and organizational factors affecting the implementation of a school-based indicated prevention program. *Health Education Research, 23*(2), 238–248. doi:10.1093/her/cym025.

Thapa, A., Cohen, J., Guffey, S., & Higgins-D'Alessandro, A. (2013). A review of school climate research. *Review of Educational Research, 83*(3),357–385.doi:10.3102/0034654313483907.

Trickett, E. J., & Rowe, H. L. (2012). Emerging ecological approaches to prevention, health promotion, and public health in the school context: Next steps from a community psychology perspective. *Journal of Educational and Psychological Consultation, 22*(1–2), 125–140. doi:1 0.1080/10474412.2011.649651.

Unnever, J. D., & Cornell, D. G. (2003). The culture of bullying in middle school. *Journal of School Violence, 2*(2), 5–27. doi:10.1300/J202v02n02_02.

Waasdorp, T. E., Pas, E. T., O'Brennan, L. M., & Bradshaw, C. P. (2011). A multilevel perspective on the climate of bullying: Discrepancies among students, school staff, and parents. *Journal of school violence, 10*(2), 115–132. doi:10.1080/15388220.2010.539164.

Wilson, D. (2004). The interface of school climate and school connectedness and relationships with aggression and victimization. *Journal of School Health, 74*(7), 293–299. doi:10.1111/j.1746-1561.2004.tb08286.x.

Yee, G. & Cuban, L. (1996). When is tenure long enough? A historical analysis of superintendent turnover and tenure in urban districts. *Educational Administration Quarterly, 32*(1 suppl), 615–641. doi:10.1177/0013161X960321003.

Ziebarth, T. (2002). *The roles and responsibilities of school boards and superintendents: A state policy framework.* Denver, CO: Educational Commission of the States. http://www.ecs.org/html/Document.asp?chouseid=4126. Accessed 14 Jan 2015.

Chapter 4
Professional Counselors' Impact on Schools

Amy Nitza, Kerrie R. Fineran and Brian Dobias

Prevention is inherently embedded in the profession of school counseling. On a daily basis, counselors find themselves juggling a variety of prevention-related tasks. Academic failure and dropping out, substance abuse, violence, and bullying are among the many problems that counselors work to prevent at individual, classroom, and school-wide levels.

Prevention in schools can be conceptualized as enabling academic success by removing potential barriers to learning. Many of the learning, behavioral, and emotional problems seen in schools stem from situations where external barriers to learning are not addressed. These problems then become exacerbated as struggling students internalize the frustrations of trying to navigate these hurdles to development and learning compounded by the resulting effects of performing poorly at school (Roysircar 2006). A prevention framework can enable school counselors to address the wide range of factors that may become barriers to young people's learning.

The American School Counselor Association (ASCA 2009) described professional school counselors as:

> certified/licensed educators with a minimum of a master's degree in school counseling, making them uniquely qualified to address all students' academic, personal/social and career development needs by designing, implementing, evaluating and enhancing a comprehensive school counseling program that promotes and enhances student success.
> Professional school counselors serve a vital role in maximizing student success (Lapan et al. 2007; Stone and Dahir 2006). Through leadership, advocacy and collaboration, professional school counselors promote equity and access to rigorous educational experiences

A. Nitza (✉) · K. R. Fineran · B. Dobias
Indiana University–Purdue University Fort Wayne, Fort Wayne, USA
e-mail: nitzaa@ipfw.edu

K. R. Fineran
e-mail: finerank@ipfw.edu

B. Dobias
e-mail: dobibf01@ipfw.edu

© Springer Science+Business Media New York 2015
K. Bosworth (ed.), *Prevention Science in School Settings*,
Advances in Prevention Science, DOI 10.1007/978-1-4939-3155-2_4

for all students. Professional school counselors support a safe learning environment and work to safeguard the human rights of all members of the school community (Sandhu 2000) and address the needs of all students through culturally relevant prevention and intervention programs that are part of a comprehensive school counseling program (Lee 2001) (paras. 1–2).

This description of counselors' roles in a school makes it clear that they can and should be key contributors to the implementation of school-based prevention programming. A range of prevention services exist in numerous school districts, many of which involve school counselors directly or indirectly. Yet, despite the time and effort counselors put into these activities, in many cases, prevention has not been made central to the work of the school. School-based prevention programs are often not sustained, not supported by systemic or contextual interventions, and not well integrated into the educational practices of a school (Payton et al. 2000). The ultimate result of this marginalization is that prevention is neither as efficient nor as effective as it has the potential to be. Reviewers of prevention programming efforts in schools have noted that such programs have been utilized in a fragmented and disjointed manner; as a result, despite evidence that prevention programming can be successful, the efficacy of such programs may be significantly limited by a lack of comprehensive implementation (Payton et al. 2000).

For example, suicide prevention is an important issue in schools. Although many schools participate in specific efforts such as National Depression Screening Day, they may not necessarily follow through with targeted attention to the mental health needs of students identified as at risk during such screenings. Additionally, some schools may focus specifically on suicide prevention programming. However, most do not take this full circle by preparing a plan for responding to students returning to school after a suicide attempt or completed student suicide; preparing for postvention is a significant part of prevention in this area.

Counselors are skilled professionals with the training and expertise necessary to be prevention specialists within a school. With sufficient administrative and teacher support and opportunity within their job expectations, counselors can lead the way in overcoming some of the barriers to implementation of comprehensive, school-wide, and effective prevention programming. This chapter will review the profession of school counseling and highlight how counselors can best contribute to the overall prevention efforts of any school system.

4.1   The Role of Professional School Counselors

School counseling is a subspecialty of the general counseling profession. The Council for Accreditation of Counseling and Related Educational Programs (CACREP) accredits graduate programs in school counseling as well as clinical mental health counseling, marriage and family counseling, college counseling and student affairs, and addictions counseling, among other specialties. CACREP (2009) has established a set of core counseling standards that include developmental, preventive, and wellness emphases to be infused in didactic and clinical coursework alongside general counseling theories and practical skills. Students in all accredited counseling programs must meet these standards in addition to specialty-specific standards. School counselors thus have a thorough general counseling orientation, with a scope of practice in school settings.

Prevention is emphasized in school counselor training. The current CACREP (2009) standards assert that prevention is an important value of the counseling profession. These standards state that all counseling students should have experiences that emphasize "an orientation to wellness and prevention as desired counseling goals" (p. 12). The school-counseling-specific standards in the category "Counseling, Prevention, and Intervention" include the requirement that school counseling trainees understand and be able to implement "prevention and intervention plans related to the effects of atypical growth and development, health and wellness, language, ability level, multicultural issues, and factors of resiliency on student learning and development" (p. 41). Other training standards focus on truancy and dropout prevention, emergency management and crisis preparation as prevention strategies, and substance use prevention. Clearly, the practice of prevention is an integral aspect of the practicing school counselor's role; training standards are increasingly highlighting the importance of prevention as vital to counselor preparation.

Even as they operate from within a counseling orientation, on a day-to-day basis, school counselors function in an environment shaped by educational philosophies and priorities. Additionally, unlike counselors in most other specialties, school counselors are typically licensed as educators through state departments of education. In fact, until recently, many states required school counselors to have held a teaching license for a certain number of years before being eligible for a school counseling license. This requirement still exists in some states, such as Oregon, Texas, Nebraska, and the District of Columbia, where school counselors must have 2 years of full-time teaching experience to earn licensure as a school counselor (ASCA n.d.). Other states, such as Louisiana, North Dakota, and Kansas, require school counselors to hold or be pursuing a teaching license, despite the very different professional roles they play in the lives of students.

The training and orientation that counselors bring to a school allow them to offer unique perspectives and contributions to school leadership and culture. Yet, this unique position within a school can at times present a challenge as school counselors define their own roles and clarify their professional identity externally. School counselors' potential value and contributions to a school's mission may not be well understood by other school professionals, including principals, teachers, superintendents, and school board members. Counselors may be underutilized by being assigned duties that are non-counseling related.

Compounding the potential for role confusion and underutilization of counselors' skills are the differing job descriptions of counselors across school levels (that is, elementary, middle, and high school), as well as possibly conflicting job descriptions among counselors of the same level between buildings or districts. Because the school counselor's specific role requirements (both formal and informal) are often defined by the school principal and thus may differ, for example, between schools within the same district, the time, support, and expectations regarding prevention programming may be inconsistent.

Within this context, a number of important questions have emerged about the appropriate functions of professional school counselors, including whether they should focus primarily on educational and academic issues, vocational and career issues, or personal and social issues, and mental health concerns that interfere with students' academic success (ASCA 2012). Other questions have centered on the delivery of services and whether counselors should focus on direct services to students or utilize an indirect, leadership- and consultation-oriented approach. The use of data by school counselors also has become a more prominent issue, both as a means of identifying students' needs and as a measure of accountability for counseling programs. Additionally, the need to provide an increasingly large range of services to students has necessitated a shift from an orientation based on a school counselor *position* to one based on a school counseling *program*. Attempts to respond cohesively to these issues became the basis for the development of comprehensive school counseling programs as a way to organize and manage school counseling responsibilities.

4.2 The ASCA National Model: A Comprehensive Vision for the Role of School Counselors

One major effort to help define the role of school counselors and counseling in schools has been the development of the ASCA National Model, a comprehensive framework for school counseling programs. In 1997, ASCA published the National Standards for School Counseling Programs (Campbell and Dahir 1997). Nine standards were identified in three domains of student development: academic, career, and personal/social. Each of these standards was accompanied by suggested student competencies. The inclusion of all three domains emphasized the need for counseling programs to be well rounded and balanced in promoting student success. Together, the National Standards provided an initial foundation for the creation of comprehensive, developmental, preventive school counseling programs by outlining what students should be able to know and do as a result of such programs (Erford 2011).

The publication of the National Standards was followed in 2003 by the publication of the *ASCA National Model: A Framework for School Counseling Programs*. Currently in its third edition (ASCA 2012), the National Model provides additional structure for the development and implementation of comprehensive school counseling programs. The ASCA National Model is built on four primary program components: foundation, delivery system, management, and accountability. Collectively, the components convey the intended comprehensive nature of school counseling programs. Individually, they effectively categorize various elements within the program. As described by Erford (2011), the National Model addresses "how" to achieve the "what" outlined in the National Standards.

Foundation The first of the four components, the foundation, identifies what the program is designed to achieve. This includes a program's beliefs, philosophies, and mission statement, which should be aligned with and support the overall mission of the school in which the program operates. The foundation also specifies what all students will know and be able to do as a result of the program and identifies the student standards and competencies to be achieved in the academic, career, and personal/social domains.

Delivery System The second component of the model, the delivery system, identifies the methods and strategies to be used in providing services to students and other stakeholder groups, including parents and teachers. The delivery system itself can be divided into four program components: guidance curriculum, individual student planning, responsive services, and systems support. Guidance curriculum includes developmental counseling/guidance lessons taught in classrooms and sequenced across grade levels. Individual student planning refers to activities that assist all students in planning for and achieving their educational, career, and personal goals. Responsive services are all activities that support a student with immediate or crisis concerns and may involve counseling either individually or in small groups. Finally, systems support refers to the activities necessary to manage the comprehensive school counseling program; specifically, "program management and operations involve planning and connecting the numerous initiatives of service delivery, as well as data analysis and 'fair share' responsibilities within a school" (Erford 2011, p. 50).

School counselors implement the delivery system through both direct and indirect services. Direct services, those provided by counselors directly to students, include classroom guidance lessons, small-group counseling, and individual counseling. However, an important aspect of the ASCA National Model is that school counselors are not limited to delivering the school counseling program solely through direct services. Counselors can work on behalf of students through the provision of indirect services that affect students, such as coordination and collaboration, consultation, leadership and advocacy, and training and team building. To be most effective in the delivery of a comprehensive school counseling program, counselors must be skilled in both direct and indirect service delivery. Notably, the ASCA National Model recommends that 80 % of a school counselor's time be spent in providing direct or indirect services.

Management System The management system component of the model provides guidelines and tools for assessing student needs and monitoring the ongoing operation of the school counseling program. This structure helps ensure that school counseling priorities are aligned with identified student needs and that the counseling program is addressing those needs in an effective manner. The management system may include, among other things, management agreements between school administrators and counselors about the school counseling program, the school counseling program calendar, programmatic strategic plans, and a school counseling advisory council.

Accountability System The final component of the ASCA National Model is the accountability system. This section articulates the need for school counselors to design and implement prevention and intervention programs based on structured assessment and data analysis. Additionally, the accountability system component reinforces the expectation that the effectiveness and impact of a comprehensive school counseling program should be evaluated using measurable outcomes in areas such as student achievement, attendance, and behavior (ASCA 2012). In other words, the accountability system is intended to answer the question, "How are students different as a result of the program?" In an era of school reform, accountability, and budget cuts, the importance of school counselors being able to answer this question can hardly be overestimated.

The four components of foundation, delivery, management, and accountability provide the framework outlining the elements of a comprehensive school counseling program. Additionally, the model emphasizes four themes woven throughout these components: leadership, advocacy, collaboration, and systemic change. These themes highlight an important shift in the role of school counselors from ancillary support personnel who work on an individual, problem-focused basis to comprehensive professionals who are integral to the success of not only individual students but also the complex systems that form school communities. Driven by school reform, counselors' leadership and orientation toward systemic change at the school level are becoming increasingly valued as multiple stakeholder groups within a school collaborate in supporting each student's academic, career, and personal/social success (Stone and Dahir 2007).

4.3   Integrating Prevention Science into School Counseling

As stated previously, prevention efforts are embedded within the work of school counselors. To most effectively implement prevention programming within schools, current best practices in prevention science should be clearly and purposefully integrated into comprehensive school counseling programs. Doing so provides a framework for strengthening school counselors' contributions to successful prevention programming.

In a review of prevention programming with school-age youth, Vera and Reese (2000) summarized the important aspects of the design and implementation of such programs:

> One must begin with a thorough understanding of the risk and protective factors involved in the development of specific problems. Because risk and protective factors come from within the child as well as the social context, multiple-level interventions seem to hold the greatest promise. Also the interrelatedness of many types of problematic behaviors must be considered and addressed in a systematic way. Cultural and developmental appropriateness are also critical to the design of successful prevention programs. (p. 414)

This review highlights several prevention principles that are important for school counselors to consider. First, prevention programs are likely to be most effective when they address both risk and resilience; that is, when they focus on reducing risk factors as well as promoting the development of protective factors (Kenny et al.

2002). Prevention science has moved from a focus on specific problems or risk factors to a comprehensive approach that addresses multiple, interacting factors that put children at risk for a number of different problematic outcomes or disorders (Greenberg et al. 1999). First, best practices thus suggest that programs should address those underlying risk and protective factors that are related to a number of different potential problems. These might include, for example, reducing poor interpersonal problem-solving skills and building self-efficacy and positive coping skills.

Second, prevention efforts are most successful when they address both the individual and systemic or contextual levels. Prevention in schools is most likely to be effective when classroom-based skill development programs are supported by simultaneous efforts to promote changes in children's environments (Kenny et al. 2002). For example, in their comprehensive text on bullying prevention, Orpinas and Horne (2006) addressed two major themes: developing children's social competence and creating a positive, caring school environment. These two goals are derived from a thorough review of the multiple risk and protective factors for bullying and aggressive behaviors at the individual and contextual levels.

Finally, to be most effective, prevention programs should address these goals in a comprehensive, developmental manner. In schools, this principle suggests that such programs take into account the biological, cognitive, emotional, and social development of each student. Programs should be sustained over a number of years and focus on the sequential acquisition of skills in a developmentally and culturally appropriate way (Walsh et al. 2002).

4.4 School Counselors as Implementers of Prevention Programming

Counselors can and should be leaders of prevention efforts in schools. Multicomponent preventive interventions, which incorporate both universal and selected prevention elements, fit well within the framework of a comprehensive, developmental school counseling program. Such programs can thus serve as a school-wide foundation on which to build prevention programming. Counselors can contribute to all aspects of prevention programming, from the identification of schools' and students' needs and potential programs to implementation of various prevention program components and thorough evaluation of the effectiveness of programming.

4.4.1 Needs Assessment and Program Identification

The use of data to identify program goals and select interventions is a component of the accountability system of the ASCA National Model. The use of tools to evaluate prevention programming is thus a natural fit for school counselors. With their systemic, school-wide perspective, and their management of the comprehensive counseling program structure, counselors can lead the process of data-informed decision making in addressing their schools' prevention needs.

A public health approach to the process of identifying and implementing prevention programs provides a model for counselors to utilize in schools. As described by Orpinas and Horne (2006), this model involves four tasks: describing the problem, identifying the factors that influence the development of the issue, deciding what is effective in reducing the problem or preventing its occurrence, and implementing selected programming.

Defining the Problem The first task is to clarify the problem and its parameters. Through the use of school performance data along with survey data and other assessments of important stakeholders, including students, teachers, parents, and administrators, counselors work to clearly define the target of their prevention efforts. This means understanding how, where, when, and how frequently the problem occurs.

Identifying Risk and Protective Factors The focus of task 2 is on understanding what factors increase or decrease the probability that the problem will occur. This step refers to identifying those established risk and protective factors that are potentially modifiable within the school context. Although some risk and protective factors may be outside the realm of influence of the school, identifying goals based on factors that are likely to be effectively addressed within the school is important for success. It is essential to consult relevant prevention science literature; simply identifying factors that appear at face value to be related to the problem can result in erroneous assumptions and the adoption of inappropriate or ineffective interventions.

Planning In step 3 of the model, the emphasis is on determining what interventions work to prevent and reduce the problem. Therefore, this step involves identifying available programs and interventions. Many of these programs have been evaluated to determine their level of effectiveness, resulting in an increase in the availability of evidence-based practices. Evidence-based practices provide research results regarding the factors contributing to the problem, as well as effective interventions and an established outcome base. It is essential that counselors be aware of the available effectiveness information for any prevention program under consideration at their schools. National databases of effective prevention programs for a broad range of problems have been established by the Center for School Mental Health at the University of Maryland School of Medicine (http://csmh.umaryland.edu/), the Blueprints for Violence Prevention project of the Center for the Study and Prevention of Violence at the University of Colorado, Boulder (http://www.blueprintsprograms. com/), and Substance Abuse and Mental Health Services Administration's (SAMSHA's) National Registry of Evidence-based Programs and Practices (http://www. nrepp.samhsa.gov/). Additionally, the Ronald H. Fredrickson Center for School Counseling Outcome Research & Evaluation (CSCORE, http://www.umass.edu/ education/research/centers/center-for-school-counseling) at the University of Massachusetts, Amherst, disseminates information about evidence-based school counseling practices, including prevention programming in the career, social/emotional, and academic domains.

Often, schools or even school districts implement prevention programs in response to a mandate from a local, state, or federal legislative body. At times, counselors are "handed" programs selected by district or building administrators and told to implement them, or are given responsibility for only specific parts of a school-wide program. There is a need for school counselors to take the lead in advocating for the adoption of evidence-based practices whenever possible. Despite the proliferation of evidence-based approaches and their documentation in various databases, these programs may not be being utilized to their potential in schools. For example, a 2005 survey found that only 10.3 % of school districts with at least one high school reported administering any of the substance use prevention curricula rated as effective by either SAMSHA or the Blueprints for Violence Prevention project (Ringwalt et al. 2008).

The limited utilization of evidence-based approaches in schools is likely related to several practical and structural factors within schools. As with all school professionals, counselors are often stretched thin and pressed for time. As such, they continually find themselves balancing systematic planning with responding to immediate needs as they arise. The utilization of empirically supported approaches could be increased if materials on evidence-based programs were easily identified and readily accessible to counselors. Another very important issue is the time and resource allocation necessary to implement research-based programs with fidelity. Even once counselors identify potential programs with empirical support, they may or may not have the authority to allocate the resources and time necessary to implement them as intended. Particularly, when such programs either require the use of classroom instructional time or pull counselors away from other administrative tasks (scheduling and so on), they can be met with resistance unless buy-in is obtained from principals and other administrators. Thus, counselors can benefit from prevention specialists advocating for and supporting the importance of investing educational time and resources into empirically driven prevention work. Using data to demonstrate to school administrators the academic value associated with such programs can be of particular value.

Implementation of Programming The fourth step of the model addresses dissemination of the effective intervention. Once an evidence-based program has been identified, school counselors can lead the development of a plan for implementing the program within the school, using the established comprehensive school counseling program as a starting point. The implementation plan is likely to include different roles for the counselor, including direct delivery of some program components; training, support, and consultation for other school professionals assigned to implement program components; and school-wide program coordination and leadership. Counselors' multiple contributions to program delivery will be discussed further in the next section.

4.4.2   Program Delivery

Program delivery is possibly the most commonly recognized role school counselors play in prevention efforts. Professional school counselors are trained in the methodologies for delivery of universal and targeted prevention interventions, expertise which can help ensure that programs are implemented thoroughly and effectively.

4.4.2.1   Universal Prevention

The implementation of a comprehensive developmental school counseling program is a *universal* prevention effort. As described by ASCA, a comprehensive guidance program promotes overall student success by addressing students' academic, personal/social, and career development needs. Through this programming, school counselors can work within the risk and resilience framework that is at the heart of successful prevention efforts.

An essential function for school counselors, and a primary means through which they deliver universal prevention programming, is by facilitating the developmental classroom guidance curriculum. The ASCA National Model recommends that at the elementary school level, 35–45 % of counselor time be committed to implementing the curriculum; at the middle school level, 25–35 % of counselor time; and at the high school level, 15–25 %. In many cases, counselors will be responsible for the direct teaching of classroom guidance lessons. In other cases, prevention programs may be designed for delivery by classroom teachers, or prevention content may be incorporated into other classroom curricular units, with counselors providing consultation and collaboration to support the teachers.

Regardless of who is delivering the content, counselors have an important role to play in the facilitation and success of the guidance curriculum (Goodnough et al. 2011). This involves program coordination to ensure that the curriculum is delivered using a school-wide, systemic approach. It is also vital that counselors engage teachers and staff in supporting and reinforcing the program components. This function may include providing consultation, training, and support for teachers as well as working to ensure generalizability of the program content. Because skills learned in one setting do not necessarily transfer spontaneously to other settings, counselors can provide school-wide leadership in providing opportunities for students to apply the skills learned in the program throughout their school day.

When implemented in a thorough and sustained manner across grade levels, universal guidance programs can and should promote the development of social competence and other protective factors that prevent difficulties. However, some students may need additional services to overcome barriers to success. The implementation of a universal prevention program allows school personnel to identify students who are at higher risk or may need more support.

4.4.2.2 Selected and Indicated Prevention

As noted earlier, a comprehensive approach to prevention is multimodal and incorporates universal prevention with selected prevention services that offer more intensive assistance. Risk factors for a particular problem may be concentrated within identifiable subgroups of students who could benefit from these more focused services (Roysircar 2006). With a carefully planned identification and referral process in place, school counselors can then develop and implement selected prevention programming to students identified as being at higher risk or to those who do not respond to universal prevention (Mason and Nakkula 2008). Such services may include small-group counseling, individual counseling, and targeted crisis intervention strategies.

Group Counseling Small-group counseling has frequently been identified as a selected prevention approach (Mason and Nakkula 2008). The small-group format is ideal in school settings for a number of reasons. Groups are a good fit for the developmental needs of children and adolescents. They can provide opportunities to practice new skills and behaviors, to both give and receive support, to learn from the differing ideas and opinions of others, to learn about oneself through feedback from others, and to improve one's reasoning skills through discussions with peers (Akos et al. 2007).

ASCA has recognized the potential fit and value of groups in schools, and the use of small groups for prevention is well supported in the professional literature. As defined by Conyne and Wilson (2001), prevention groups are targeted for individuals at risk for the development of an identified difficulty. In such groups:

> members interact with each other focusing on an appropriate blend of content (e.g., social skills development; psychoactive substance use and abuse information) and process (e.g., cognitive clarification, interpersonal feedback, consciousness raising, group decision making) consistent with the focus and structure of the group. The general purpose is to gain knowledge and skills that will empower them to avoid future harmful events and situations and to live their lives more meaningfully and productively. (p. 10)

A review of the literature on prevention groups has documented their effectiveness (Conyne and Horne 2001); in schools, successful prevention groups have focused on academic success such as study skills, social skills such as problem solving, and life transitions such as coping with parents' divorce.

Conyne (2004) highlighted the processes through which prevention groups can be successfully implemented. Successful groups provide a balance of information delivery, skill development, and group processes. As Conyne noted, well-intended groups can become unbalanced, with an overemphasis on didactic information delivery over interaction; in such cases, the power of the group process and, consequently, the opportunity for change are diminished.

Individual Counseling Individual counseling is a form of indicated or targeted prevention for students needing the most intensive support. The ASCA National Model lists individual counseling as a responsive service within its delivery system component. Individual counseling cannot be used to meet the needs of every student in a school; decisions about providing individual counseling should be consistent with the educational mission of the school and the objective of supporting the success of all students (Erford 2011).

Individual counseling interventions should be anchored within a comprehensive prevention framework. That is, the most symptomatic students receive support in the form of individual counseling to help prevent even more extensive challenges from developing (Mason and Nakkula 2008). A comprehensive school counseling program should have procedures in place for identifying such students and providing targeted services that are appropriate to their needs. Individual counseling as a targeted prevention service may look similar to, and overlap with, mental health counseling. The ASCA National Model clearly states that school counselors do not provide traditional, ongoing mental health therapy. For students who are identified as being in need of individual counseling in the school setting, counselors work within a developmental framework toward specific goals related to the broader school-wide prevention goals and the student's educational success (ASCA 2012). Brief, solution-focused, and cognitive-behavioral models of individual counseling intervention are frequently utilized in schools.

An important role of the school counselor is to ensure that students who need an intensive level of intervention have access to such services. For students who are involved in multiple systems of care, collaboration across these systems is necessary. School counselors work to develop relationships with numerous treatment providers to support effective referrals and can provide leadership and coordination of services to ensure that all relevant agencies are working together to remove barriers to students' success and prevent further difficulties. School counselors also work with parents and guardians to help them become aware of and access services to improve the health and well-being of students and the families in which they are embedded.

The prevalence and wide range of problems that children and adolescents bring to school make a sole reliance on responsive services, such as group and individual counseling, inefficient in part because they are likely to draw counselors' time away from a systemic, school-wide approach. Furthermore, it is unreasonable to expect such efforts to succeed in the absence of a clear, school-wide commitment to universal prevention. Targeted work with individual students is often necessary and effective, but these activities should be conceptualized as part of a coordinated universal prevention plan.

4.4.3   Evaluation of Prevention Programming

The accountability system of the ASCA National Model establishes that school counselors should use data to answer the question, "How are students different as a result of this program?" Although a full discussion of program evaluation is beyond the scope of this chapter, it is essential for counselors to include an evaluation strategy as part of the overall planning and implementation of any prevention program. This includes both process evaluation to ensure that the program is being implemented as intended and to guide adjustments along the way as necessary, and outcome evaluation to assess the degree to which the program is meeting its established objectives. In both these processes, school counselors provide leadership to ensure that an appropriate evaluation plan is developed, as well as coordination and management efforts to ensure that relevant data are collected, and perhaps most importantly, that the results are fed back into a decision-making process.

4.5   Summary and Case Examples

With their systemic, school-wide perspective and their developmental counseling expertise, school counselors are uniquely positioned to provide leadership in prevention programming within schools. In collaboration with administrators and other education professionals, counselors can implement prevention programming through direct service delivery, as well as indirectly through coordination, consultation, advocacy, and training.

Comprehensive school counseling programs can include prevention efforts that cover universal, selected, and indicated prevention levels. To ensure that current best practices in prevention science are clearly and purposefully integrated into school counseling programs, prevention specialists and other school personnel can support school counselors by ensuring that evidence-based programs are readily accessible and well documented and by advocating for the time and resources necessary to implement programs at each of these levels. Efforts toward individual skill development should be combined with and supported by systemic efforts targeting the whole school environment.

The following sections provide examples of school counselors' contributions to a range of prevention efforts: The development and implementation of a universal prevention program aimed at all freshmen in a high school, a selected prevention group for students identified as being at high risk for contracting human immunodeficiency virus (HIV), and comprehensive school-wide suicide prevention that includes universal and selected prevention strategies as well as targeted crisis intervention.

4.5.1   Universal Prevention in a High School

School counselors at a high school in the US Midwest with an enrollment of approximately 2200 students set out to use student evaluations of the freshman orientation day to improve that program (B. Dobias, personal communication, August 1, 2013).

Researchers found that freshmen considered the 40-min discussion with junior and senior volunteers to be the most useful part of the day. During this panel, these upperclassmen shared their insights and experiences on a variety of topics related to the high school culture, including academic expectations and homework, extra-curricular activities and social life, and cliques and bullying, all presented through a largely unstructured dialogue. Using data from evaluations, the counselors found that creating further opportunities for upperclassmen to work directly with fresh-men could be an effective means of delivering additional components of the school counseling curriculum.

This experience resulted in the formation of the Spartan Mentor Program (SMP), a group-based peer mentoring program designed and facilitated by the school coun-selors in collaboration with school faculty, administrators, and parents. Using a small-group format, upperclassmen were trained to colead freshman discussion groups that covered such guidance curriculum content as study skills, career ex-ploration, and bullying, among other topics. At the same time, the small discussion group design was intended to promote overall school connectedness by promoting the development of peer connections and support. The program combined the es-tablished effectiveness of group-based interventions and the influential role of peer social relationships in adolescence to accomplish these goals. This format offered the greatest flexibility in offering possible topics to discuss and opportunities for generating conversation, answering questions, and delivering the guidance curricu-lum in an experiential manner.

As a universal prevention effort, the SMP included all incoming freshmen. In-creasing students' connectedness to school was chosen as the overall goal to en-hance a protective factor against dropping out of school (Manning 2005). Addition-ally, the group sessions were designed with the goal of promoting specific resiliency factors, such as study skills, communication skills, and career planning skills.

The school counselors largely played indirect roles in the implementation of this program, including leadership, collaboration, training, and supervision, while much of the direct service was provided by the upperclassmen to the freshmen. Counsel-ors designed the program by adapting the guidance curriculum to a format that up-perclassmen could deliver in the small groups. They also identified and trained the upperclassmen to serve as peer mentors and provided ongoing supervision during program implementation. The development of the SMP also required counselors to engage in a great deal of leadership, advocacy, and collaboration with admin-istrators, faculty, and parents. Implementing a new school-wide program required investment and cooperation from faculty and administrators. Making scheduling changes to allow time for the groups, offering course credit to students serving as peer mentors, and cooperating with teachers who assisted in both training the peer mentors and supervising the peer-led groups were all essential to the successful implementation of the SMP.

An additional important component of the SMP as a universal prevention pro-gram was the establishment of a policy and protocol through which students who needed services beyond what the peer mentoring program could provide were re-ferred to school counselors for more targeted interventions. As part of their training, mentors were taught when and how to refer student concerns to program facilitators. Counselors' ongoing supervision and training of mentors allowed opportunities for discussion of any concerns, and a norm was set that when in doubt mentors should always err on the side of reporting concerns.

A final step in strengthening the sustainability and success of the program was the ongoing use of data to monitor its effectiveness. Particularly, with such a large-scale program that involved many school personnel and other resources, it was crucial that counselors be able to document that the SMP was achieving its goals. Feedback from students revealed they were becoming invested in not only their own individual success but also that of their peers. The systemic focus of this program benefited both the mentors and the mentees and provided a prevention emphasis to the school culture.

4.5.2   Targeted HIV/Acquired Immunodeficiency Syndrome (AIDS) Prevention with At-Risk Adolescent Girls

Nitza et al. (2010) described a targeted HIV/AIDS prevention group developed and implemented in a secondary school in Botswana, where universal HIV/AIDS prevention was already an established part of the guidance curriculum. The group originated from the school counselor's identification of a need for more intensive prevention efforts targeted to students who were at particular risk for contracting HIV due to a number of identified risk factors. First, the group was designed for adolescent girls, who in Botswana are at significantly increased risk of infection over adolescent boys (Botswana AIDS Impact Survey II 2005) due to a number of economic, social, and cultural influences (Green 2003). Second, inclusion criteria for the group identified girls at higher risk of infection due to one or more risk factors; specifically, having a disability, being orphaned, or having extremely limited economic means based on school report. The school counselor used these established risk criteria to identify and recruit group members.

The goals of the targeted prevention group were to assist members in naming barriers girls face as a result of a restrictive gender context in the country, identifying how these barriers have affected adolescent girls in general and group members as individuals, and developing and practicing collective and individual strategies for overcoming these barriers. Based on the existing literature regarding risk and protective factors surrounding HIV/AIDS for adolescent girls in Botswana, the specific objectives of the group were (a) to examine and deconstruct cultural practices and traditions that may negatively influence girls' sexual decision making, (b) to develop efficacy, skills, and strategies for dealing with barriers that impede members' success, and (c) to develop a supportive peer network for coping with present and future challenges.

Consistent with Conyne and Wilson's (2001) description of prevention groups, the interventions used to achieve the aforementioned goals promoted both knowledge and skill development. Knowledge was addressed through activities designed to heighten members' awareness of the many cultural messages that influence gender roles and relationships. Individual members then established goals for themselves, and skill development in areas such as assertiveness, conflict resolution, and self-esteem was tailored toward those goals. An important aspect of the group was a balance of content and process; an emphasis was placed on the development of a safe and collaborative atmosphere in which girls felt comfortable discussing these sensitive topics. Content-related topics were infused with opportunities for discussion and sharing of personal stories and experiences.

During the closing session, members identified goals for themselves relative to applying what they had learned to their lives outside the group. The school counselor conducted informal outcome evaluation by following up with the students to determine the extent to which they were able to achieve their goals. She reported that members requested permission to share what they had learned in the group to the rest of the school during an assembly and that all members demonstrated increased assertiveness skills in a variety of ways, such as singing a solo in the school choir for the first time. As the group members went on to share what they had learned from the program with other students, the targeted prevention program led to enhanced universal prevention.

4.5.3   Comprehensive Suicide Prevention in Schools

Child and adolescent suicide is a significant public health problem (Bridge et al. 2006). According to the Centers for Disease Control and Prevention (CDC) (CDC 2008), suicide is the third leading cause of death for youth. The CDC reported a study of US adolescents (grades 9–12) which indicated that 15 % of the students surveyed had considered suicide, 11 % had formed a plan to complete suicide, and 7 % had actually attempted suicide in the preceding year. Clearly, prevention of youth suicide is a concern for many mental health professionals, including school counselors (Chap. 16 for detail on suicide prevention). School counselors can be an integral part of school-based suicide prevention, crisis intervention and management, and postvention efforts (Capuzzi 2002; Eschbach 2005), and they may be the only professionals with counseling training available in a particular school. School counselors, as professionals who are familiar with the school system, have skills in leadership and coordination, are knowledgeable about available community resources, and are positioned to connect with other mental health professionals who could assist in crisis situations and should be instrumental in developing procedures for crisis intervention (ASCA 2013; Eschbach 2005; Fineran 2012; Siehl 1990). The ASCA position statement on dealing with crises in schools states that professional school counselors should respond proactively by taking a leadership role in planning and implementing prevention, intervention, and postincident crisis plans in schools (ASCA 2013, p. 12).

Most school counselors are trained specifically to respond to crisis situations. In fact, the CACREP standards for school counseling programs require that school counselors understand the potential effects of disasters and crises on the school community and that they have the knowledge and skills necessary to manage emergency situations (CACREP 2009).

Although preventing students from attempting suicide is of primary concern, completed youth suicides do occur. (See Chap. 16 for a discussion of suicide prevention.) Of equal importance is that school counselors be prepared to design, implement, and manage postvention efforts in the wake of student suicide as a preventive measure in and of itself. *Suicide postvention,* a term initially coined by Edwin Shneidman, has been defined by the American Association of Suicidology (1998, p. 1) as "the provision of crisis intervention, support, and assistance for those affected by a completed suicide." Strategically implemented procedures can assist in improving the emotional environment of the school after the death of a student by suicide. Action plans for quick and strategic responses can help minimize the emotional upheaval and confusion that may delay important interventions in the aftermath of a suicide and may help lessen long-term negative effects on survivors (ASCA 2013; Laux 2002; Westefeld et al. 2000). Therefore, the goals of suicide postvention in schools are (a) to provide support to minimize the emotional distress of survivors (Kerr et al. 2006), (b) to reduce the likelihood of contagion resulting in additional imitation or cluster suicides (CDC 2008), and (c) to help return the school to normal routines (Kerr et al. 2006). Numerous authors have advised that schools have postvention strategies in place well in advance of any student death and have noted that this is particularly important in the case of student suicide (Kerr 2009; King 1999; Siehl 1990). Such a protocol should include written guidelines for dealing with at-risk students, suicide attempts, and the student body returning to school following a completed suicide (Kalafat 1990; Kerr et al. 2006; McGlothlin 2008).

Beyond providing guidelines for crisis intervention, another primary purpose for the postvention plan is to arrange for preventive education (King 1999). The school counselor may conduct workshops that educate faculty, staff, students, and parents about adolescent suicide. Such workshops may focus on empirically identified risk factors, symptoms of depression, resources available to help a suicidal student, suicide risk assessment, and the school plan in place should a student complete suicide. Schools counselors may also partner with outside suicide prevention organizations to provide training and ongoing support.

Another aspect of the school counselor's role is to advocate for school transformation and systemic change at all levels: local, state, regional, and national (Kaffenberger et al. 2006). Promoting the role of the school counselor in developing, implementing, and evaluating effective and efficient suicide prevention, intervention, and postvention plans for all schools is a matter of advocacy that could influence the training of school counselors, public opinion of school counseling programs, and resources provided to schools for suicide prevention programs and postvention efforts. Many suicide interventions need to take place at an individual level. For example, to meet the three aforementioned postvention goals, the school counselor may implement macro-level interventions, but individual sessions will likely also be necessary with students, teachers, and administrators who were close to the deceased student. School counselors may need to proactively encourage survivors to participate in postvention activities, as some individuals, especially adolescents, may fear a social stigma attached to seeking out mental health assistance (Slate and

Scott 2009). Ongoing monitoring of individual students during and in the wake of the crisis is necessary. Particular attention should be paid to those who were close associates of the student, are currently in treatment for mental health issues, have a personal or family history of issues such as depression, anxiety, and substance abuse disorders, have a history of prior suicide attempts, or have been identified by concerned others, such as parents and teachers (Kerr 2009; Parrish and Tunkle 2005).

The school counselor may meet individually or in groups with teachers, administrators, parents, and family members of a deceased student. It may be necessary to contact the deceased student's family to determine their wishes for disclosure, obtain information on funeral arrangements, identify siblings and close friends who may be in need of assistance, discuss the school's postvention response, return personal items from a desk or locker, and offer any support that the school may be able to provide. This personal contact in such a tragic situation must be managed sensitively and privately and certainly requires individual counseling skills. Because school counselors may be the first mental health contact for the family after a student's death, they should be prepared to offer parents the names of mental health agencies and survivor support groups and assist the family in making connections with these outside groups for ongoing counseling outside the school setting.

In the area of youth suicide, both universal and selected prevention is necessary to prevent suicide and to respond to completed suicide in a preventive manner. Universally, all members of a school community need to be screened for depression and suicide risk, be aware of warning signs and risk factors, and be knowledgeable about relevant resources. On the selected prevention level, school counselors work to identify students who may be at heightened risk for suicide due to mental health disorders, prior suicide attempts, substance use problems, recent losses, or other factors. After a suicide occurs, plans must be in place to respond to the crisis in a way that is preventive and proactive. Students, families, teachers, administrators, and school staff must have access to resources and services, and school staff needs to have a plan in place to respond supportively to all members of the school community. A carefully planned identification and referral process is important for identifying vulnerable students and others in need of additional support, including group and individual crisis counseling. School counselors can then proceed to develop and implement selected-level prevention programming to assist students identified as being at higher risk or to those who do not respond to the universal prevention measures.

4.6 Implications and Future Directions

Professional school counselors have an important role to play in the success of school-wide prevention efforts. The establishment, implementation, and evaluation of a comprehensive developmental guidance program within a school serves as the basis for universal and targeted prevention efforts.

For prevention efforts to be successful, school counselors must provide leadership and advocacy in their areas of expertise and continue to develop systemic, school-wide approaches to their work that are linked directly to the mission of the school. School administrators can contribute to this success by authorizing school counselors to implement school counseling programs as intended as well as minimizing counselor time spent in non-counseling activities. Positioning collaboration and a school-wide commitment to prevention efforts as integral parts of a school's mission is also essential for supporting the success of all students.

References

Akos, P., Hamm, J. V., Mack, S., & Dunaway, M. (2007). Utilizing the developmental influence of peers in middle school groups. *Journal for Specialists in Group Work, 32*(1), 51–60. doi:10.1080/01933920600977648.

American Association of Suicidology. (1998). *Suicide postvention guidelines: Suggestions for dealing with the aftermath of suicide in the schools.* Washington, DC: American Association of Suicidology.

American School Counselor Association (ASCA). (2009). The role of the professional school counselor. http://www.schoolcounselor.org/school-counselors-members/careers-roles/the-role-of-the-professional-school-counselor. Accessed 13 July 2013.

American School Counselor Association (ASCA). (2012). *The ASCA national model: A framework for school counseling programs* (3rd ed.). Alexandria: American School Counselor Association (ASCA).

American School Counselor Association (ASCA). (2013). The professional school counselor and crisis/critical incident response in the schools. http://www.schoolcounselor.org/files/Position-Statements.pdf. Accessed 13 July 2013.

American School Counselor Association (ASCA). (n.d.). State certification requirements. http://www.schoolcounselor.org/school-counselors-members/careers-roles/state-certification-requirements. Accessed 4 Aug 2013.

Botswana AIDS Impact Survey II: Popular report. (2005). Gaborone, Botswana: Central Statistics Office and National AIDS Coordinating Agency.

Bridge, J. A., Goldstein, T. R., & Brent, D. A. (2006). Adolescent suicide and suicidal behavior. *Journal of Child Psychology & Psychiatry, 47,* 372–394. doi:10.1111/j.1469-7610.2006.01615.x.

Campbell, C., & Dahir, C. (1997). *The national standards for school counseling programs.* Alexandria: ASCA.

Capuzzi, D. (2002). Legal and ethical challenges in counseling suicidal students. *Professional School Counseling, 6,* 36–45.

Centers for Disease Control and Prevention (CDC). (2008). Suicide. http://www.cdc.gov/ncipc/dvp/suicide/youthsuicide.htm. Accessed 16 Aug 2013.

Conyne, R. (2004). Prevention groups. In J. L. DeLucia-Waack, D. A. Gerrity, C. R. Kalodner, & M. T. Riva (Eds.), *Handbook of group counseling and psychotherapy* (pp. 620–629). Thousand Oaks: Sage.

Conyne, R., & Horne, A. (Eds.). (2001). The use of groups for prevention [Special issue]. *Journal for Specialists in Group Work, 26,* 205–292.

Conyne, R., & Wilson, F. R. (2001). Division 49 position paper: Recommendations of the task force for the use of groups for prevention. *Group Psychologist, 11,* 10–11.

Council for Accreditation of Counseling and Related Educational Programs (CACREP). (2009). *CACREP accreditation standards and procedures manual.* Alexandria: Council for Accreditation of Counseling and Related Educational Programs (CACREP).

Erford, B. T. (2011). The ASCA national model: Developing a comprehensive, developmental school counseling program. In B. T. Erford (Ed.), *Transforming the school counseling profession* (pp. 44–57). Upper Saddle River: Pearson.

Eschbach, L. (2005). School-based crises. In B. G. Collins & T. M. Collins (Eds.), *Crisis and trauma: Developmental-ecological intervention* (pp. 407–463). Boston: Lahaska Press.

Fineran, K. R. (2012). Suicide postvention in schools: The role of the school counselor. *Journal of Professional Counseling: Practice, Theory, & Research, 39*(2), 14–21.

Goodnough, G. E., Perusse, R., & Erford, B. T. (2011). Developmental classroom guidance. In B. T. Erford (Ed.), *Transforming the school counseling profession* (pp. 154–177). Upper Saddle River: Pearson.

Green, E. C. (2003). *Rethinking AIDS prevention: Learning from successes in developing countries.* Westport: Praeger.

Greenberg, M. T., Domitrovich, C., & Bumbarger, B. (1999). *Preventing mental disorders in school-age children: A review of the effectiveness of prevention programs.* Washington, DC: U.S. Department of Health and Human Services, Substance Abuse Mental Health Services Administration, Center for Mental Health Services.

Kaffenberger, C. J., Murphy, S., & Bemak, F. (2006). School counseling leadership team: A statewide collaborative model to transform school counseling. *Professional School Counseling, 9,* 288–294.

Kalafat, J. (1990). Adolescent suicide and the implications for school response programs. *School Counselor, 37,* 359–369.

Kenny, M. E., Waldo, M., Warter, E. H., & Barton, C. (2002). School-linked prevention: Theory, science and practice for enhancing the lives of children and youth. *Counseling Psychologist, 30,* 726–748. doi:10.1177/0011000002305004.

Kerr, M. M. (2009). *School crisis prevention and intervention.* Columbus: Pearson.

Kerr, M. M., Brent, D. A., McCain, B., & McCommons, P. S. (2006). *Postvention standards manual: A guide for a school's response in the aftermath of a sudden death* (5th ed.). Pittsburgh: University of Pittsburgh, Services for Teens at Risk (STAR-Center).

King, K. (1999). High school suicide postvention: Recommendations for an effective program. *American Journal of Health Studies, 15,* 217–223.

Laux, J. M. (2002). A primer on suicidology: Implications for counselors. *Journal of Counseling & Development, 80,* 380–384. doi:10.1002/j.1556-6678.2002.tb00203.x.

Manning, D. (2005). *Connected students: The key to school-initiated graduate rate improvement.* Oroville: Bridges Transitions.

Mason, M. J., & Nakkula, M. J. (2008). A risk and prevention counselor training program model: Theory and practice. *Journal of Primary Prevention, 29,* 361–374. doi:10.1007/s10935-008-0148-6.

McGlothlin, J. M. (2008). *Developing clinical skills in suicide assessment, prevention, and treatment.* Alexandria: American Counseling Association.

Nitza, A., Chilisa, B., & Makwinja-Morara, V. (2010). Mbizi: Empowerment and HIV/AIDS prevention for adolescent girls in Botswana. *Journal for Specialists in Group Work, 35,* 105–114. doi:10.1080/01933921003705990.

Orpinas, P., & Horne, A. M. (2006). *Bullying prevention: Creating a positive school climate and developing social competence.* Washington, DC: American Psychological Association.

Parrish, M., & Tunkle, J. (2005). Clinical challenges following an adolescent's death by suicide: Bereavement issues faced by family, friend, schools, and clinicians. *Clinical Social Work Journal, 33,* 81–102. doi:10.1007/s10615-005-2621-5.

Payton, J. W., Wardlaw, D. M., Graczyk, P. A., Bloodworth, M. A., Tompsett, C. J., & Weissberg, R. P. (2000). Social and emotional learning: A framework for promoting mental health and reducing risk behaviors in children and youth. *Journal of School Health, 70,* 179–185. doi:10.1111/j.1746-1561.2000.tb06468.x.

Ringwalt, C., Hanley, S., Vincus, A. A., Ennett, S. T., Rohrbach, L. A., & Bowling, J. M. (2008). The prevalence of effective substance use prevention curricula in the nation's high schools. *Journal of Primary Prevention, 29,* 479–488. doi:10.1007/s10935-008-0158-4.

Roysircar, G. (2006). A theoretical and practice framework for universal school-based prevention. In R. L. Toporek, L. H. Gerstein, N. A. Fouad, G. Roysircar, & T. Israel (Eds.), *Handbook for social justice in counseling psychology: Leadership, vision, and action* (pp. 130–145). Thousand Oaks: Sage.

Siehl, P. M. (1990). Suicide postvention: A new disaster plan—what a school counselor should do when faced with suicide. *School Counselor, 38,* 52–58.

Slate, C. N., & Scott, S. A. (2009, March). A discussion of coping methods and counseling techniques for children and adults dealing with grief and bereavement. Paper based on a program presented at the American Counseling Association Annual Conference and Exposition, Charlotte, NC.

Stone, C. B., & Dahir, C. A. (2007). *School counselor accountability: A measure of student success* (2nd ed.). Upper Saddle River: Pearson Merrill/Prentice Hall.

Vera, E. M., & Reese, L. E. (2000). Prevention interventions with school-age youth. In S. D. Brown & R. W. Lent (Eds.), *Handbook of counseling psychology* (pp. 411–434). New York: Wiley.

Walsh, M. E., Galassi, J. P., Murphy, J. A., & Park-Taylor, J. (2002). A conceptual framework for counseling psychologists in schools. *Counseling Psychologist, 30,* 682–704. doi:10.1177/0011000002305002.

Westefeld, J. S., Range, L. M., Rogers, I. R., Maples, M. R., Bromley J. L., & Alcorn, J. (2000). Suicide: An overview. *Counseling Psychologist, 28,* 445–510. doi:10.1177/0011000000284002.

Chapter 5
Teachers on the Front Line of Prevention Science

Nancy Fichtman Dana and Angela Hooser

To implement prevention with fidelity, teachers had to learn the content of the social competence lessons, utilize behavioral techniques, and do other activities that may be outside the normal scope of academic instruction. Thus, the most direct role for a classroom teacher in prevention work is the implementation of universal-level prevention programs or curricula because school is the most efficient place to reach a "captive audience" of children. As McVey et al. (2004) pointed out with regard to a life-skills promotion program designed to improve body image satisfaction and reduce predisposing factors for eating disorders in sixth-grade girls, providing the information during the girls' regular school health class "provides wider access to the information. It also helps to prevent students from feeling stigmatized about their concerns, a potential problem if students have to seek support outside of the class or school setting" (p. 9).

The roles classroom teachers play within the delivery of particular intervention programs can vary considerably. A comprehensive meta-analysis of drug prevention programs (including tobacco and alcohol) showed that interactive programs are dramatically more effective than knowledge-focused programs delivered by didactic lecture and adult-led discussion, a finding "consistently reproduced across a multitude of diverse categories and breakout variables" (Tobler et al. 2000, p. 300). "Interactive" programs are characterized by activities such as role-plays that rehearse refusal skills and peer-led discussions. Teachers are often called upon to become trained in and implement such curricula. Finally, Tobler and colleagues reported that the most effective program type was system-level interventions, such as those influencing school climates to promote student attachment to school. These involve

N. F. Dana (✉)
School of Teaching and Learning, University of Florida, 2215 Norman Hall,
PO Box 117056, Gainesville, FL 32611, USA
e-mail: ndana@coe.ufl.edu

A. Hooser
Department of Teaching and Learning, University of South Florida,
4202 East Fowler Ave. MAIL STOP EDU 105, Tampa, FL 33620, USA
e-mail: hoosera@usf.edu

© Springer Science+Business Media New York 2015
K. Bosworth (ed.), *Prevention Science in School Settings*,
Advances in Prevention Science, DOI 10.1007/978-1-4939-3155-2_5

teachers focusing on positive and supportive everyday interactions with students and practicing consistency in their classroom management practices (Chap. 13).

Because current federal guidelines require that school-based prevention practices be evidence-based, prevention specialists typically conduct research in schools to demonstrate the effectiveness of newly designed prevention curricula (Chap. 11). Wilson and colleagues (2003) found that 92 % of the violence prevention studies reported in the literature involved demonstration projects rather than routine practice and may not be as effective as system-level routine interventions. For newly designed curricula to become a part of everyday interactions, collaboration between prevention specialists and the teachers or school staff implementing the program is needed, along with support for educators to learn new skills and content outside their established knowledge base. In order to design school-based programs that are feasible for implementation in routine practice, and to collaborate fruitfully with school personnel, it is imperative for prevention specialists to understand the day-to-day work in classrooms. As Han and Weiss (2005) underscore, the successful dissemination and scaling up of evidence-based prevention programs cannot occur without attention to "understanding the complexity of program implementation under 'real world' conditions" (p. 665). Hence, the purpose of this chapter is to provide a glimpse into the life of teachers, their frontline work with students, and the ways prevention specialists can best work in schools given the reality of the work teachers do. We begin our glimpse into the work of a teacher by providing a basic overview of the knowledge base for teaching, teachers' educational preparation for the profession, and the ways teachers engage in professional development throughout their careers to continue to build this knowledge.

5.1 Overview of the Knowledge Base for Teaching

The literature on teaching emphasizes that it is much more than "personal style, artful communication, knowing some subject matter, and applying the results of research on effective teaching" (Shulman 1987, pp. 5–6). Rather, it is a complex art requiring multiple types of knowledge derived from four major sources: (a) scholarship in content disciplines; (b) materials and settings of the institutionalized educational process; (c) research on schooling, social organizations, human learning, teaching and development, and the other social and cultural phenomena that affect what teachers do; and (d) the wisdom of practice itself (Shulman 1987). In a seminal article entitled "Knowledge and Teaching: Foundations of the New Reform," Shulman (1987) drew upon these sources to identify and describe seven connected types of knowledge teachers must master to meet the diverse needs of the students they teach: (a) content knowledge, (b) curriculum knowledge, (c) pedagogical knowledge, (d) pedagogical content knowledge, (e) knowledge of learners, (f) knowledge of educational contexts, and (g) knowledge of educational purpose.

First, *content knowledge* and *curriculum knowledge* require the teacher to master the underlying principles of a subject area as well as understand how to use resources such as standards documents and textbooks to create coherent lessons. Yet, content and curriculum knowledge alone do not lead to effective teaching. In addition, a teacher must understand pedagogy, that is, the planning, delivery, and assessment of learning activities within a classroom setting. Classroom management and organization of students for instruction are interwoven within *general pedagogical knowledge,* defined as understanding and selecting from a range of approaches to instruction and assessment. Connected to the attainment of general pedagogical knowledge, teachers also need to develop pedagogical knowledge related to the specific content they teach. Shulman (1987) coined the term *pedagogical content knowledge* (PCK) to describe this notion. PCK refers to the teacher's ability to connect specific subject matter to students with diverse backgrounds and academic needs. The development of PCK often requires teachers to deepen their understanding of the subject matter and subsequently think about this academic content from students' varying perspectives, to make it meaningful and relevant to them.

For PCK to develop, teachers must possess *knowledge of learners.* This knowledge includes understanding child development, cultural differences, and the ways students may perceive instruction differently based on their culture and developmental levels. Knowledge of learners is built not in a vacuum, but rather within specific settings, necessitating *knowledge of educational contexts* as well. Shulman describes this knowledge as ranging from "the workings of the classroom, and the governance and financing of school districts, to the character of communities and cultures" (Shulman 1987, p. 7). Finally, related to understanding their individual learners and the contexts within which teaching takes place, educators must possess *knowledge of educational purposes,* which includes the philosophical and historical grounds for a teacher's daily work.

Hence, each school day, educators draw upon multiple types of knowledge while striving to select the most appropriate methods for the students in their care. Adding prevention programing to the teacher's workday asks teachers for far more than simply carving out the time to implement the requisite curriculum. Doing so demands that teachers connect the prevention program to classroom learning. Understanding the ways teachers acquire the fundamental knowledge necessary for teaching can help prevention specialists support teachers as they implement intervention programs in the classroom.

5.2   Educational Preparation for the Teaching Profession

Although a variety of pathways exist for entering the teaching profession, and certification requirements and regulations vary from state to state, the most traditional pathway to acquire the fundamental background knowledge base for teaching that Shulman discusses is through earning a degree at a university, either a bachelor's or a master's, depending on the program. In general, teacher education programs contain four components: (a) arts and sciences coursework in the subject matter fields the prospective teacher plans to teach as well as courses taken as electives to fulfill general education requirements; (b) foundations of education coursework in areas such as history of education, sociology of education, philosophy of education, and educational psychology; (c) education coursework in teaching methods; and (d) field experience/clinical practice.

Arts and sciences coursework is a logical and commonsense component of teacher education programs as teachers need to understand the central concepts in the subject areas they will teach. Deep understanding of one's content (what Shulman coined content knowledge) is critical to enable teachers to create multiple approaches to teaching a concept when some learners do not grasp the material the way it is first presented, a common occurrence during lessons. Deep understanding of their subject matter empowers teachers to respond flexibly and effectively when students ask questions or misunderstandings occur (Ball 1997; McDiarmid et al. 1989).

Foundations of education coursework "uses theories and results from psychology, sociology, history, and philosophy to address issues of how children learn, how schooling connects to broad social issues, how U.S. education has changed since Colonial times, and how ethical issues arise in instruction" (Floden and Meniketti 2005, p. 262). Because many of these courses focus on learning and development, most states require some coursework in educational foundations as a part of licensure requirements. The goal of such coursework is to cultivate teaching candidates' *knowledge of educational purposes,* to use Shulman's term.

Coursework in teaching methods seeks to develop teacher candidates'

- intellectual command of the concepts and schemata of teaching (characterized by the ability to comprehend, develop, and articulate models of basic approaches to teaching practice);
- interpretation of the complexities of content and context (specifically, understanding how the ways one conceptualizes the purposes of subject matter and views curricular outcomes influences unit and lesson planning);
- socialization into the professional role of the teacher (characterized by use of the words, theories, and points of view associated with "becoming a professional"); and
- demonstration of skillful teaching practice (characterized by acquisition of appropriate skills and application of these skills in instructional settings) (Stengel and Tom 1996).

Within methods coursework, teacher candidates practice teaching skills through multiple mechanisms (e.g., microteaching, case study, simulation), with the most prevalent avenue being structured experiences in schools and classrooms (field experience). In a review of research on methods courses and field experiences, Clift and Brady (2005) report, "in many instances, methods courses and fieldwork have become inseparable" (p. 329).

As the final and most critical aspect of educational preparation for the teaching profession, field experience or clinical practice has received heightened attention in recent years (National Council for Accreditation of Teacher Education 2010).

Most states require that a specific minimum number of hours be spent in clinical settings throughout the teacher preparation program, culminating with a semester-long student teaching experience or yearlong internship in a public school setting. It is the interaction between methods coursework and field experiences that enables teaching candidates to develop the remaining knowledge bases Shulman discusses: curriculum knowledge, pedagogical knowledge, pedagogical content knowledge, knowledge of learners, and knowledge of educational contexts.

5.3 Professional Development Throughout the Teaching Career

Complicating teacher preparation for the profession is the fact that the knowledge base for teaching is "not fixed and final" (Shulman 1987, p. 12). Because multiple types of knowledge are necessary for effective teaching, and the knowledge base for teaching continually evolves, teachers participate in continual professional learning throughout their careers, through either or both graduate programs or professional development offered within their school or district. The research on teacher professional development is of particular relevance to prevention specialists who aspire to partner with teachers to work in the best interest of children.

In a review of research on teacher professional development, Desimone (2009) states, "a research consensus [exists] on the main features of professional development that have been associated with changes in knowledge, practice, and, to a lesser extent, student achievement" (p. 183). These features form the basis of a conceptual framework for use in professional development programs to "move the field forward in terms of building a consistent knowledge base" (p. 184). These core features of effective professional development are content focus, active learning, coherence, duration, and collective participation.

Content-focused activities increase teachers' subject matter knowledge and understanding of how students acquire knowledge of particular content. This aspect is important in any professional development but particularly in the context of a prevention program. Not only is the content of prevention programs new to most teachers, but the goal of implementing them is to go beyond teaching students new knowledge and influence their current and future behavior. Thus, the "how" of student skill acquisition is different. *Active learning* involves teachers in observing expert teachers, being observed and receiving interactive feedback and discussion on their teaching, or reviewing student work rather than listening to a lecture. In the context of prevention, Han and Weiss (2005) point out that combining classroom practice with performance feedback during teacher training produces the strongest effects in terms of teacher willingness to implement the program and the fidelity of their implementation. *Coherence* reflects the extent to which the material taught in the professional development event aligns with state and district goals and standards for student learning. Another aspect is the extent to which the content of professional development is consistent with teachers' knowledge and beliefs

(Desimone 2009). Han and Weiss (2005) review research suggesting that teachers' judgments of whether an intervention program is acceptable hinge on three factors including whether the program targets a serious student problem, the nature of the intervention, and how much time is required. In turn, "teachers' judgments of the acceptability of an intervention program significantly influence their interest and willingness to implement a program and the degree to which they implement the program with fidelity" (p. 669). In terms of *duration* of professional development, research suggests that programs include at least 20 hour of contact time, either spread out over a semester or in an intensive training with follow-up over a semester (Desimone 2009). Similarly, research suggests that teachers need both adequate initial training and ongoing consultation support to ensure sustained implementation of a prevention program (Han and Weiss 2005). *Collective participation* refers to teachers working together during professional development sessions, which can be a powerful form of teacher learning. These research-based core features of teacher professional development provide important areas of consideration for prevention specialists who work with teachers.

In addition to understanding the knowledge base for teaching, initial preparation for the teaching career, and components of effective teacher professional development programs, understanding the lived experience of the classroom teacher can also help the prevention specialist form working partnerships with teachers. The next section of this chapter illuminates the life of a teacher through the story of a middle school teacher, Susan James, and her introduction to implementing a prevention program at her school.

5.4 The Life of a Teacher

Susan James always wanted to be a teacher. Her parents tell stories of how as a child she used to "play school" by lining up her stuffed animals and teaching them. Susan loved science and was inspired to teach science by her ninth-grade environmental science teacher, who engaged Susan in an investigation-based curriculum. Susan could not wait to finish high school and enroll in science teacher education at a local university.

As she pursued her bachelor's degree, Susan quickly realized how limited her childhood perceptions of teaching were, frequently chuckled at the simplistic view of teaching she held when playing school with her stuffed animals, and marveled at how easy her ninth-grade science teacher had made teaching seem. As she completed her first student teaching placement at a middle school, she realized that teaching was more difficult than she had ever imagined, but she remained passionate about science and the profession she had chosen to enter, and thoroughly enjoyed spending time with young adolescents.

She found that teaching to meet the needs of middle school children was both challenging and exhilarating. Middle school students have entered an age of sociability and activity, exploration and risk-taking (Sizer and Meier 2006). Furthermore, as middle school teachers well know, most young adolescents find traditional schooling—which often involves solitary reading, poring over text, and passively exploring the world of the mind—does not match the energy, passion, adventurousness, romanticism, and yearning to be grown up that characterizes the early teen years (Sizer and Meier 2006).

As she experienced this unique age group, Susan decided she wanted to teach at the middle school level and secured her first teaching position at Oakview Middle School, where she has now been teaching for 10 years. Susan's typical day as an eighth-grade science teacher begins at 5:30 a.m., when she wakes up to get her own family ready for the day, then commutes 25 min to Oakview for the 7:30 a.m. start of the school day. She teaches five science classes, each with approximately 25 students. She has one period designated for planning, which she often ends up using for tasks such as making parent phone calls, meeting with colleagues about student issues, or sometimes to substitute teaching in other classes when her school is unable to secure coverage for a teacher who is ill. Often Susan has no time during the day for lesson planning or providing students feedback on their assignments. Often she leaves these tasks until the evening hours after her own young children have gone to bed. It is not unusual for her to spend 1–2 hour each evening preparing for her next teaching day.

Each of her five classes covers similar content, but the individual needs of the students in each class are very different, so her day is never routine. Susan works hard to personally connect with her students, but with being responsible for teaching 125 students, whom she usually sees for only one period a day, getting to know her students well is a never-ending challenge.

To help her students become scientifically literate, Susan has always focused on investigation-based teaching, including scientific questioning and analysis (Anderson 2002; Bransford and Donovan 2005; Crawford 2000; Olson and Loucks-Horsley 2000). A member of the National Science Teachers Association (NSTA), Susan regularly reads this organization's newsletter and the professional journal it publishes—*Science Scope,* one of her favorites—to stay abreast of the latest approaches to teaching science. She also attends professional development seminars each summer. The most recent was a workshop on understanding and implementing the Common Core State Standards.

Common Core is the latest in a long line of innovations Susan's district has undertaken in her 10 years teaching at Oakview. The introduction of new initiatives has always been challenging for Susan and her colleagues, but the Common Core State Standards loom larger than any initiative they had seen come and go at Oakview before. Intended to "provide a clear and consistent framework to prepare our children for college and the workforce," these standards have been adopted by Susan's state, as well as 44 others, the District of Columbia, four territories, and the Department of Defense Education Activity (National Governors Association 2012).

One feature of the Common Core that intrigued Susan was its emphasis on literacy development as a shared responsibility among all educators (Calkins et al. 2012). She recognized how important it was for her to help her students develop as readers and writers, but she could not help but feel a little concerned that she now needed to spend time developing her students' literacy in addition to their knowledge of science. As it was, there was never enough time to do all the rich science investigations she wanted to engage her students with each year, and Susan often agonized over the curriculum decisions she was forced to make.

One aspect of the Common Core State Standards that really excited Susan and her colleagues was that they seemed to necessitate a departure from the mind-set of the previous high-stakes testing era, where teachers were often handed teacher editions to textbooks and pacing guides that prescribed every detail of a lesson (Dana et al. 2013). Fortunately, Susan and her colleagues worked for a principal who kept her eye on test scores but was not consumed by them. Although Susan had never felt boxed in by the Basic Science Skills Test (BSST) administered to all eighth-grade students statewide at the end of the school year, she could not help but experience some stress about her students' performance on this exam. Those students who did not perform well would have limited options for which science courses they would be allowed to take in high school (Handwerk et al. 2008). Furthermore, her own yearly evaluation and effectiveness rating, which directly affected her salary, was tied to the scores her students were able to achieve on this single exam (US Department of Education 2009).

In the upcoming school year, Susan would need to find a balance between covering the content knowledge that was tested on the BSST and preparing her students for college and the workforce as described in the Common Core. To this end, Susan planned to begin the year by taking a historical look at the work of various scientists and how each contributed to both technological advances and our understanding of the way the natural world works. Her students would be assigned roles within collaborative groups and would search for information on different websites she had identified over the summer. She planned to ask them critical questions, not just about the scientists' discoveries but also about how that work affected students' lives today. The standards for reading science would be addressed as they followed multistep procedures in their web quest, drew conclusions from the information they gained, and cited evidence to support their arguments. Simultaneously, students would hone their writing in history and science as they built arguments based on scientific knowledge and wrote and presented an essay on their research.

As Susan planned this first lesson to kick off the school year, she also needed to keep behavior management issues in mind. Some of the seventh-grade teachers had given her a heads up that the incoming class of eighth-graders was prone to frequent off-task behavior. If Susan's lessons were to be successful, she would need to manage the students' behavior effectively.

She also knew that her students were beginning to experiment with risk-taking behavior, such as smoking, drinking, or early sexual experimentation. Several students had been suspended for smoking, and she had heard a few talking about drinking over the weekend. One student had asked her if they could analyze the chemicals in marijuana, which led to a discussion of medical marijuana. Having grown up with an alcoholic parent, Susan knew that some of her students were likewise challenged by the unpredictability of such an environment. These issues spilled into classrooms and created barriers to learning.

At the end of every Tuesday and Thursday, Susan took her post outside for bus duty, her "other duty as assigned" for the year. Susan did not mind this responsibility, because she often saw and could briefly reconnect with her students as they headed home. One Thursday, after the last bus pulled out of the schoolyard, Susan's principal approached her to ask if she would meet with a health educator from the County Health Department about a prevention initiative for eighth-graders the Health Department wished to implement at Oakview. Because of her concern over how risky behaviors affected her students, Susan was glad to learn more about this possibility. At the meeting the next week, the Health Department representative, Jason Garcia, described the evidence-based prevention curriculum to Susan and the other science teachers and outlined the summer training opportunities. The teachers would be learning not only neuroscience content about how various substances affect the brain but also facilitation skills for supporting students in role-plays practicing assertiveness skills. She was familiar with various types of active learning, but behavioral role-playing would be new territory for her. Susan knew this program would be important and relevant to her students' lives, but she already struggled to cover all of the science content that appeared on the BSST at the end of the year. Even though the program involved teaching students about the neuroscience of how the brain works and is affected by various substances, this was not a topic covered on the BSST. What science lessons would she need to skip over or curtail to make time for the prevention program and at what cost? On the other hand, what would be the cost to her students if she did not address this important topic with them at their vulnerable age?

These days, everything at her school revolved around Common Core. She and the entire eighth-grade team were working diligently to better understand the standards and approach all of their teaching with those standards in mind. The prevention program, developed and researched before the advent of Common Core, did not easily align with those standards, and Susan worried that it might feel apart *from* instead of a part *of* their work to build the higher-order, critical thinking, and literacy skills associated with the Common Core. Garcia had emphasized that as an evidence-based program, the prevention curriculum needed to be implemented as written to accomplish its proven outcomes. Susan feared she would not have any flexibility to integrate this program with the content and standards she was responsible for teaching and on which her job performance would be evaluated. Despite the myriad of concerns swirling in her brain, Susan assured her principal she would be happy to take the lead on the program and looked forward to learning all of the details associated with her participation in it.

5.5   The Complexity of Teaching

As Shulman's (1987) discussion of the knowledge base for teaching and Susan James's story begin to reveal, teaching is an incredibly complex act. Effective teachers must know their content deeply, know pedagogy, know human development, develop relationships with the 25 (in elementary school) to 100-plus students (in secondary schools) they interact with each day. After identifying each of these learners' academic, social, and emotional needs, they must attend to all of these unique and varied needs simultaneously during each instructional moment of the day. Teachers must understand lesson planning and understand that every lesson taught will produce a unique outcome that results from the interaction of the context, the timing of the teaching, the teacher him- or herself, and the learners in the classroom. Then, they must attend to managing the behavior and transitions of large groups of learners before, during, and after each lesson. Teachers are bombarded with decision-making each minute of their day, ranging from determining how to modify a planned lesson when it is not progressing productively to deciding whether Johnny, who just asked to use the bathroom for the third time that day, should be given permission to leave the room. In addition, teachers constantly assess their students' learning and progress, both formally and informally. Among their contributions to the running of the school are managing such tasks as collecting lunch money, taking lunch counts, and rotating on bus and lunch duties. They must communicate and collaborate with parents and other education professionals, such as guidance counselors, the principal, school psychologists, and other teaching colleagues. In their spare time, they serve on committees, attend faculty meetings, and read professional journals and books to stay abreast of latest developments in their field. They do all of this while simultaneously keeping an eye on high-stakes testing and their students' performance, balancing preparation for test-taking and the teaching of test-taking skills with the teaching and learning of real content.

This picture we have painted of a teacher's work is by no means complete, but we believe it sufficiently complete to illustrate the inherently complex nature of teaching. Superimpose upon all of this complexity the numerous issues contemporary teachers must grapple with, such as implementation of a new set of standards (Common Core), and constantly being asked to do more with shrinking budgets. Teaching has many inherent stresses and pressures often unseen by outsiders who do work within schools and must depend on teachers to support their work.

When Susan's principal approached her to lead the implementation of a prevention program, she knew it was important and wanted this program for her students, whom she cared deeply about, but at the same time she could not help but experience some pause and trepidation over how this new duty would affect her daily teaching practice as well as the totality of her work as a teacher. So, given the "real-world" conditions of a teacher's life, what is a prevention specialist to do?

5.6   The Prevention Specialist and the Teacher: Principles for Successful Collaboration

We end this chapter with three simple, but very important, lessons prevention specialists can learn from the story of Susan James and the real-world conditions that contextualize teachers' work.

5.6.1 Empathize

Teaching is challenging, demanding work. Teacher burnout, characterized by emotional exhaustion and a low sense of personal accomplishment from one's work, is well documented as a common condition often associated with somatic problems (Belcastro and Gold 1983; Jackson et al. 1986; Maslach et al. 1996). Teachers are tired, and many leave the profession after only a few years. The National Commission on Teaching and America's Future (2003) reports that "after just 3 years, it is estimated that almost a third of new entrants to teaching have left the field, and after 5 years almost half are gone" (p. 19). In more challenging contexts, such as rural areas and inner cities, these rates are often dramatically higher. Studies show that professional burnout leads teachers to have less positive evaluations of their students and more negative attitudes about implementing a new program. Low job satisfaction may also reduce their sense of self-efficacy in implementing the new program, willingness to invest effort in it, or recognition of improvements in students' behavior (Han and Weiss 2005). For all these reasons, prevention experts are wise to be sensitive to and supportive of teachers' mental states.

It is important for prevention specialists to understand the intensity and overwhelming demands of teaching. Like Susan, teachers appreciate the need for prevention programs, particularly during the high-risk period of early adolescence. At the same time, they wonder how prevention programs—no matter how needed and important—can fit on their already overflowing plates. Acknowledging the hard work teachers already do goes a long way in helping the prevention specialist connect with and relate to teaching professionals and work in partnership with them to figure out a way to seamlessly weave prevention programming into the already overcrowded school day.

5.6.2 Provide Ongoing Support

Learning about and implementing new content and activities is never an easy task. As noted earlier in this chapter, solely attending trainings is an ineffective approach to teacher learning and successful application of that new learning to classroom practice (Desimone 2009). As Killion and Harrison (2006, p. 8) point out, "Traditional professional development usually occurs away from the school site, separate from classroom contexts and challenges in which teachers are expected to apply what they have learned, and often without the necessary support to facilitate transfer of learning."

It is important for prevention specialists to provide teachers with long-term and ongoing support as they begin prevention program implementation, keeping in mind the five core features of effective professional development described by Desimone (2009): content focus, active learning, coherence, duration, and collective participation. Similarly, with regard to sustaining teacher implementation of school-based mental health programs, Han and Weiss (2005) reported that teachers' implementation fidelity was better and more sustained when training provided them with opportunities for direct classroom practice with performance feedback to produce deep understanding of the skills the program targeted (Farmer-Dougan et al. 1999; Jones et al. 1997; Mortenson and Witt 1998). Ongoing support provides the encouragement and reinforcement teachers need as they integrate new knowledge about prevention into their teaching practice. Additionally, the fidelity of teachers' program implementation inevitably degrades over time. Therefore, arranging a cost-effective means of refresher training or long-term support from a master teacher contributes to keeping teachers' confidence and commitment high (Han and Weiss 2005).

Finally, acknowledging and recognizing teachers' contributions is important for relationship building. For example, sending a letter to the principal documenting the extra effort and time a teacher gave to support implementation of a prevention program and how students benefitted as a result can both recognize the teacher and promote administrator support. Similarly, with permission of school administration, schools and teachers can be acknowledged in reports and publications regarding the prevention program.

5.6.3   Be Flexible

Teaching practice is unpredictable and ever-changing. Teachers respond to their students collectively and adjust lessons accordingly when they are not going as planned. Additionally, teachers work to differentiate instruction to meet the learning needs of individuals, and no two classes are the same. Finally, teachers adjust their practice in response to new initiatives mandated at the school, district, and state levels.

The teacher has the ongoing responsibility for adapting prevention lessons in real time to ensure they are relevant for students, feasible to implement within the schedules and other parameters of their individual school, and in harmony with their classroom teaching practices. For example, having the flexibility to align a prevention program with the goals and objectives of Common Core would support teaching. For teachers to make successful adaptations that enhance, rather than detract from, program delivery, they need to understand the core principles of the intervention, recognize how these principles are effective in changing behavior, and believe that the effort they invest is commensurate with the benefits students receive (Han and Weiss 2005). Recognizing the complexity of teaching and teachers' need for a deep understanding of both the theory and practice of the intervention they are to implement will go far in promoting collaboration between teachers and prevention specialists, as well as long-term sustainability of the intervention. Two things are required for teachers to adapt a program according to changing circumstances:

1. The program must be developed and structured with sufficient flexibility such that it can be adapted to changing circumstances.
2. Teachers must understand the program well enough so that they are able to modify it without sacrificing the core principles and central intervention techniques (Han and Weiss 2005 p. 673).

Keeping these two things in mind will help prevention specialists and teachers adapt to real-world circumstances without sacrificing the benefits of prevention work.

5.7 Conclusions

Educators today are called upon to do much more than provide academic learning experiences for students; they are also charged with the social and emotional development of our youth. Often, teachers are asked to lead that charge by implementing school-based prevention programs. For teachers and prevention specialists to partner, an understanding of a teacher's work on the front lines of education is vital. Empathy for the complexity of teaching, ongoing support in classroom application, and flexibility to meet students' needs are necessary to enable teachers to successfully implement prevention programs. When the ideals of a prevention program can withstand the inherently demanding day-to-day life in schools, children reap the rewards, and the needs of the whole child can be met.

References

Anderson, R. D. (2002). Reforming science teaching: What research says about inquiry. *Journal of Science Teacher Education, 13*(1), 1–12. doi:10.1023/A:1015171124982.

Ball, D. L. (1997). Developing mathematics reform: What don't we know about teacher learning-but would make good working hypotheses? In S. N. Friel & G. W. Bright (Eds.), *Reflecting on our work: NSF teacher enhancement in K-6 mathematics* (pp. 77–111). Lanham: University of Press of America.

Belcastro, P. A., & Gold, R. S. (1983). Teacher stress and burnout: Implications for school health personnel. *Journal of School Health, 53,* 404–407. doi:10.1111/j.1746-1561.1983.tb03148.x.

Bransford, J. D., & Donovan, M. S. (2005). Scientific inquiry and how people learn. In National Research Council (Ed.), *How students learn: History, mathematics, and science in the classroom* (pp. 397–420). Washington, DC: National Academies Press.

Calkins, L., Ehrenworth, M., & Lehman, C. (2012). *Pathways to the common core: Accelerating achievement.* Portsmouth: Heinemann.

Clift, R. T., & Brady, P. (2005). Research on methods courses and field experiences. In M. Cochran-Smith & K. M. Zeichner (Eds.), *Studying teacher education: The report of the AERA panel on research and teacher education* (pp. 309–424). Mahwah: Lawrence Erlbaum Associates.

Crawford, B. A. (2000). Embracing the essence of inquiry: New roles for science teachers. *Journal of Research in Science Teaching, 37*(9), 916–937. doi:10.1002/1098-2736(200011)37:9<916:: AID-TEA4>3.0.CO;2-2.

Dana, N. F., Burns, J. B., & Wolkenhauer, R. (2013). *Inquiring into the common core*. Thousand Oaks: Corwin Press.

Desimone, L. M. (2009). Improving impact studies of teachers' professional development: Toward better conceptualization and measures. *Educational Researcher, 38*, 181–199. doi:10.3102/0013189×08331140.

Farmer-Dougan, V., Viechtbauer, W., & French, T. (1999). Peer-prompted social skills: The role of teacher consultation in student success. *Educational Psychology, 19*(2), 207–219. doi:10.1080/0144341990190207.

Floden, R. E., & Meniketti, M. (2005). Research on the effects of coursework in the arts and sciences and in the foundations of education. In M. Cochran-Smith & K. M. Zeichner (Eds.), *Studying teacher education: The report of the AERA panel on research and teacher education* (pp. 261–308). Mahwah: Lawrence Erlbaum Associates.

Han, S. S., & Weiss, B. (2005). Sustainability of teacher implementation of school based mental health programs. *Journal of Abnormal Child Psychology, 33*(6), 665–779. doi:10.1007/s10802:005-7646-2.

Handwerk, P., Tognatta, N., Coley, R. J., & Gitomer, D. H. (2008). *Access to success: Patterns of advanced placement participation in U.S. high schools (Policy Information Report)*. Princeton: Educational Testing Service.

Jackson, S. E., Schwab, R. L., & Schuler, R. S. (1986). Toward an understanding of the burnout phenomenon. *Journal of Applied Psychology, 71*, 630–640. doi:10.1037/00219010.71.4.630.

Jones, K. M., Wickstrom, K. F., & Friman, P. C. (1997). The effects of observational feedback on treatment integrity in school based behavioral consultation. *School Psychology Quarterly, 12*, 316–326. doi:10.1037/h0088965.

Killion, J., & Harrison, C. (2006). *Taking the lead: New roles for teachers and school-based coaches*. Oxford: National Staff Development Council.

Maslach, C., Jackson, S. E., & Schwab, R. L. (1996). Maslach burnout inventory educators survey (MBI-ES). In C. Maslach, S. E. Jackson, & M. P. Leiter (Eds.), *Maslach burnout inventory (MBI) manual* (3rd edn.). Palo Alto: Consulting Psychologists Press.

McDiarmid, G. W., Ball, D. L., & Anderson, C. A. (1989). Why staying one chapter ahead doesn't really work: Subject-specific pedagogy. In M. C. Reynolds (Ed.), *Knowledge base for the beginning teacher* (pp. 193–205). New York: Pergamon.

McVey, G. L., Davis, R., Tweed, S., & Shaw, B. F. (2004). Evaluation of a school based program designed to improve body image satisfaction, global self-esteem, and eating attitudes and behaviors: A replication study. *International Journal of Eating Disorders, 36*(1), 1–11. doi:10.1002/eat.20006.

Mortenson, B. P., & Witt, J. C. (1998). The use of weekly performance feedback to increase teacher implementation of a prereferral academic intervention. *School Psychology Review, 27*, 217–234.

National Commission on Teaching and America's Future. (2003). *No dream denied: A pledge to America's children*. New York: National Commission on Teaching and America's Future.

National Council for Accreditation of Teacher Education. (2010). *Transforming teacher education through clinical practice: Report of the blue ribbon panel on clinical preparation and partnerships for improved student learning*. Washington, DC: National Council for Accreditation of Teacher Education.

National Governors Association Center for Best Practices & Council of Chief State School Officers. (2012). Common core state standards initiative: About the standards. http://www.corestandards.org/aboutthe-standards.

Olson, S., & Loucks-Horsley, S. (Eds.). (2000). *Inquiry and the National Science Education standards: A guide for teaching and learning*. Washington, DC: National Academies Press.

Shulman, L. S. (1987). Knowledge and teaching: Foundations of the new reform. *Harvard Educational Review, 57*(1), 1–23.

Sizer, T., & Meier, D. (2006). Foreword. Education Alliance at Brown University and EEI Communication (Ed.), *Breaking ranks in the middle: Strategies for leading middle level reform* (pp. vii–viii). Reston: National Association for Secondary Principals.

Stengel, B. S., & Tom, A. R. (1996). Changes and choices in teaching methods. In F. B. Murray (Ed.), *The teacher educator's handbook: Building knowledge base for the preparation of teachers* (pp. 593–619). Mahwah: Lawrence Erlbaum Associates.

Tobler, N. S., Roona, M. R., Ochshorn, P., Marshall, D. G., Streke, A. V., & Stackpole, K. M. (2000). School-based adolescent drug prevention programs: 1998 meta-analysis. *Journal of Primary Prevention, 20*(4), 275–336. doi:10.1023/A:1021314704811.

U.S. Department of Education. (2009). *Race to the top program: Executive summary.* Washington, DC: U.S. Department of Education. http://www2.ed.gov/programs/racetothetop/executive-summary.pdf.

Wilson, S. J., Lipsey, M. W., & Derzon, J. H. (2003). The effects of school based intervention programs on aggressive behavior: A meta-analysis. *Journal of Consulting and Clinical Psychology, 71*(1), 136–149. doi:10.1037/0022:006X.71.1.136.

Chapter 6
Health Services and Health Education

Diane DeMuth Allensworth

6.1 Introduction

Health and education are intertwined. Healthy children are better learners (Suhrcke and de Paz Nieves 2011). Students distracted by a chronic disease, a toothache, or an unintended pregnancy will not benefit from the instructional process whereas those with no health problems will. Estimates are that 15–35 % of adolescents currently have one or more chronic diseases (van der Lee et al. 2007). Certain health conditions can directly affect cognitive function and reduce student's achievement; examples are diabetes, sickle cell anemia, epilepsy (Taras and Potts-Datema 2005), and lead poisoning (Barton and Coley 2009). Students living in poverty—approximately 20 % of all students—experience more chronic disease (Currie and Lin 2007; Flores and Committee on Pediatric Research 2010), infectious disease, childhood injury, social-emotional and behavioral problems, and violence and death than their more affluent peers (Currie and Lin 2007). School-based and school-linked health services (SBHCs) can help ensure that students' learning is not compromised by poor health status.

In addition to those students who have health conditions that impede learning, many students engage in health-risk behaviors. Consistently engaging in even one type of risky health behavior can undermine a student's progress toward graduating on time from high school (Terzian et al. 2011). Approximately 40 % of premature illness and death in both adolescents and adults is attributable to adopting health-risk behaviors (Schroeder 2007). The leading causes of mortality and morbidity among all age groups from adolescents to the elderly are related to six categories of behavior that are often established during youth, extend into adulthood, and are frequently interrelated; namely, unhealthy dietary choices, physical inactivity, tobacco use, alcohol and other drug use, behaviors leading to injuries or violence, and sexual behaviors that contribute to unintended pregnancy and sexually transmitted

D. DeMuth Allensworth (✉)
Kent State University, 3053 Pointe Court, Snellville, GA 30039, USA
e-mail: Dimaster6@gmail.com

© Springer Science+Business Media New York 2015
K. Bosworth (ed.), *Prevention Science in School Settings*,
Advances in Prevention Science, DOI 10.1007/978-1-4939-3155-2_6

diseases. Chronic diseases in adults, such as heart disease, cancer, and stroke, are closely related to three behaviors that are often established in youth: tobacco use, physical inactivity, and poor diet. Eighteen percent of high school students smoke tobacco; only 29% of students routinely engage in the recommended 60 min of physical activity everyday, and 14% do not participate in any physical activity on any day; only 28% of students eat vegetables two or more times per day; and only 30% of students eat fruit two or more times per day. The US Department of Agriculture recommends at least two servings of fruit and three servings of vegetables a day. Alcohol use is a major factor in the three leading causes of death for teenagers—automobile crashes, homicide, and suicide. A 2012 national survey found that more than 20% of high school students have had five or more drinks of alcohol in a row (CDC 2012). Unprotected intercourse can lead to unintended pregnancy, which is one of the major reasons young women drop out of school. Among teens, 34% are sexually active, but only 9.5% used both a condom to protect against a sexually transmitted disease and a birth control method at their last sexual encounter (CDC 2012). Many adolescents engage in multiple health-risk behaviors. Fox et al. (2010) assessed high school students' participation in 12 health-risk behaviors and found that 53% reported engaging in two or more; 36% reported engaging in three or more; and 15% reported engaging in five or more risk behaviors. Quality health education programs assist students in adopting health-enhancing behaviors.

This chapter describes how a quality health services program and a quality health education course of study can improve health and educational outcomes for students. The research establishing the value of these services is outlined, along with the extent to which they are available nationwide and illustrative examples of programs. According to the Centers for Disease Control and Prevention (CDC) Division of Adolescent and School Health (DASH), a quality school health approach contains eight components: they are health education and health services; physical education; a healthy school environment; nutrition services; psychological, counseling, and social services; health promotion for faculty and staff; and family and community involvement. The CDC has identified the priority actions for coordinating these services and disciplines, a process that school-level practitioners wanting to improve an individual component can also follow.[1] The CDC (2013a) recommended priority actions for schools are as follows:

1. Securing administrator support and commitment.
2. Organizing a school health team.
3. Appointing a team leader at the school level.
4. Planning for continuous improvement using a program-planning process.

---

[1] DASH was organized when education was the only response available to prevent the spread of the HIV/AIDS epidemic among adolescents. The first director of DASH authored the eight-component school health model. At the height of its funding, DASH/CDC provided HIV prevention funding for all states and territories and funding for their state Departments of Education and Departments of Health to address the prevention of chronic diseases among youth by reducing health-risk behaviors.

5. Implementing multiple strategies (instruction, policy mandates, environmental changes, social support, media, screenings, and referrals) through multiple components.
6. Addressing both students' health protective factors and their health-risk factors.
7. Engaging students through such activities as peer education, peer advocacy, cross-age mentoring, and service learning as a part of the continuous improvement initiative.
8. Providing professional development opportunities for faculty and staff to aid them in becoming more committed and skilled at improving student health and well-being, and consequently their academic success (CDC 2013b).

6.2   Health Services

Medical inspections of children for specific infectious diseases were established shortly after Lemuel Shattuck's 1850 report for the Sanitary Commission of Massachusetts. This report, which became a classic in the field of public health, also had a significant impact on school health. Both the health-care and public health sectors began to recognize the role that schools could play in controlling communicable disease among their "captive audience" of students (Allensworth et al. 1997). Lillian Wald, a pioneer in nursing research, demonstrated in 1902 that if schools employed a school nurse, they could reduce absenteeism by 50 %. By 1911, more than 100 schools nationwide employed a cadre of school nurses to conduct daily medical inspections, treat minor health conditions, instruct students in self-care, and visit families to provide information on available medical and financial resources (Connolly 2013). Although medical inspections by school physicians continued until the 1930s, the White House Conference on Child Health and Protection in 1930, which called for the elimination of medical treatments in schools, ultimately ensured that the primary providers of health services in the school would become school nurses. For the next 50 years, the nurses' role in promoting student health (in those schools that had school nurses) was to refer students in need of medical care to their private physicians. It was not until 1986, when the Robert Wood Johnson Foundation began its work to support school-based clinics, that medical services began returning to a few schools (Allensworth et al. 1997). The need for both curative and preventative student health services was supported by results of both school-based and school-linked health services.

Currently, several prominent professional health and educational organizations have identified the value of health services in supporting learning, particularly for poor and vulnerable students. Two leading health organizations—the American Public Health Association (membership 25,000) and the Society for Public Health Education (membership 4000)—have resolutions calling for the linking of schools and communities to ensure that health services are provided to students in order to improve the health of the overall population and reduce health disparities. These two organizations have identified that dropping out of school is a major health-risk factor and that providing health-care access enables students to focus on learning. The Association for Supervision and Curriculum Development (ASCD), a professional organization of 150,000 educators and administrators, has also called for schools to address the whole child and ensure that all students are safe, healthy, engaged, supported, and challenged. Being healthy includes both curative and preventative services (ASCD 2007).

The CDC has recently defined the scope of school health services as being:

> designed to ensure access or referral to primary health care services or both, foster appropriate use of primary health care services, prevent and control communicable disease and other health problems, provide emergency care for illness or injury, promote and provide optimum sanitary conditions for a safe school facility and school environment, and provide educational and counseling opportunities for promoting and maintaining individual, family, and community health. (CDC 2013b)

Currently, the most common provider of health services to students nationwide is the school nurse, who provides day-to-day health-care management for all students. Physicians, nurses, dentists, and other allied health personnel may provide health services in schools. However, most schools do not employ all of these professionals. Some schools have available school-based or school-linked health services that provide students access to primary health-care services. Other schools have contracted with community agencies or individual professionals in the community to provide physical, mental, or dental health-care services for students. Many schools, however, do not ensure that all students have access or referral to primary health-care services. Those schools that do promote access to primary health-care services have found improved student learning outcomes (Allison et al. 2007; Bryk et al. 2010; City Connects 2012; CIS 2011; Council on School Health 2012).

6.2.1 School Nursing

A 2006 survey found that whereas 86.3 % of schools nationwide had at least a part-time nurse to oversee standard school health services, only 31.5 % of these schools had a registered nurse providing health services full time to students. Furthermore, the recommended ratio of 1 nurse to 750 students was achieved in only 48 % of those schools (Brener et al. 2007). Not having the appropriate ratio means that even though a school nurse is available, the nurse may not have time to provide all the health services that students in the school need. Data from the same national survey also revealed that the higher the proportion of racial/ethnic minority students in a school, the less likely school-based health services were to be offered (Balaji et al. 2010).

The role of the school nurse, according to the National Association of School Nurses (NASN 2011), includes but is not limited to the following responsibilities:

- School nurses facilitate normal development and positive student responses to interventions. As the health-care expert within the school, the nurse develops plans for student care based on the nursing process. Seventy-four percent of schools provide case management for students with chronic health conditions (e.g., asthma or diabetes) and 45 % of schools provide case management for students with disabilities (Brener et al. 2007).

- School nurses provide leadership in promoting health and safety, including a healthy environment. These responsibilities include monitoring student immunizations, managing communicable diseases, assessing the school environment for safety, consulting with other school professionals, and providing health-related education to students and staff in individual and group settings (NASN 2011). Seventy-nine percent of schools provide instruction on self-management for students with chronic health conditions, 55 % provide nutrition and dietary behavior counseling, 56 % provide injury prevention and safety counseling, and 44 % provide HIV prevention services (Brener et al. 2007).
- School nurses provide quality health care and intervene with actual and potential health problems. Providing care for chronically and acutely ill students, as well as those injured at school, involves the administration of medication, the provision of health-care procedures, and the development of health-care plans (NASN 2011). Sixty-one percent of schools provide first aid, 48 % assist with accessing benefits for students with disabilities, 48 % assist with enrolling students in Medicaid or the Children's Health Insurance Program, and 36 % assist with enrolling students in Special Supplemental Food Programs (Brener et al. 2007).
- School nurses use clinical judgment in providing case management services. In collaboration with physicians, school nurses implement medical orders by developing Individualized Healthcare Plans (IHPs) that direct nursing care for individual students (NASN 2011). Thirty-five percent of all schools have medically fragile students requiring advanced nursing procedures. During 2005 in those schools with at least one such student, 24 % provided catheterizations, 24 % provided tube feedings, 16 % performed stoma care, 15 % performed suctioning, 12 % provided respirator care, and 10 % provided tracheostomy care (Brener et al. 2007).
- School nurses actively collaborate with others to build student and family capacity for adaptation, self-management, self-advocacy, and learning. The school nurse has health expertise that is essential for coordinating the linkages among medical professionals; home and family; and school educational teams, including the Committee on Special Education, the Individualized Education Plan (IEP) team, and the Section 504 team (NASN 2011). In 71 % of all schools, a school nurse participated in the development of IEPs when indicated; in 74 % of schools, the school nurse participated in the development of IHPs; and in 65 % of all schools, the nurse participated in the development of 504 plans when indicated (Brener et al. 2007).

Evidence of the Effectiveness of Having a School Nurse Having a full-time nurse in a school has been shown to improve (a) attendance of poor and minority students (Lwebuga-Mukasa and Dunn-Georgiou 2002; Tellejohn et al. 2004), (b) case management of chronic diseases (Engelke et al. 2008), (c) attendance of all students (Weismuller et al. 2007), and (d) immunization rates (Salmon et al. 2005). An example where school nurses can improve case management of a chronic disease and consequently students' school attendance is asthma. Asthma is one of the most common chronic diseases of childhood, affecting 14% of students (Basch 2010). The school nurse can develop asthma plans and offer asthma education classes for all students known to have the disease. Further, the school nurse can lead a team in using the Environmental Protection Agency's Healthy School Environments Assessment Tool to identify and minimize asthma triggers within the school environment (EPA 2011).

6.2.2 School-Based Health Services

SBHCs provide accessible, low-cost medical and mental health-care services specifically designed for students. As of 2007–2008, almost 2000 SBHCs were operating in 48 US states and territories, with 57% located in urban communities, 16% in suburban communities, and 27% in rural communities (Strozer et al. 2010). However, the School-Based Health Alliance (n.d.) estimates that 5808 SBHCs would be needed to serve all uninsured children and youth aged 6–17 years.

In 2007–2008, approximately 24% of SBHCs were located in elementary or middle schools, 33% in high schools, and 43% in alternative schools or schools with a combination of grade levels (Council on School Health 2012). More than half of these SBHCs were sponsored and managed by community health-care institutions, including community health centers (28%), hospitals (25%), local health departments (15%), or other community organizations such as universities and mental health agencies. Only 12% of SBHCs were sponsored by a school system (Strozer et al. 2010). Although services at SBHCs did vary from clinic to clinic, 97% offered health assessments, 96% offered treatment of acute illness, 96% provided prescriptions for medications, 92% conducted vision and hearing screenings, 92% provided sports participation examinations, 91% provided nutrition counseling, and 90% provided anticipatory guidance (Strozer et al. 2010).

Evidence of Effectiveness of School-Based Health Care Students using SBHCs, in comparison with non-users:

- Receive more preventative care visits (Allison et al. 2007; Council on School Health 2012), and more primary care visits (Allison et al. 2007)
- Receive more screening for high-risk behaviors (Council on School Health 2012)
- Receive more mental health services (Guo et al. 2008)
- Have fewer emergency room visits (Allison et al. 2007; Council on School Health 2012; Guo et al. 2005)
- Experience less hospitalization and better outcomes for treatment of asthma (Council on School Health 2012; Guo et al. 2005)
- Have reduced school absenteeism rates (Walker et al. 2010)
- In those, SBHC sites providing dental care services have improved access to dental care (Council on School Health 2012)

6.2.3   School-Linked Health Services and Community Schools

According to the Coalition for Communities in Schools, "community schools are both a place and a set of partnerships between the school and other community resources. There are a number of national models and local community school initiatives that share a common set of principles: fostering strong partnerships, sharing accountability for results, setting high expectations, building on the community's strengths, and embracing diversity and innovative solutions" (www.communityschools.org). Early in its history, the Coalition for Community Schools, an alliance organized in 1997, coined the term *full-service schools* to describe public schools that were linked with community agencies to ensure that the physical, social, and emotional needs of students and families were met. This organization and the nationwide Communities in Schools (CIS) network both promote access to community support and health-care services for students—and in some sites, for their family members as well. Both organizations have a similar focus on addressing the prerequisite conditions necessary for student learning but articulate slightly different strategies.

The Coalition for Community Schools (2014) identifies five necessary conditions:

- The school has a core instructional program with qualified teachers, a challenging curriculum, and high standards and expectations for students.
- Students are motivated and engaged in learning—both in school and in community settings during and after school.
- The basic physical, mental, and emotional health needs of young people and their families are recognized and addressed.
- There is mutual respect and effective collaboration among parents, families, and school staff.
- Community engagement, together with school efforts, promotes a school climate that is safe, supportive, and respectful and that connects students to a broader learning community.

CIS began in 1977 and by 2009–2010 served students in approximately 3000 schools in 25 states, focusing on the following five basic strategies (CIS 2011):

- A one-on-one relationship with a caring adult
- A safe place to learn and grow
- A healthy start and a healthy future (through access to health and dental care, food programs, and counseling services)
- A marketable skill to use upon graduation
- A chance to give back to peers and community

Evidence of the Effectiveness of Community Schools By meeting students' health and social needs, community schools produce a variety of positive educational outcomes, including improvements in test scores, graduation rates, behavior, and attendance (Blank et al. 2012). Evaluation results showed that CIS produced the largest reduction in dropout rates of any existing, fully scaled dropout prevention program identified by the US Department of Education in its "What Works" listing (CIS 2011). The more fully and faithfully the model is implemented, the stronger the effects. The annual evaluation by CIS of the programming of their affiliate organizations identified the following successes for the 2009–2010 academic year:

- 82 % of students met their goals for reduction in high-risk behavior.
- 77 % of students met their goals for attendance improvement.
- 88 % of students met their goals for behavior improvement.
- 79 % of students met their goals for reduced suspensions.
- 82 % of students met their goals for academic improvement.
- 83 % of students met their goals for improving attitude and commitment to school.
- 98 % of students being monitored as potential dropouts remained in school at the end of 2009–2010 school year. Of those students being monitored for promotion risk, 88 % were promoted to the next grade and 87 % of monitored seniors graduated (CIS 2011).

A number of researchers and organizations have made a case for the need to address students' health status and health behaviors as a prerequisite to ensuring learning (APHA 2010; ASCD 2007; Basch 2010; Bryk et al. 2010; Rothstein 2011; Ruglis and Freudenberg 2010; SOPHE 2008). Teachers and support staff in schools recognize their students' health needs. MetLife's 2011 survey of American teachers found that a majority of teachers (64 %) reported that over the previous year, the number of students and families needing health and social support services had increased, while 35 % of teachers also reported that the number of students coming to school hungry had increased. At the same time, many teachers (28 %) had seen health or social services be reduced or eliminated (MetLife 2012).

6.3   Health Education

Health education courses can help students become health literate and adopt a health-enhancing lifestyle. Approximately 50 % of premature death is due to living an unhealthy lifestyle (Schroeder 2007). Six high-risk behaviors in youth and adults are related to two thirds of premature deaths and illness: sedentary lifestyle, poor nutrition behaviors, smoking, alcohol or other drug abuse, behaviors leading to intentional or unintentional injury, and behaviors leading to sexually transmitted disease (CDC 2012). Many adolescents engage in multiple health-risk behaviors (Fox et al. 2010; Lowry et al. 1996). Quality health education can reduce health-risk behaviors, improve academic behaviors, and improve health literacy. According to the CDC (2013b), instruction in health education:

> address[es] a variety of topics such as alcohol and other drug use and abuse, healthy eating/nutrition, mental and emotional health, personal health and wellness, physical activity, safety and injury prevention, sexual health, tobacco use, and violence prevention. Health

education curricula should address the National Health Education Standards (NHES) and incorporate the characteristics of an effective health education curriculum. Qualified, credentialed teachers teach health education.

Most public schools provide some instruction in health. Many states mandate health education, and at least 87% of states and 71% of districts have adopted standards for elementary, middle, and high school health education that specifically incorporate each of the National Health Education Standards (NHES; Kann et al. 2013). These national standards provide a framework for curriculum development and selection, instruction, and student assessment, as follows:

- Students will comprehend concepts related to health promotion and disease prevention to enhance health.
- Students will analyze the influence of family, peers, culture, media, technology, and other factors on health behaviors.
- Students will demonstrate the ability to access valid information, products, and services to enhance health.
- Students will demonstrate the ability to use interpersonal communication skills to enhance health and avoid or reduce health risks.
- Students will demonstrate the ability to use decision-making skills to enhance health.
- Students will demonstrate the ability to use goal-setting skills to enhance health.
- Students will demonstrate the ability to practice health-enhancing behaviors and avoid or reduce health risks.
- Students will demonstrate the ability to advocate for personal, family, and community health.

Although the majority of states and districts nationwide subscribe to the content of the NHES, they do not meet the established time requirement. The NHES calls for 80 h of instruction annually for grades 3–12 and 40 h annually for grades K–2 (Joint Committee on National Health Standards 2007). In actuality,

- 7.5% schools nationwide provide the 360 cumulative hours of health education for students in grades K–5.
- 10.3% schools nationwide provide the recommended 240 cumulative hours for grades 6–8.
- 6.5% of high schools provide the recommended 320 cumulative hours of health instruction (N. D. Brener, personal communication, January 29, 2010).
- The percentage of students receiving mandatory health instruction in each grade is less than 35% in grades 9–12, 60% in grades 4–8, and less than 50% in grades K–3 (Kann et al. 2007).

The goals for health education extend beyond the goals of reducing health-risk behaviors and promoting health-enhancing behaviors. Health instruction provides students with an understanding of their body and how it works, and with personal and social skills. Students learn how to recognize and understand the practices related to health as well as how to access health information.

Health literacy is the ability to make appropriate health decisions based upon understanding basic health information (Ratzan and Parker 2000). It requires both literacy skills (being able to read) and health knowledge skills (understanding how a healthy body functions, how to keep it healthy, and how to make healthy choices). Although no national survey of children's health literacy levels exists, a national survey of adults found only 12% were proficient and only 53% had intermediate health literacy (Kutner et al. 2006). Health illiteracy is estimated to cost the USA between $100 and 200 billion a year in increased medical costs (Vernon et al. 2007). The National Plan to Improve Health Literacy (U.S. Department of Health and Human Services 2010b) has as one of its seven goals to incorporate accurate, standards-based, and developmentally appropriate health and science information and curricula in childcare, elementary and secondary, and university levels of education. The report also notes that adherence to the NHES can build health knowledge and skills that are critical to achieving proficient health literacy. The need to increase health education in schools was also noted in *Healthy People 2020*, 10-year agenda of science-based national objectives for improving the health of all Americans, issued in 2010. This agenda is the latest installment in a three-decadelong, joint public–private initiative organized by the federal government (http://www.healthypeople.gov/2020/topicsobjectives2020/objectiveslist.aspx?topicID=11). Among the various objectives is:

ECBP-2 Increase the proportion of elementary, middle, and senior high schools that provide comprehensive school health education to prevent health problems in the following areas: unintentional injury; violence; suicide; tobacco use and addiction; alcohol or other drug use; unintended pregnancy, HIV/AIDS, and STD infection; unhealthy dietary patterns; and inadequate physical activity. (U.S. Department of Health and Human Services 2010a)

Evidence of the Effectiveness of Health Education and Health-Promotion Initiatives Effective and evidence-based health education programs do exist and can reduce the incidence of health-risk behaviors. As an example, COPE (Creating Opportunities for Personal Empowerment) Healthy Lifestyles TEEN (Thinking, Emotions, Exercise, Nutrition) Program is a 15-week intervention focused on empowering secondary students to engage in a healthy lifestyle. A randomized controlled trial found that immediately post-intervention, participating students took a greater number of steps per day ($p=0.03$), had a lower body mass index ($p=0.01$), and used less alcohol ($p=0.04$). Further, the intervention students scored higher in cooperation, assertion, and academic competence than did the control students (Melnyk et al. 2013).

In contrast to this generic approach to reducing health-risk behaviors, many evidence-based programs focus on a single behavior, such as preventing tobacco use (Dent et al. 1995; Griffin et al. 2003), reducing heavy drinking (Botvin et al. 2001; Hawkins et al. 1999), decreasing risky sexual behavior (Coyle et al. 2001), preventing dating aggression (Foshee et al. 1998), preventing violence (Botvin et al. 2006; Hawkins et al. 1999), and increasing physical activity (Luepker et al. 1996). The NHES also lists standards for instruction in social-emotional skills, namely, communication, decision-making, and goal-setting skills. The teaching of age-appropriate social-emotional skills has been shown to improve students' academic behavior, including increasing motivation and positive attitude toward school (Zins et al. 2004), reducing absenteeism (Christenson and Havsy 2004), reducing conduct problems within the classroom (Flay et al. 2001), and improving scores on achievement tests (Durlak et al. 2011) as well as high school graduation rates (Hawkins et al. 1999). Several registries of effective and evidence-based school health interventions are available. Among the programs listed on the various registries are ones that utilize strategies in addition to health instruction and could be implemented at sites other than schools:

- Child Trends "What Works" Listings: http://www.childtrends.org/what-works/
- SAMHSA's National Registry of Evidence-Based Programs and Practices: www.nrepp.samhsa.gov
- Institute of Education Sciences What Works Clearinghouse: http://ies.ed.gov/ncee/wwc/
- Office of Juvenile Justice and Delinquency Prevention Model Programs Guide: http://www.ojjdp.gov/mpg/
- Guide to Community Preventive Services: http://www.thecommunityguide.org/index.html

Many of the most effective health education programs use strategies in addition to instruction, including environmental change, social support, screening and referral, and policy mandates. Effective programs may also have strategies that engage not just students, but also their caregivers or teachers in the same behavior(s).

6.4 Case Study: HealthMPowers

Childhood obesity is a major problem in Georgia. Both parents and school staff are concerned about this issue and its implications for children's health and learning. With research showing that increased physical activity does not detract from learning and may even contribute to improving achievement, an initiative called HealthMPowers is gaining momentum in Georgia schools. The approach has demonstrated success in improving nutrition and physical activity.

HealthMPowers (http://www.healthmpowers.org/), a nonprofit organization established in 2000 by two parents, has implemented a comprehensive whole-school model to improve physical activity and nutrition programming in pre-K–8 schools. Illustrating its rapid expansion, HealthMPowers extended its services from eight Georgia elementary schools in 2002–2003 to 90 schools in 28 districts in 2011–2012 (reaching 57,457 students along with school staff and family members). Over the course of the organization's history, it has served more than 200 elementary schools, each for an implementation period of 3–5 years, utilizing CDC (2013a) priority actions for schools. Alumni schools continue to have access to technical assistance as needed. Participating schools are located in urban, rural, and suburban communities and range across all socioeconomic levels, but the average free and reduced lunch rate for the 2011–2012 school year was 78%, indicating that a large proportion of the participating schools are in underserved areas.

The mission of HealthMPowers is to promote healthy behaviors and environments by empowering students, school staff, and families to improve their health and students' academic achievement. In addition to assessing and promoting healthy student nutrition and physical activity, the agency also provides physical activity and programming to school staff and families. Schools commit to participate for a 3-year time period, during which HealthMPowers provides whole-school intervention involving student assemblies, classroom physical activity DVDs, supplemental health education and physical education lessons, worksite wellness programs for staff, and family engagement activities around nutrition and physical activity. To ensure sustainability after 3 years, HealthMPowers organizes a school health team and facilitates the use of annual data on student knowledge and behavior, school policy, and program effects to promote a climate of continuous improvement. Additional programs and initiatives are available and promoted, such as a pedometer math challenge, family fun fitness activities, student health advocates, and family newsletters promoting specific healthy behaviors with activities parents and students can do together. Each school receives an annual report on its activities, to guide it in setting physical activity and nutrition objectives for the upcoming school year.

A few examples documenting HealthMPowers success during 2011–2012 follow.

Student-Level Outcomes
- Sixty percent of students improved their score on the Progressive Aerobic Cardiovascular Endurance Run (PACER), a test measuring aerobic fitness.
- Students in all grades showed a statistically significant increase in health knowledge from baseline (average increase of 4–5% from pre- to posttest).
- Improvements in health behavior were statistically significant among both boys and girls, and across all grade levels.

School-Level Outcomes By their third (final) year of participating in HealthMPowers, schools showed these improvements:

- Eighty-five percent of schools were offering daily physical activity for students, a 43% increase from the baseline.
- The number of functional and effective school health teams increased by more than sixfold over baseline.
- Participating schools provided 273% more health education instruction hours to students annually than they did at baseline.

Lessons Learned HealthMPowers staff have developed several principles for successful dissemination of school health programming from their experience:

- Base the initiative on theory and best practices.
- The principal's approval and ongoing support are critical.
- It is important to organize, support, and utilize a school health team to undertake a whole-school approach to change, focusing on continuous improvement.

- Collecting, analyzing, and using data on students' behavior, health knowledge, and physical fitness, along with data on school policies and programming, drive priority actions for a school's changes in programming and activities.
- Flexibility and options in programming encourage school involvement and engagement at a pace that school staff can handle.
- Environmental change and policy change result in long-term, sustainable, and systemic change within the school.
- Provide ongoing professional development to motivate and engage school staff.
- Engage students as partners in the process of change.
- Create a communication plan outlining how the school health team can engage students, staff, and families in more activities, as well as spread the word about the need for continuous improvement in students' health and learning.
- It takes 3 years or more in a process of continuous improvement to bring about systemic change.

6.5   Summary

Students who have health problems (Basch 2010; Rothstein 2011; Ruglis and Freudenberg 2010) and those who are abused, neglected, or homeless (Bryk et al. 2010) often have issues that reduce their capacity to learn and increase the number of days that they are absent from school—which also impedes learning. Chronic absenteeism can lead to failing courses and ultimately failing to graduate (Allensworth and Easton 2007). Students who fail to graduate have numerous negative outcomes, including a shorter life span (Wong et al. 2002). In addition, many students engage in health-risk behaviors that can jeopardize their current learning and future health status. Schools that link school-based health services with those in the community, and those that focus on promoting a healthy lifestyle through a sequential K–12 health education curriculum that adheres to both the content and time recommendations in the NEHS will have students who are absent less often, engage in fewer health-risk behaviors, engage in more health-enhancing behaviors, and achieve more academically.

References

Allensworth, E., & Easton, J. Q. (2007). *What matters for staying on track and graduating in Chicago public high schools*. Chicago: University of Chicago Consortium on Chicago School Research. http://ccsr.uchicago.edu/content/publications.php.

Allensworth, D. D., Wyche, J., Lawson, E., & Nicholson, L. (Eds.). (1997). *Schools and health: Our nation's investment. Final report of the Committee on Comprehensive School Health Programs in Grades K–12*. Washington, DC: National Academies Press.

Allison, M. A., Crane, L. A., Beaty, B. L., Davidson, A. J., Melinkovich, P., & Kempe, A. (2007). School-based health centers: Improving access and quality of care for low-income adolescents. *Pediatrics, 120*(4), e887–e894. doi:10.1542/peds.2006-2314.

American Public Health Association (APHA). (2010). *Public health and education: Working collaboratively across sectors to improve high school graduation as a means to eliminate health disparities* (Policy statement 20101, November 9, 2010). Washington, DC: American Public Health Association (APHA). http://www.apha.org/advocacy/policy/policysearch/default. htm?id=1395.

Association for Supervision and Curriculum Development (ASCD). (2007). *The learning compact redefined: A call to action* (Report of the Commission on the Whole Child). http://www.ascd. org/ASCD/pdf/Whole%20Child/WCC%20Learning%20Compact.pdf.

Balaji, A. B., Brener, N. D., & McManus, T. (2010).Variation in school health policies and programs by demographic characteristics of U.S. schools, 2006. *Journal of School Health, 80*(12), 599–613. doi:10.1111/j.1746-1561.2010.00547.x.

Barton, P. E., & Coley, R. J. (2009). *Parsing the achievement gap II* (Policy Information Report). Princeton: Educational Testing Service. http://www.ets.org/Media/Research/pdf/PICPARSINGII.pdf.

Basch, C. (2010). *Healthier students are better learners: A missing link in school reforms to close the achievement gap* (Equity Matters Research Review No. 6). http://www.equitycampaign. org/i/a/document/12557_EquityMattersVol6_Web03082010.pdf.

Blank, M. J., Jacobson, R., & Melaville, A. (2012, Jan.). *Achieving results through community school partnerships: How district and community leaders are building effective, sustainable relationships*. Washington, DC: Coalition for Community Schools. http://www.americanprogress.org/issues/2012/01/pdf/community_schools.pdf.

Botvin, G. J., Griffin, K. W., Diaz, T., & Ifill-Williams, M. (2001). Preventing binge drinking during early adolescence: One- and two-year follow-up of a school-based preventive intervention. *Psychology of Addictive Behaviors, 15*(4), 360–365. doi:10.1037/0893:164X.15.4.360.

Botvin, G. J., Griffin, K. W., & Nichols, T. R. (2006). Preventing youth violence and delinquency through a universal school-based prevention approach. *Prevention Science, 7*(4), 403–408. doi:10.1007/s11121:006-0057-y.

Brener, N. D., Wheeler, L., Wolfe, L. C., Vernon-Smiley, M., & Caldart-Olson, L. (2007). Health services: Results from the School Health Policies and Programs study, 2006. *Journal of School Health, 77*(8), 464–485. doi:10.1111/j.1746:1561.2007.00230.x.

Bryk, A., Sebring, P. B., Allensworth, E., Luppesca, S., & Easton, J. Q. (2010). *Organizing schools for improvement: Lessons from Chicago*. Chicago: University of Chicago Press.

Centers for Disease Control and Prevention (CDC). (2012). Youth risk behavior surveillance—United States, 2011. *MMWR, 61*(4). http://www.cdc.gov/mmwr/pdf/ss/ss6104.pdf.

Centers for Disease Control and Prevention (CDC). (2013a). *Components of coordinated school health*. Atlanta, GA: Author. http://www.cdc.gov/healthyyouth/cshp/components.htm.

Centers for Disease Control and Prevention (CDC). (2013b). *How schools can implement coordinated school health*. Atlanta: Centers for Disease Control and Prevention (CDC). http://www. ced.gov/healthyyouth/cshp/schools.htm.

Christenson, S., & Havsy, L. H. (2004). Family-school-peer relationships: Significance for social, emotional, and academic learning. In E. Zins, R. P. Weissberg, M. C. Wang, & H. J. Walberg (Eds.), *Building academic success on social and emotional learning* (pp. 59–75). New York: Teachers College Press.

City Connects. (2012). *The impact of City Connects: Progress report 2012*. Boston: Boston College Center for Optimized Student Support. http://www.bc.edu/content/dam/files/schools/lsoe/ cityconnects/pdf/CityConnects_ProgressReport_2012.pdf.

Coalition of Community Schools. (2014). Frequently asked questions about community schools. http://www.communityschools.org/aboutschools/faqs.aspx#_7.

Communities in Schools (CIS). (2011). *2009–2010 results from the Communities in Schools Network*. Arlington: Communities in Schools (CIS). http://www.communitiesinschools.org/media/uploads/attachments/Network_Results_2009:2010.pdf.

Connolly, C. A. (2013). *A history of the Commonwealth Fund's child development and preventive care program*. New York: Commonwealth Fund. http://www.commonwealthfund.org/~/media/Files/Publications/Fund%20Report/2013/Aug/1693_Connolly_history_Commonwealth_ Fund_child_devel_prog_v2.pdf.

Council on School Health. (2012). School-based health centers and pediatric practice. *Pediatrics, 129*(2), 387–393. doi:10.1542/peds.2011-3443.

Coyle, K., Basen-Engquist, K., Kirby, D., Parcel, G., Banspach, S., Collins, J., Baumler, E., Carvajal, S., & Harrist, R. (2001). Safer choices: Reducing teen pregnancy, HIV and STDs. *Public Health Reports, 116*(Suppl. 1), 82–93. doi:10.1093/phr/116.S1.82.

Currie, J., & Lin, W. (2007). Chipping away at health: More on the relationship between income and child health. *Health Affairs, 26,* 331–344. doi:10.1377/hlthaff.26.2.331.

Dent, C. W., Sussman, S., Stacy, A. W., Craig, S., Burton, D., & Flay, B. R. (1995). Two-year behavior outcomes of project towards no tobacco use. *Journal of Consulting and Clinical Psychology, 63*(4), 676–677. doi:10.1037/0022-006X.63.4.676.

Durlak, J. A., Weissberg, R. P., Dymnicki, A. B., Taylor, R. D., & Schellinger, K. B. (2011). The impact of enhancing students' social and emotional learning: A meta-analysis of school-based universal interventions. *Child Development, 82*(1), 405–432. doi:10.1111/j.1467-8624.2010.01564.x.

Engelke, M., Guttu, M., & Warren, M. (2008). School nurse case management for children with chronic illness: Health, academic, and quality of life outcomes. *Journal of School Nursing, 24,* 205–214. doi:10.1177/1059840508319929.

Environmental Protection Agency (EPA). (2011). *Healthy School Environments Assessment Tool (HealthySEAT)* (version 2). Washington, DC: Environmental Protection Agency (EPA). http://epa.gov/schools/healthyseat/.

Flay, B., Allred, C. G., & Ordway, C. (2001). Effects of the Positive Action program on achievement and discipline: Two matched-control comparisons. *Prevention Science, 2*(2), 71–89. doi:10.1023/A:1011591613728.

Flores, G., & Committee on Pediatric Research. (2010). Racial and ethnic disparities in the health and health care of children. *Pediatrics, 125*(4), e979–e1020. doi:10.1542/peds.2010-0188.

Foshee, V. A., Bauman, K. E., Arriaga, X. B., Helms, R. W., Koch, G. G., & Linder, G. F. (1998). An evaluation of Safe Dates, an adolescent dating violence prevention program. *American Journal of Public Health, 88*(1), 45–50. doi:10.2105/AJPH.88.1.45.

Fox, H. B., McManus, M. A., & Arnold, K. N. (2010, March). *Significant multiple risk behaviors among U.S. high school students* (National Alliance to Advance Adolescent Health Fact Sheet No. 8). http://osbhcn.org/files/Risk%20Behaviors%20and%20HS%20Students.pdf.

Griffin, K. W., Botvin, G. J., Nichols, T. R., & Doyle, M. M. (2003). Effectiveness of a universal drug abuse prevention approach for youth at high risk for substance use initiation. *Preventive Medicine, 36,* 1–7. doi:10.1006/pmed.2002.1133

Guo, J. J., Jang, R., Keller, K. N., McCracken, A. L., Pan, W., Cluxton, R. J. (2005). Impact of school-based health centers on children with asthma. *Journal of Adolescent Health, 37*(4), 266–274.

Guo, J. J., Wade, T. W., & Keller, K. N. (2008). Impact of school-based health centers on students with mental health problems. *Public Health Reports, 123,* 768–780. http://www.ncbi.nlm.nih.gov/pmc/articles/PMC2556722/.

Hawkins, J., Catalano, R., Kosterman, R., Abbott, R., & Hill, K. (1999). Preventing adolescent health-risk behaviors by strengthening protection during childhood. *Archives of Pediatric Adolescent Medicine, 153,* 226–234. doi:10.1001/archpedi.153.3.226.

Joint Committee on National Health Standards. (2007). *National health education standards* (2nd ed.). Atlanta: American Cancer Society.

Kann, L., Telljohann, S. K., & Wooley, S. F. (2007). Health education: Results from the school health policies and programs study, 2006. *Journal of School Health, 77*(8), 408–434. doi:10.1111/j.1746-1561.2007.00228.x.

Kann, L., Telljohann, S., Hunt, H., Hunt, P., & Haller, E. (2013). Health education. In *Results from the school health policies and practices study 2012*. Atlanta: CDC. http://www.cdc.gov/healthyyouth/shpps/2012/pdf/shpps-results_2012.pdf#page=27.

Kutner M., Greenberg, E., Jin, Y., & Paulsen, C. (2006). *The health literacy of America's adults: Results from the 2003 National Assessment of Adult Literacy* (NCES 2006-483). Washington, DC: National Center for Education Statistics, U.S. Department of Education. http://nces. ed.gov/pubs2006/2006483.pdf.

Lowry, R., Kann, L., Collins, J. L., & Kolbe, L. J. (1996). The effect of socioeconomic status on chronic disease risk behaviors among U.S. adolescents. *Journal of the American Medical Association, 276*(10), 792–797. doi:10.1001/jama.1996.03540100036025.

Luepker, R. V., Perry, C. L., McKinlay S. M., Nader, P. R., Parcel, G. S., Stone, E. J., Webber, L. S., Elder, J. P., Feldman, H. A., Johnson, C. C., Verter, J. (1996). Outcomes of a field trial to improve children's dietary patterns and physical activity: The child and adolescent trial for cardiovascular health (CATCH). *Journal of the American Medical Association, 275*(10), 768–776. doi:10.1001/jama.1996.03530340032026.

Lwebuga-Mukasa, J., & Dunn-Georgiou, E. (2002). A school-based asthma intervention program in the Buffalo, New York schools. *Journal of School Health, 72*(1), 27–32. doi:10.1111/j.1746-1561.2002.tb06508.x.

Melnyk, B. M., Jacobson, D., Kelly, S., Belyea, M., Shaibi, G., Small, L., O'Haver, J., Marsiglia, F. F. (2013). Promoting healthy lifestyles in high school adolescents: A randomized controlled trial. *American Journal of Preventive Medicine, 45*(4), 407–415. doi:10.1016/j.amepre.2013.05.013.

MetLife. (2012, March). *The MetLife survey of the American teacher: Teachers, parents and the economy.* New York: MetLife. http://www.metlife.com/assets/cao/contributions/foundation/american-teacher/MetLife-Teacher-Survey-2011.pdf.

National Association of School Nurses (NASN). (2011). *Role of the school nurse: Position statement.* Silver Spring: National Association of School Nurses (NASN). http://www.nasn.org/Portals/0/positions/2011psrole.pdf.

Ratzan, S. C., & Parker, R. M. (2000). Introduction. In C. R. Selden, M. Zorn, S. C. Ratzan, & R. M. Parker (Eds.), *National library of medicine current bibliographies in medicine: Health literacy* (NLM Pub. No. CBM 2000-1). Bethesda: National Institutes of Health.

Rothstein, R. (2011). *A look at the health-related causes of low student achievement.* Washington, DC: Economic Policy Institute. http://www.epi.org/publication/a_look_at_the_health-related_causes_of_low_student_achievement/.

Ruglis, J., & Freudenberg, N. (2010). Toward a healthy high schools movement: Strategies for mobilizing public health for educational reform. *American Journal of Public Health, 100*(9), 1565–1571. doi:10.2105/AJPH.2009.186619.

Salmon, D. A., Omer, S. B., Moulton, L. H., Stokley, S., deHart, M. P., Lett, S., Norman, B., Teret, S., Halsey, N. A. (2005). Exemptions to school immunization requirements: The role of school-level requirements, policies, and procedures. *American Journal of Public Health, 95,* 436–440. doi:10.2105/AJPH.2004.046201.

School-Based Health Alliance. (n.d.). *Location of existing programs & number of SBHCs needed to serve children living in designated health professional shortage areas.* Washington, DC: School-Based Health Alliance. http://www.nasbhc.org/atf/cf/%7BB241D183:DA6F-443F-9588-3230D027D8DB%7D/EQ_HPSAmap.pdf.

Schroeder, S. A. (2007). We can do better—Improving the health of the American people. *New England Journal of Medicine, 357,* 1221–1228. doi:10.1056/NEJMsa073350.

Society for Public Health Education (SOPHE). (2008). *Resolution: Improving population health by improving graduation rates.* Washington, DC: Society for Public Health Education (SOPHE). http://www.sophe.org/Resolutions.cfm.

Strozer, J., Juszczak, L. & Ammerman, A. (2010). *2007–2008 National school-based health care census.* Washington, DC: National Assembly on School-Based Health Care. http://www.nasbhc.org/atf/cf/%7Bcd9949f2-2761-42fb-bc7a-cee165c701d9%7D/SNAPSHOT%20OF%20SBHCS.PDF.

Suhrcke, M., & de Paz Nieves, C. (2011). *The impact of health and health behaviours on educational outcomes in high-income countries: A review of the evidence.* Copenhagen: WHO Regional Office for Europe.

Taras, H., & Potts-Datema, W. (2005). Chronic health conditions and student performance at school. *Journal of School Health, 75,* 255–266. doi:10.1111/j.1746:1561.2005.tb06686.x.

Tellejohn, S. K., Dake, J. A., & Price, J. H. (2004). Effect of full-time versus part-time school nurses on attendance of elementary students with asthma. *Journal of School Nursing, 20,* 331–334. doi:10.1177/10598405040200060701.

Terzian, M. A., Andrew, K. M., & Moore, K. A. (2011). *Preventing multiple risky behaviors among adolescents: seven strategies.* Child Trends Results-to-Practice Brief (Publication #2011-24). Washington, DC: Child Trends. http://www.childtrends.org/wp:content/uploads/2011/09/Child_Trends-2011_10_01_RB_RiskyBehaviors.pdf.

U.S. Department of Health and Human Services, Office of Disease Prevention and Health Promotion. (2010a). *Healthy People 2020 topics & objectives: Educational and community-based programs.* Washington, DC: U.S. Department of Health and Human Services, Office of Disease Prevention and Health Promotion. http://www.healthypeople.gov/2020/topicsobjectives2020/objectiveslist.aspx?topicId=11.

U.S. Department of Health and Human Services, Office of Disease Prevention and Health Promotion. (2010b). *National action plan to improve health literacy.* Washington, DC: U.S. Department of Health and Human Services, Office of Disease Prevention and Health Promotion.

van der Lee, J. H., Mokkink, L. B., Grootenhuis, M. A., Heyman, H. S., & Offringa, M. (2007). Definitions and measurement of chronic health conditions in childhood: A systemic review. *Journal of the American Medical Association, 297,* 2741–2751. doi:10.1001/jama.297.24.2741.

Vernon, J., Trujillo, A., Rosenbaum, S., & DeBuono, B. (2007). *Low health literacy: Implications for national health policy.* Washington, DC: School of Public Health and Health Services, George Washington University. http://sphhs.gwu.edu/departments/healthpolicy/CHPR/downloads/LowHealthLiteracyReport10_4_07.pdf.

Walker, S. C., Kerns, S. E., Lyon, A. R., Bruns, E. J., & Cosgrove, T. J. (2010). Impact of school-based health center use on academic outcomes. *Journal of Adolescent Health, 46,* 251–257. doi:10.1016/j.jadohealth.2009.07.002.

Weismuller, P. C., Grasska, M. A., Alexander, M., White, C. G., & Kramer, P. (2007). Elementary school nurse interventions: Attendance and health outcomes. *Journal of School Nursing, 23,* 111–118. doi:10.1177/10598405070230020901.

Wong, M. D., Shapiro, M. F., Boscardin, W. J., & Ettner, S. L (2002). Contribution of major diseases to disparities in mortality. *New England Journal of Medicine, 347,* 1585–1592. doi:10.1056/NEJMsa012979.

Zins, J. E., Bloodworth, M. R., Weissberg, R. P., & Walberg, H. J. (2004). The scientific base linking social and emotional learning to school success. In J. E. Zins, R. P. Weissberg, M. C. Wang, & H. J. Walberg (Eds.), *Building academic success on social and emotional learning: What does the research say?* New York: Teachers College Press.

Part II
Prevention Science

Chapter 7
Prevention Science 1970–Present

Kris Bosworth and Zili Sloboda

7.1 Growth of Prevention Science

Research has led to a growing recognition of the relevance of a variety of strategies aimed at preventing harmful lifestyles and behaviors that affect many aspects of the public's health. Prevention approaches and research have expanded beyond substance abuse to embrace a number of risk factors for premature mortality and morbidity. The Office of Behavioral and Social Science Research at the USAs' National Institutes of Health (NIH 2007) recognized that "… about 70 % of the quality of our health and health care comes from malleable behavioral, sociocultural, and environmental determinants…." including "smoking, poor diet, stress, inactivity, hypertension, violence, accidents, alcohol and substance abuse, and mental illness." Furthermore, the highly prestigious US Institute of Medicine (IOM) of the National Academies of Science has issued reports on the successes accrued over the past 30 years in addressing violence (IOM 1993), mental disorders including substance use (IOM 1994, 2009), underage drinking (2003), and tobacco use (IOM 2007). Support for prevention also comes from economic interests such as the World Bank (Bloom and Canning 2008), which issued a statement about the relationship of health, safety, and well-being of populations to national economic growth and cited, for example, the importance of prenatal and early childhood health and physical and cognitive development.

The growth of prevention science can be attributed largely to the success of prevention efforts in a number of areas (Greenberg 2010; Hale et al. 2014). For example, the great strides in slowing the spread of HIV and the reduction in tobacco

K. Bosworth (⊠)
Educational Policy and Practice, University of Arizona, 1430 E 2nd Street, Tucson, AZ 85721, USA
e-mail: boswortk@email.arizona.edu

Z. Sloboda
Applied Prevention Science, Inc., Akron, USA
e-mail: zsloboda255@gmail.com

© Springer Science+Business Media New York 2015
K. Bosworth (ed.), *Prevention Science in School Settings,*
Advances in Prevention Science, DOI 10.1007/978-1-4939-3155-2_7

use and related diseases are recognized as the outcomes of effective prevention interventions and policies that integrate behavioral strategies that target individual and group decision-making regarding harmful behaviors and environmental strategies that target access and availability (Petras and Sloboda 2014). Meta-analyses and reviews (e.g., Greenberg et al. 2003; Gottfredson and Wilson 2003 Tobler 1992) have shown that prevention interventions for adolescents are effective in curbing violence and antisocial behavior (Bosworth et al. 2000; Durlak et al. 2001; Elliot and Mihlaic 2004; Fagan and Catalano 2013; Wilson et al. 2001), substance abuse (Blitz et al. 2002; Tobler 1992), and mental health (Calear and Christiansen 2010; Hoagwood et al. 2007; Tenant et al. 2007).

This chapter provides an overview of the events, legislation, and research that have defined the field of prevention science in the past 40 years with special emphasis on prevention related to alcohol, tobacco, and other drugs (ATOD). These factors that have shaped the public responses to ATOD prevention, policy, and legislation that facilitated development of an infrastructure supportive of prevention science will be explored. A discussion of the research that provided the foundation for prevention science is the focus of the final section of this chapter.

7.2 Defining Events

The evolution of prevention and the steps taken to develop an infrastructure for prevention are marked by defining public events. Several events with national significance focused national attention and galvanized action for preventing misuse of alcohol and abstinence from illicit drug use: the temperance movement and the passage of the Eighteenth Amendment (Prohibition) in 1919; The 1964 US Surgeon General's Report on Smoking and Health, which first documented the cumulative health risks of smoking; and the1986 death of college basketball superstar Len Bias from a cocaine overdose, which led to legislation that supported implementation of prevention curricula in public schools. All of these events had implications for public schools and were the stimulus for legislative solutions to health and social concerns.

7.2.1 Temperance Movement—US Constitutional Amendments 18 and 21

Concerned about the evils of "spirits," the temperance movement in the USA started early in the nineteenth century and reached a crescendo after the turn of the twentieth century. Supporters of the movement campaigned for strong controls of hard spirits and sanctions on public drunkenness but not total abstinence. There was a political and societal undertone to the movement, which was based in rural protestant areas, and might have been in part a response to the newer European immigrants who settled in the cities and whose religion (Catholicism) and drinking habits were perceived as a moral threat (Mosher and Yanagisako 1991).

Legislative initiatives became the predominant strategy to lower rates of drinking. Kansas was the first state to outlaw alcoholic beverages in 1881, and the prohibition crusade took root in other states and municipalities before and eventually reached the national theater. The Eighteenth Amendment to the Constitution originated in the Senate and became Constitutional law in January 1919. The amendment prohibited the production, transportation, and sale of "intoxicating" beverages. As a result, the country "went dry" on January 16, 1920. After passage, courts were overloaded with criminal cases related to violations of the amendment and prisons became jammed with violators. Additionally, the amendment is viewed as giving rise to expansion of organized crime and other illegal activities to include bootlegging. Although it survived several court challenges, prohibition was very unpopular in much of the country, where many otherwise law-abiding citizens had enjoyed alcoholic beverages. This legislative attempt to control access to alcohol proved politically unsuccessful and had damaging effects in terms of corruption and disrespect for law. The Eighteenth Amendment was repealed by the Twenty-first Amendment in 1933.

By reducing access to alcohol, the Eighteenth Amendment had some positive outcomes. Death rates from cirrhosis and alcoholism, alcoholic psychosis hospital admissions, and drunkenness arrests declined (Blocker 2006). In the 14 years the amendment stood, for example, there was a reduction of between 10% and 20% in cirrhosis of the liver (Dills and Miron 2004). This legislative attempt to control access to alcohol proved politically unsuccessful and resulted in damaging effects in terms of corruption and disrespect for the law.

During the same era, education was a parallel approach to reducing drinking problems. In 1886, President Cleveland signed a bill that required all public schools to offer "scientific temperance instruction" to students as a part of hygiene instruction. Publishers and authors were persuaded to stress total abstinence in their text books (Zimmerman 1999). However, Mezvinsky (1961) reported that although temperance instruction was part of textbooks for about 50 years, "Annual alcoholic beverage consumption increased between 1880 and 1920, leading to questioning of the impact of this instruction." At the onset of the prohibition era, both legislation and education were the tools to prevent the social and health harm caused by alcohol consumption.

7.2.2   Surgeon General's Report on Smoking and Health— Cigarette Labeling and Advertising Act of 1965

While the temperance movement gained momentum from its grass roots citizen organizers—and had a moral as well as a health component, the fight against tobacco originated with researchers and health organizations such as the American Cancer Society, the American Heart Association, and the American Lung Association and was driven primarily by health issues. Two now famous articles were published in 1950 documenting the negative health impact of smoking. The first, authored by the US research team, Wynder and Graham (1950), showed a possible link between smoking and lung cancer. The second, an independent study by a British research team, Doll and Hill (1954), also established a connection between smoking and lung cancer. It took 14 years before the health field publicly acted on the results of these studies, but during that period thousands of other studies indicating similar outcomes were published. In 1964, the then Surgeon General, Dr. Luther Terry, published *Smoking and Health: Report of the Advisory Committee to the Surgeon General of the Public Health Service*. In an unusual move, the Surgeon General Dr. Luther Terry announced the findings in a two hour press conference. The report provided an analysis of existing scientific studies. It concluded that cigarette smoking was: (a) a cause of lung cancer and laryngeal cancer in men, (b) a probable cause of lung cancer in women, and (c) the most important cause of chronic bronchitis. The findings from the report made immediate front page news, and tobacco sales dropped sharply, only to rebound months later (Garfinkel 1997; Housman 2001). "Luther Terry's famous announcement marked an important turning point in the antismoking movement, precipitating a decline in smoking that has lasted to the present day" (Housman 2001, p. 118).

The Surgeon General's report spawned the Federal Cigarette Labeling and Advertising Act in 1965. A key provision of the act was to require warning labels to be placed on all cigarette packages. The warning label: "Caution: Cigarette Smoking May Be Hazardous to Your Health" represented a bold declaration in its time. The Public Health Cigarette Smoking Act of 1969 represented stronger legislation aimed at reducing smoking. The warning label was required to read: "Warning: The Surgeon General has determined that Cigarette Smoking is Dangerous to your health." Additionally, cigarette advertising was prohibited on radio and television, and the Department of Health and Human Services was required to report annually to Congress on the health consequences of smoking.

Labeling cigarette packaging and reducing exposure to mass advertising provided an opportunity for people to learn the risks of tobacco use from science rather than from an advertising spin. Concurrently, increased taxation, campaigns to ban smoking in public places, and counter advertising that revealed the duplicity of tobacco companies became strategies in a synergistic, multidisciplined effort to reduce smoking and tobacco use. Rates of tobacco use have been drastically reduced; however, the challenge of preventing youth from starting to use tobacco remains.

Even before the Surgeon General's Report was issued, school-based programs were being developed to educate students about the dangers of tobacco use. These programs generally were in two broad categories. The first school campaigns consisted of multi-method approaches that included a combination of discussions, lectures, demonstrations, assemblies, and posters. The second category was youth-to-youth programs in which secondary students would plan activities based on a specified curriculum for younger students. In a meta-analysis, Thompson (1977) found that the latter category of programs showed little reduction in smoking in the participants.

7.2.3 Len Bias—Drug Free Schools and Communities Act

Hours after the University of Maryland's Len Bias, the most celebrated college basketball player of the year 1986, signed a dream contract with the Boston Celtics, he died of cardiac arrest as a result of cocaine overdose. The news of Len Bias' death spread throughout the country and created conditions that focused the public's attention on drug prevention, accelerated legislations, and shaped the tone of prevention for the next decades. The event triggered a media explosion of coverage of drug problems, especially cocaine (Orcutt and Turner 1993).

The year 1986 was an election year, and politics played a major role in the legislative response to the public outcry (Orcutt and Turner 1993). The Speaker of the House was Democrat Tip O'Neill from Boston who responded to the citizen's concerns by pushing to move legislation forward that had been at the edges of the legislative process. Dan Baum in his book, *Smoke and Mirrors: The War on Drug and the Politics of Failure,* described events as follows: Immediately upon returning from the July 4 recess, Tip O'Neill called an emergency meeting of the crime-related committee chairmen and said:

Write me some **** legislation, he thundered. All anybody up in Boston
is talking about is Len Bias. The papers are screaming for blood. We need
to get out front on this now. This week. Today. The Republicans beat us to
it in 1984 and I don't want that to happen again. I want dramatic new initiatives for dealing with crack and other drugs. If we can do this fast enough,
he said to the Democratic leadership arrayed around him, we can take the
issue away from the White House.

In life, Len Bias was a terrific basketball player. In death, he became the Archduke Ferdinand of the Total War on Drugs. What came before had been only skirmishing; the real Drug War had yet to begin. Within weeks, the country would be marching, bayonets fixed. (Baum 1997, p. 225).

Speaker O'Neill knew that the legislation had to be out of Congress by October to have any impact on the fall elections. The comprehensive bill that emerged included law enforcement, education, and research and advocacy provisions, yet it was lacking the opportunity for extensive hearings and background research. The resulting bill—Anti-Drug Abuse Act of 1986, included mandatory minimum sentences, asset forfeiture, and other provisions that provided the impetus for the label, "War on Drugs." Title IV of the act contained the Drug-Free Schools and Communities Act of 1986 that was focused on prevention with the funding for:

- State and local drug abuse education and prevention programs
- Institution of higher education or consortia for drug abuse education and prevention programs

Several federal agencies were given specific responsibilities in the legislation. The Secretary of Education was directed to carry out federal education and prevention activities on drug abuse. The Secretary of Health and Human Services was required to establish an alcohol and drug abuse information clearinghouse and also to make grants for prevention, treatment, and rehabilitation demonstration projects for high-risk youth. The Public Health Service was urged to take certain actions regarding the health consequences of alcohol abuse.

For the next 30 years, this legislation would shape the role of schools in prevention by providing consistent funding on a per pupil basis for prevention activities. Funds were directed to state departments of education to develop training and support for district-initiated prevention programming. Research funded under Title IV would provide a bevy of evidenced-based curricula and programs that could be implemented in schools across the country.

7.3   Creating an Infrastructure for Evidence-Based Strategies

Building on Success—Reductions in Smoking Prevention scientists point to reductions in smoking as the major accomplishment of prevention. This success is a result of a combination of factors including research, legislation, and education.

The next epidemiologic studies that impacted public policy on smoking were the work of a Japanese scientist, Hirayama, who showed that one did not have to be a smoker to get lung cancer and that nonsmokers who lived with heavy smokers were also at risk (2000). Two other studies, one conducted in the USA and the other in Greece, replicated these findings. Hirayama's publication in 1981 was followed by the 1986 Surgeon General's Report on the Health Consequences of Involuntary Smoking—popularly known as secondhand smoke (SHS). That report led to a number of other federal, state and local community laws, and ordinances banning smoking in a variety of places including restaurants, bars, offices, and casinos.

Two other major pieces of legislation were the Racketeer Influenced and Corrupt Organizations (RICO) Act. This statute was used to prosecute the tobacco industry; plaintiffs used it to charge the industry with fraud and deceit regarding the knowledge of harmful ingredients in cigarettes and hiding that information from the public. The Congressional hearings in which tobacco company executives testified brought to the public's attention how the tobacco companies withheld information regarding additives to tobacco products and manipulated the public, particularly women and young people, to enhance sales. And most recently in 2009, the Family Smoking Prevention and Tobacco Control Act became law. It gives the Food and Drug Administration (FDA) the authority to regulate the manufacture, distribution, and marketing of tobacco products to protect public health.

As prevention programming has matured, updated and more effective school-based prevention interventions have been developed (Flay 2009; McClellan and Perera 2013). The problem preventing the use of ATOD, especially among teens can be approached from several different paradigms, each of which could lead logically to a different approach to reducing harmful behaviors. For some, it is an issue of morals: A person who uses illegal drugs or abuses alcohol is morally deficient. Moreover, the use of drugs harms others; therefore, people who use drugs should be punished through the criminal justice system. Another approach is based in the belief that alcohol and other drug abuse is a medical issue that requires medical and psychological treatment once addiction manifests itself such as methadone therapy. Drug abuse as a public health issue precipitated using the multitiered public health model that based interventions on the level of risk of the recipient. Regardless of the response to the abuse or use itself, there has been consensus on the need for prevention so that individuals (particularly adolescents) do not initiate drug use, or at least delay starting to use a substance and thereby reduce the harm. In preventing young people from starting any use of alcohol, tobacco, or other drugs, the federal government took the lead to develop an infrastructure that supported the development and implementation of prevention strategies and programs.

7.3.1   Federal Reports and Responses

Since 1938, the National Institute of Mental Health (NIMH) in the US Department of Health Education and Welfare (the now Department of Health and Human Services) had been charged with treatment of narcotics users. However, as the number of users of all drugs steadily increased, especially among youth, a call for prevention came from many stakeholders. In 1975, Dr. Bertram S. Brown, the Director of NIMH, expressed the growing concern for prevention:

> All workers in the field of drug abuse would agree that the preferred first priority in drug abuse programs is to prevent, not to treat causalities after they occur. The fact of the matter is, however, that today our ability to conduct primary prevention is severely limited both by inadequate knowledge of the etiology of drug abuse and by the lack of prevention approaches with demonstrated effectiveness (Brown 1995, p. 199).

A major assumption of the research effort that Brown outlined was that research should inform public policy as well as program development and implementation for the prevention of drug abuse. Thus, the focus on prevention moved drug use or abuse from the justice and punishment paradigm to a public health three-fold focus model: (a) the agent or drug; (b) the environment, including attitudes and organizational culture; and (c) the host—the user or potential user, initially seen as a "high-risk adolescent." Changing the agent and the environment was relegated to policy makers, whereas researchers nationwide focused on preventing drug use totally or delaying onset (Coie et al. 1993).

In 1970, as American involvement in the Vietnam War was nearing its end, policy makers and treatment providers feared that a significant number of returning soldiers would need drug treatment. Thus, there was a great deal of activity at the national level aimed at addressing the treatment and prevention of drug use. The Drug Abuse Education Act of 1970 stated that "drug abuse diminishes the strength and vitality of the people of our Nation…" (H.R. 15252, pg. 1) and authorized the allocation of funds for grants and contracts to support research demonstration and pilot projects designed to educate the public on problems related to drug abuse. Regional centers were established to provide training for education in the public schools and the community (Bukoski 1990).

Also in 1970, the National Institute on Alcohol Abuse and Alcoholism (NIAAA) joined the Mental Health (NIMH) under the umbrella organization Alcohol, Drug Abuse, and Mental Health Administration (ADAMHA; Brown 1975). Congress created a lead drug prevention agency, the National Institute on Drug Abuse (NIDA), in 1974. Within NIDA, a prevention branch was created with the singular focus to support primary prevention research and to provide a primary prevention focus within the drug treatment system. Thus, within these new organizational structures, an infrastructure at the federal level was created to provide support for researchers and program developers to build, one study at a time, the foundation for the field of prevention science.

Previously, the prevention branch at NIDA took on two strategic approaches. The first was program evaluation, and the second was longitudinal studies of children and adolescents. For program evaluation, competitive grants were required to have a methodologically sound evaluation of any strategy, program or curriculum. The National Prevention Evaluation Research Network (NPERN) was formed as a collaborative of four states under contract to NIDA to advance evaluation skills of prevention providers nationally (N. J. Kaufman, personal communication, January 24, 2014). The requirement for early prevention researchers to have rigorous evaluations was a step on the road to developing evidenced-based practice (Brown 1975; Bukoski 1986). With more rigorous evaluations in place, many of the early approaches to prevention were found to be ineffective.

As a second strategy, longitudinal studies of children were undertaken to document factors or characteristics that differentiated those that initiated the use of drugs from those who did not. Up to that time, no database existed to measure actual adolescent drug use. The University of Michigan was given a grant to conduct an annual survey of alcohol and other drug use in high schools. In 1975, the first High School Senior Survey (now called *Monitoring the Future Study*) was used to survey seniors attending a representative sample of public and private high schools on their drug use. The results have been reported to Congress annually. Later, the adolescent population survey was expanded to include students in the 8th and 10th grades. Annual Congressional reports continued to be provided. The data from this survey remain relevant for describing trends of the common (e.g., alcohol and marijuana) and the less common drugs (e.g., PCP, Meth, inhalants); for identifying factors that correlate with increases and decreases in drug use, such as perceptions of harm associated with use; and for providing prevention program developers with a better understanding of the motivation of students who use drugs (Johnston et al. 1979), which informs prevention strategies.

As several federal agencies focused on the prevention of ATOD use in adolescents, the foundation for building a scientific base for prevention research and program development was established within the framework of other scientific endeavors in health. The availability of a national database of youth ATOD use and precursors enabled researchers, policy makers, educators, and the general public to judge progress and examine trends.

Private Sector Funding Foundations also provided support for prevention evaluation and research during the post-Vietnam era. These organizations were able to supplement federal funding for research and support the translation of research into practice with a more flexible grant review process and fewer restrictions on funds available while adhering to the rigorous research and evaluation standards set by the federal agencies. Thus, foundations contributed to the national and local infrastructure that set the stage for evidence-based practice in alcohol, tobacco, and drug use prevention. Further, they set standards for research that became the accepted level of quality. In this section, two examples of the role of foundation funding and support are described.

One of the largest contributors was the Robert Wood Johnson Foundation. Robert Wood Johnson, one of the founders of the Johnson & Johnson company known for pharmaceuticals and first aid supplies, began a small community foundation that was "dedicated to the public's health." (About RWJF 2014). In 1992, this foundation began investing millions of dollars in efforts to combat drug abuse and other addictions (Bornemeier 2009). In its quest to impact public policy on substance use or abuse through research findings, the foundation was able to fund ideas that do not fit well into federal priority-based funding. The foundation could "push the envelope" and fund cutting edge ideas (N. J. Kaufman, personal communication, January 29, 2014). Several different prevention models were developed and evaluated with varying degrees of success. Funding priorities included establishing community coalitions, creating a research and advocacy unit at Columbia University, and supporting groups that provided technical assistance to policy makers and service providers.

On a smaller scale, an evaluated prevention program with both school and community components tapped into a local community foundation to support community-wide implementation and evaluation. Project Star Students Taught Awareness and Resistance (STAR) was one of the first school-based prevention interventions to move beyond the school walls to include parent education, multimedia events, and community organizing (Pentz et al. 1989). A local Kansas City foundation, Ewing Marion Kauffman Foundation, funded the evaluation of Project STAR from 1984 through 1987. Through inclusion of all the public middle and junior high schools in the city, this rigorous, comprehensive evaluation established community involvement in addition to a school-based curriculum as an important model for prevention.

While the federal government provided various avenues of support for prevention through funding and resources, private foundations were able to contribute to the infrastructure through policy coordination and resources. Large national foundations provided support for projects with policy significance. Local foundations funded prevention activities that impacted local prevention efforts. Prevention scientists took advantage of both sources of funding and other support, and used them to further the advancement of prevention science.

7.4 Schools and Prevention Initiatives

The second decade of an individual's life is logically the ideal time for prevention activities, because it is in this period of experimentation that risky behaviors could lead to future health and social problems. Almost all adolescents were in schools. Thus, schools appeared to be the optimal venue for prevention activities. However, the results of early school-based prevention endeavors were discouraging. Lueke-field and Moskowitz (1983) summarized the state of prevention research in a *NIDA Research Monograph (47)*:

> ...Research on prevention interventions is in its infancy due to theoretical and method-ological inadequacies. Few interventions are theoretically based... Most evaluations have suffered from weak designs.... The result of these shortcomings is that there is little knowl-edge regarding (a) how prevention programs actually operate; (b) which programs have been effective; (c) why certain programs have been effective; and (d) whether these pro-grams are likely to be effective in other settings and with other populations. (p. 253)

In response, the 1980s and the early 1990s saw an explosion of research on a variety of school-based prevention approaches. These can be categorized as: (a) informa-tion, (b) affective education or values clarification, and (c) social influences.

Early school-based prevention interventions were deficit oriented and often em-ployed scare tactics in the guise of information to youth to guide decision-making. Prevention specialists theorized that if youth knew the dangers of using drugs, then that information would deter them from ever trying drugs (Evans 1998; Kohn et al. 1982). However, the information approach did not deter teens from using and in some cases, actually may have increased use (Evans 1976; Swisher and Hoffman 1975).

Since this information approach did not seem to have the desired effect, preven-tion developers alternatively approached drug use as a product of individual values in the belief that students who had goals for their future or values counter to the use of drugs would be less likely to try or use drugs. This values clarification approach did not take into account adolescent developmental stages. At the time when adoles-cents are most vulnerable to using drugs, they are also more frequently in environ-ments with less adult supervision and less contact with adult values. The desire to fit in with peers places teens susceptible to pressures to use drugs, in spite of their core values or long-term goals in which the use of drugs is counterproductive. In values clarification approach to drug prevention, teens often expressed a desire to fit in with friends. Since drug use was seen as something that would reduce social anxiety, it was proved not to be a very effective prevention approach (Goodstadt and Sheppard 1983; Tobler 1986).

In response to the neutral or negative evaluations of these prevention approach-es, a prominent smoking prevention researcher, Dr. Richard Evans at the University of Houston, convened focus groups of teens to gain a better understanding of the dynamics of youth cigarette use. From their data, Evans and colleagues, in recogni-tion of the fact that smoking and other drug use was a social phenomenon for ado-lescents, shifted the focus of prevention interventions to information about social pressures, bolstering the current information with skills to resist pressures (Evans et al. 1978). This approach dominated several decades of smoking and other drug prevention interventions.

With a theoretically justified model to guide program development, three key elements were now in place for the field of ATOD use to establish evidence-based practices. First, federal agencies such as NIDA, NIMH, US Department of Education, and Centers for Disease Control and Prevention (CDC) began requiring increasingly rigorous evaluations with any competitive grant or contract. Second, prevention researchers were publishing small but positive outcomes of success in widely read and respected academic journals such as the *Journal of the American Medical Association, Science, Journal of the American Public Health Association, and Preventive Medicine* (Bukoski 1986; Perry and Kelder 1992). Finally, there was a mechanism to distribute these evidence-based programs to states and local school districts through Title IV of the Anti-Drug Abuse Act.

7.5 The Next Generation Prevention Science in the 1990s

The infrastructure that was established in the 1970s and 1980s led to several seminal studies, papers, reports, and events in the 1990s that coalesced prevention research from a variety of disciplines to a coherent field of prevention science. Additionally, two key organizations essential to the development of the science came into being in this decade: Substance Abuse Mental Health Services Administration (SAMH-SA) and the Society for Prevention Research (SPR). This section lays the research foundation for understanding the science that is the basis of evidence-based prevention, the progress that has been made over the past 40 years in developing this science, and the opportunities and challenges that the field confronts. The two new organizations and their role in the development of prevention science are described.

7.5.1 Defining Prevention Science

The term "prevention science" was coined by John Coie and a group of researchers from seven American universities in a seminal paper published in *American Psychologist* in 1993. In this paper, prevention science was envisioned as a field that examines the biomedical and social processes that influence the incidence and prevalence of mental illness (Coie et al. 1993). The paper established two theoretical underpinnings for the field that have guided curriculum and program development since then. First, prevention should look at the precursors of the problem behavior. These precursors are identified as either risk factors that predispose a person to a higher probability of participating in risky, unhealthy behavior, or protective factors that provide a buffer from risk factors. Both risk and protective factors can be found within the individual (e.g., cognitive skills, a diagnosis of attention deficit disorders) or within the environment (e.g., positive school culture, poverty). The goal of a preventive intervention is, therefore, to "disrupt the processes that contribute to human dysfunction" (Coie et al. 1993, p. 1013).

Multilevel Interventions Coie et al. (1993) also advocated for multitiered interventions particularly for youth in schools. Universal approaches focus on the needs of the entire population without identifying individuals at any particular risk. These interventions are designed to reshape the environment for all children and can have a benefit for high-risk children as well. Universal interventions include such strategies as smoking bans in public places, anti-bullying policies in a school district or developmentally appropriate social skills training for all students at a certain grade.

However, prevention interventions need to be *targeted* to special needs of particular students who are vulnerable or at high risk for developing a serious problem, disease or disorder. Some of these interventions should target the most vulnerable children and adolescents, those for instance that are the children of substance abusers. In addition, other interventions are designed for those who may have initiated the use of alcohol, tobacco, or other psychoactive drugs but have not developed any serious problems. Their *indicated* needs require interventions that will prevent further escalation and/or reduce the potential for harm. For example, prevention interventions would be indicated particularly for ninth-grade students who have failed one or more core classes in their first semester or who are in an "alternatives to suspension" program for first offenders. All interventions, whether universal, selective, or indicated, need to be developmentally appropriate.

Risk and Protective Factors The year prior to the publication of the Coie et al., David Hawkins and colleagues at the University of Washington identified the risk and protective factors for alcohol and other problems in youth and early adulthood, based on an analysis of multiple studies. Noting that a large proportion of adolescents try alcohol and other drugs and do not become addicted, the Hawkins team promoted a *risk-factor approach* to drug use prevention for "eliminating, reducing or mitigating" the precursors to drug use as "the most promising route" (Hawkins et al. 1992, p. 64). They proposed that for prevention to be effective, programs or processes must focus on both reducing risk and enhancing protective factors and processes. According to Hawkins and colleagues, risk factors can be divided into two categories: contextual factors and individual or environmental factors. Examples of the latter type include personal attributes such as problem-solving skills or positive temperament and a social bond to conventional society are protective factors that can buffer or mitigate risk factors.

The study of protective factors traces its origins from resiliency research, which began in the late 1980s with the work of Garmezy (1985), Rutter (1985), and Werner (1989). Although there is no common definition of resiliency or way to measure it, it is generally seen as the capacity to adapt to risk in challenging situations (Glantz and Sloboda 1999). Resiliency is not a specific curriculum, nor is it a purely innate trait. Students can learn how to bounce back from adversity when they experience an environment that supports focused problem-solving skills and supports an individual's talents and skills. More recent research has further explicated the risk and protective factors and introduced the concept of vulnerability. This new way of examining the etiology or origins of substance use focuses on the underlying social, psychological, and environmental influences that make an individual susceptible to the use of psychoactive substances. It posits that the primary mechanism or process is inadequate or failed socialization, which is located at the intersection of individual vulnerabilities such as genetic predisposition, negative temperament or failed bonding in infancy, and the microlevel (e.g., family, school, peer, and workplace), and macrolevel (e.g., the social and physical neighborhood, community, nation) environments that define risk or protection (Sloboda 2014). Therefore, in developing prevention interventions, the interaction between individual vulnerability and environment (risk and protective factors) with the developmental stage of the youth and the social context must be considered. These interactions must be the foundation upon which any intervention is based (Petras and Sloboda 2014).

7.5.2 Prevention in the 1990s

Two organizational activities paralleled the synthesis in the research: In 1992, Congress established a "service organization," SAMHSA within the NIH (Mrazek and Haggerty 1994). SAMHSA was charged with providing information, and research on substance abuse and mental health disorders more available and accessible. It provided a conduit through which information and programs flowed to communities throughout America. Other federal agencies such as the CDC became active supporters of prevention research. In 1994, with the reauthorization of Title IV of the Drug-Free Schools and Communities Act of 1986, in response to the growing concern about youth violence, school districts were charged with "jointly addressing 'risk factors' that cut across ATOD use and violent behavior" (Cho et al. 2009, p. 447).

Another significant event in the 1990s was the formation of a research oriented professional organization that focused on prevention research, the SPR. Before SPR, researchers who focused on prevention joined together at various meetings representing the variety of backgrounds and training of the early researchers in the prevention filed—epidemiology, public health, psychology, criminology, social work, medicine, neuroscience, biostatistics, and public policy. Although the first meetings were organized by NIDA and its grantees, in 1991 the SPR became a professional organization that united researchers and policy makers from many disciplines around theories related to explaining and preventing risky and health-compromising behaviors. The range of concerns included mental health, smoking, delinquency, eating disorders, school failure, HIV/Acquired immune deficiency syndrome (AIDS), violence, and bullying. The goal was to advance "scientific investigation on the etiology and prevention of social, physical and mental health, and academic problems and on the translation of that information to promote health and well-being." (SPR 2014) The membership in the Society for Prevention Research expanded from 120 in 1994 to 747 in 2009. In 2000, SPR launched its official publication *Prevention Science* dedicated to publishing peer-reviewed articles as an interdisciplinary forum for current research in the theory and practice of prevention in the USA and internationally.

7.5.3 Documenting Evidence-Based Practice

A 1986, meta-analysis of 143 drug and tobacco prevention programs by Nan Tobler found that effective programs based on the social influences model of prevention that combined enhancement of general social skills and a focus on drug
specific situational assertiveness decreased drug use or prevented initiation by the
average adolescent who was not at risk (Tobler 1986). Several years later, another
meta-analysis critiqued Tobler on methodological grounds presented less promising
results (Bangert-Downs 1988). The author found that although students who participated in prevention programs increased their knowledge and had more negative
attitudes about drugs, this did not translate into behavior.

Hansen (1992) reviewed substance abuse prevention studies that were published
between 1980 and 1990. Although he identified many methodological weaknesses,
the body of research led him to conclude, "Social influence and comprehensive programs are most consistently effective in reducing substance abuse among students
exposed to these programs" (p. 427).

7.5.4 Research to Practice

Researchers were finding successful approaches to prevention, although the effect
sizes were small to moderate, and few programs had longitudinal data and were independently replicated (Baumberger et al. 2010; Holder 2009). Effective universal
and targeted programs could be identified in multiple risk areas such as violence
(e.g., Wilson et al. 2001), substance abuse (e.g., Blitz et al. 2002), and mental health
(Durlak and Wells 1997). Additionally, researchers were able to identify key elements across programs that were critical to success of these interventions (Dusenbury and Falco 1995; Dusenbury et al. 1997).

Guides In the 1990s, at the national level, several publications reviewed multiple
prevention programs/curricula on several dimensions from theoretical, research,
and practical levels (Bosworth and Sailes 1993). In 1996, a Washington-based nonprofit, drug strategies released *Making the Grade:A Guide to School Drug Prevention Programs*, which reviewed 15 published and publically available prevention
programs. *Safe Schools/Safe Students: A Guide to Violence Prevention Strategies*
was released 2 years later. In 1996, the University of Colorado with funding from
the state of Colorado and the US Office of Juvenile Justice and Delinquency Prevention began identifying, evaluating, and distributing prevention programs that
have strong evidence of effectiveness. In 1997, NIDA published "Drug Abuse Prevention among Children and Adolescents: A research-based guide" (NIDA 1997).
Commonly known as the "little red book," this guide laid out research-based principles of prevention. These publications were designed to assist educators in the
selection of evidenced-based programs.

In 1998, the US Department of Education adopted the "Principles of Effectiveness," which included the requirement to select a "research-based program" (Hallfors and Godette 2002). Although these principles were aimed at giving state and local entities support for selecting programs with research support, Halfors and Godette subsequently found that the most frequently implemented programs continued to be those with little evidence of effectiveness: Drug Abuse Resistance Education D.A.R.E. (D.A.R.E) and *Here's Looking at You* 2000; (2002).

Model Programs In 1999, the SAMHSA, which was established by Congress in 1992, identified 30 exemplary prevention programs. The list and descriptions of each were widely distributed. The US Department of Education identified "model" and "promising" prevention programs in 2001.

The publication of the guides, identification of model programs, and establishment of the *Principles of Prevention* provided schools and communities with guidance in selecting prevention interventions. With these publications, the gulf between research and practice was being bridged slowly (Hogan et al. 2003).

7.6 Issues with Evidence-Based Practice

Since the 1970s, the focus of prevention scientists had been on developing and testing theory-based, evidence-based, developmentally guided prevention interventions. The logic was that once these strategies were developed and funding was available to support implementation, educators and communities would be eager to adopt them. Infrastructure was created to support the research, development, evaluation, and dissemination. Currently, most of the infrastructure is focused on either creating and identifying or scaling up evidence-based practice. However, several issues have raised questions about the efficacy of this approach.

Drug Abuse Resistance Education (D.A.R.E.) Language in the 1986 Anti-Drug Abuse Act earmarked funds to be spent on prevention programs delivered by uniformed police officers. The most popular of such programs was D.A.R.E. that grew out of cooperative effort between Los Angeles schools and the police, beginning in 1983. In a 10-lesson program originally aimed at 5th and 6th graders, trained police officers provided students with information about drugs and alcohol and taught ways to resist substance abuse and violence. Students signed a pledge not to use drugs or join gangs (Harmon 1993).

Numerous evaluations of D.A.R.E. (See Ennett et al. 1994; Lynam et al. 1999) revealed mostly negative results; however, other primary prevention programs funded by NIDA and other federal agencies and foundations were shown to be somewhat more effective (8, 1996). This controversy reached the national press *(USA Today and Dateline: NBC)* when the D.A.R.E. organization allegedly attempted to thwart the publication of an evaluation study in a research journal. At that time, D.A.R.E. was the most popular prevention intervention in schools. This controversy had an impact on the confidence level of policy makers, educators, and politicians in the approach to prevention in schools.

7.6.1 Questions of Effectiveness

Both the federal government and private groups (e.g., University of Colorado *Blue-prints* and Drug Strategies, *and Making the Grade*) published guidelines for adopting "evidence-based" programs when using federal funds. Gandhi and colleagues examined the major lists of evidence-based prevention programs and found that there was "limited evidence of effectiveness of all these (programs examined) on reducing substance abuse in the long term" (Gandhi et al. 2007, p. 60).

Other researchers questioned whether some of the decreases in substance use were related to general decreases in drug use in the population at large rather than increases in federal spending and the appearance of evidence-based interventions (Gorman 1998). Gorman concluded, "… to continue to advocate the use of school-based social influence programs on the basis of selected, isolated positive findings, is in the interest of no more than a very few individuals" (p. 141).

Evaluation expert Carol Weiss and her team extensively reviewed the effects of what they called "imposed use" of evidence-based prevention interventions. Citing the limitations of research and quality of the studies, they concluded that the selection of programs designated as "evidence-based" were biased by weak evaluations and developer self-interest and might not be the utopia it was heralded to be. Reliance on lists of such programs may discourage innovation and fail to take into consideration the context in which the evidence-based intervention will be implemented (Weiss et al. 2008).

No research group had carefully defined evidence-based prevention interventions nor had a major review of the literature been undertaken to assign rigorous criteria of effectiveness to research findings. In 2012, the United Nations Office on Drugs and Crime (UNDOC) began such a project bringing together researchers and policy makers from over 80 countries. Criteria of effectiveness were developed by this large task group, which gave the highest effectiveness ratings to those studies that applied meta-analyses or a systematic review. These were followed by at least two randomized trials or appropriate experimental designs (such as time-series analyses of policy-based interventions). The framework used to categorize interventions included developmental age (infancy and early childhood, middle childhood, early adolescence, and late adolescence and adulthood) and environment (family, school, community, workplace, and health sector). The outcome was the *International Standards on Drug Use Prevention*, published in 2013. The International Standards document lays out the key principles for the content, structure, and delivery of evidence-based prevention interventions and policies (United Nations Office on Drugs and Crime 2013).

7.6.2 Scaling-Up

As discussed in Chap. 8 of this volume, diffusion of evidence prevention has been slow and uneven. Although funds through Title IV are available to all public schools and 88 % of the middle schools received those funds in 2004, only a third of the US districts used evidence-based curricula in their middle schools (Cho et al. 2009). Although these results are disappointing to preventions scientists, Elias and colleagues reported that going to scale in many other educational reforms produced similar results (Elias et al. 2003). This phenomenon spawned a branch of prevention research that focuses on translational research or scaling up (Spoth et al. 2013).

7.7 Twenty-First Century

As we moved into the twenty-first century, prevention research methodologies have become more sophisticated (MacKinnon and Lockwood 2003), the relationship between prevention and the public school system has become codified, funding through the US Department of Education has increased (Hantman and Cross 2000), and the number of professionals identifying themselves as prevention scientists has also increased.

Policy and Legislation In 2001, a bipartisan bill, now known as No Child Left Behind (NCLB) that would shape public education for the first decade of the twenty-first century was signed by President George W. Bush (NCLB 2002). Although the NCLB emphasized academic preparation in reading and mathematics and accountability as measured by standardized test scores and graduation rates, educators in public school also were charged with "establishing drug- and violence-free environments" (Cho et al. 2009, p. 448). In this process of establishing these environments, educators were charged with using only "research-based" or "evidence-based" programs. While the message about the importance of evidence-based prevention was clear, other provisions of NCLB created a high pressure climate of accountability. Given the testing requirements, many educational leaders increased time for instruction of core subjects (e.g., reading, writing, and math), leaving little room in the school day for activities such as prevention (Cho et al. 2009; Domitrovich et al. 2010). NCLB did not significantly further the adoption and expansion of prevention interventions.

Since the economic crisis in 2007 and 2008, the infrastructure for prevention science has been eroded further. NIDA funding for prevention research has decreased from US$410.4 million in 2008 to US$358.1 million in the 2015 budget (FY 2015 Budget and Performance Summary 2015). In 2009, the US Department of Education eliminated the formula grants to state departments of education and to local school districts in favor of statewide competitions. The state infrastructure that supported educators in selecting and implementing evidence-based prevention has been weakened significantly.

7.7.1 Research

After 40 years of research and intervention development, it is possible to say that the field has moved from "prevention research to prevention science" (Sloboda 2012). The Research Knowledge Task Group Society for Prevention Research: Standards of Knowledge for the Science of Prevention (2011) of the Society for Prevention Research conceptualized prevention science as follows: "The primary goal of prevention science is to improve public health by identifying malleable risk and protective factors, assessing the efficacy and effectiveness of preventive interventions and identifying optimal means for dissemination and diffusion" (p. 3). In addition to broadening the definition of "prevention science," the group outlined three major aspects that distinguish prevention science from many disciplines that inform its direction: epidemiology, intervention development, and research methodology.

Epidemiology A foundation of all prevention program development and research has been epidemiologic studies, which describe the incidence and prevalence of the predictors of positive and negative behavioral outcomes. Research needs to be continually updated, and additional studies are needed to more accurately identify how risk and protective factors vary in different populations and developmental stages. Changes in policy, such as the legalization of marijuana, may lead to changes in previously identified risk and protective factors.

Intervention Development Research has demonstrated that effective prevention interventions have several key features. They are developmentally appropriate and designed to meet the needs of a target population. They address the role of human motivation and self-efficacy while being sensitive to population subgroups. Interventions can target individuals, families, institutions (such as school), communities, and government entities. Research into the effectiveness of interventions raises questions about the key features such as how they work, what factors explain them, and how antecedents or the environment can be altered for better outcomes. An expanded discussion of intervention development can be found in Chaps. 7 and 12. Some promising opportunities for more effective prevention include integration of breakthroughs from neuroscience in the understanding of neuroscience and addiction and the implementation of integrated approaches.

Neuroscience Advances in our knowledge about how the brain functions and the possible impacts on decision-making and addiction hold promise for another avenue of prevention interventions (Bradshaw et al. 2012; Fonagy 2012). Research on the effectiveness of neuroscience-based prevention curricula has been conducted at the elementary school level. Two studies have demonstrated that teaching about adverse effects of alcohol and other drugs on the developing brain leads to preventive effects as much as a year later (Padget et al. 2006; Sigelman et al. 2004). NIDA has developed a curriculum based on the latest neuroscience information on addiction. "The Brain," a five-lesson curriculum, which is available at no cost, includes numerous supplementary materials including images of Positron emission tomography (PET) scans and other graphics that display how drugs interact with brain functioning. Although there is no formal evaluation of the impact of such a strategy, "The Brain" is designed to be integrated into the science curriculum in middle or high schools (Bosworth and Judkins 2011).

Integrated Models The interactions between individuals and their family, school, community, and sociopolitical environment are complex. Multiple pathways to risk-taking and addiction exist. Given the integrated systems that exert influence on human behavior, prevention scientists are experimenting with integrating "perspectives from diverse disciplines and sectors" (Sanson et al. 2011, p. 85).

Longitudinal studies have identified common sets of risk factors for problem behaviors that increase a young person's risk for negative outcomes (Coie et al. 1993; Jessor and Jessor 1977; Rutter 1993). Problem behavior theory (Jessor and Jessor 1977) posits that problem behaviors (e.g., alcohol use, risky sexual behavior, drunk driving, or delinquency) are interrelated positively among themselves. Young people who engage in one problem behavior are likely to engage in several. In addition, a commonality of risk factors exists for all the risky behaviors. In response, many program developers created interventions to target multiple health-risk behaviors. In a systematic review of effectiveness of interventions for multiple health-risk behaviors, Hale et al. (2014), identified 44 randomized controlled trials of interventions for multiple health-risk factors. They found that the effects overall were small and many emerged only in long-term follow up. However, the authors concluded that integrated prevention programs "… may be more efficient than discrete prevention strategies" (p. e19).

Domitrovich and colleagues (Domitrovich et al. 2010) posited that since most problem behavior is rooted in multiple risk factors, targeting only one risk factor or one problem behavior may be insufficient. They identified two categories of integration: horizontal and vertical. Horizontal integration combines two or more prevention interventions at the same level of risk (universal, targeted, or indicated). Vertical integration combines multiple interventions across risk levels. Chaparro et al. (2012) described combining a behavior support model with academic supports. Sheppard and colleagues (2012) used horizontal integration when they united the family check-up model with the Incredible Years parenting program in a Head Start setting to bolster outcomes.

These combinations carefully integrate evidence-based curricula or programs to create a synergistic prevention environment (Bosworth 2000; Bradshaw et al. 2014; Domitrovich et al. 2010; Reinke et al. 2011). Such integrated systems draw on the multitiered public health approach that was outlined by Coie and colleagues (Coie et al. 1993). In those models, Domitrovich et al. (2009) found that "intervention elements function as part of a coordinated whole" (p. 75) which build on and reinforce each other. Such synergy happens only with careful planning and monitoring. An essential practice, therefore, is to develop an infrastructure within a school or district to coordinate the integrated systems, ensure that student needs are being met, and that programs are being implemented with fidelity.

Infrastructure In an Institute of Medicine Report, Mrazek and Haggerty (1994) recommended that the definition of prevention includes only the activities occurring before a disorder is clinically diagnosed. They supported adopting the three-tiered public health model for preventive interventions as universal, selective, and indicated; and they supported the focus on risk and protective factors. The report recommended a federal infrastructure to support prevention, through research to expand the knowledge base and inform prevention interventions; and through training of new and mid-career scientists (Muñoz et al. 1996).

Research Methodology Although prevention science research methodology draws from social science, epidemiology, and biostatistics, it is differentiated from those individual methodologies because of the complexity of collecting, measuring, and analyzing nested, multilevel, multitrait longitudinal data. Although the field has long been dominated by statistical quantitative methodologies, some prevention researchers are exploring the contributions that qualitative and mixed methods designs can make to further advance the field. Discussion of various methodological issues can be found in Chaps. 10, 11 and 12 of this volume.

7.8 Conclusion

Budget cuts and shifting priorities in all sectors of the economy offer incentives for prevention science to reassess the vision, goals, and strategies that can help protect the next generation of young people. With this "new normal," stronger partnership with schools and other institutions can provide a synergy that has the potential to strengthen students.

The future of prevention science lies in accomplishing several goals. First, a stable funding base for both prevention research and prevention services is essential to capitalize on the advances in the last 40 years. Second, prevention science theories need to be refined and strengthened to make sense of the relationships between etiology and outcomes of interest (e.g., ATOD use, diet and exercise, risky sexual behaviors, school failure, juvenile delinquency, or conduct disorders). These theories must be able to guide interventions to avoid negative outcomes. Third, silos that lead to duplication of, or gaps in, services and research must be broken down. This will be facilitated by creation and support of authentic partnerships among educators, health educators, public health professionals, and policy makers. Fourth, research designs and methodologies that are specific to translation and scaling up in real world conditions must be developed.

Finally, a prevention science workforce needs to be established at several levels: local, state, regional, national, and international. Training for, and certification of, prevention specialists needs to be widespread with clear career paths for prevention specialists in both intervention and research. Existing community, state, and national organizations (e.g., American School Counselors Association, National Association of Secondary School Administrators) need to incorporate prevention into their mission, as it is linked to overall student success. These activities would produce "a new generation of skilled and knowledgeable prevention scientists who can build effective partnerships across sectors, cut across silos, and adopt systemic thinking" (Sanson et al. 2011, p. 89).

References

2015 Budget and Performance Summary. (2015). whitehouse.gov/sites/default/files/ondcp/about-content/fy2015_summary.pdf. Accessed 15 Jan 2015.

About RWJF: Our history. (2014). http://www.rwjf.org/en/about-rwjf/our-mission/our-history.html. Accessed 12 Feb 2014.

Bangert-Downs, R. L. (1988). The effects of school-based substance abuse education: A meta-analysis. *Journal of Drug Education, 18*(3), 243–264. doi:10.2190/8U40-WP3D-FFWC-YF1U.

Baum, D. (1997). *Smoke and mirrors: The war on drugs and the politics of failure*. New York: Little, Brown and Company.

Blitz, C. C., Arthur, M. W., & Hawkins, J. D. (2002). Preventing alcohol, tobacco, and other substance abuse. In L. A. Jason & D. S. Glenwick (Eds.), *Innovative strategies for promoting health and mental health across the life span* (pp. 176–201). New York: Springer.

Blocker, J. S. (2006). Did prohibition really work? Alcohol prohibition as a public health innovation. *American Journal of Public Health, 96*(2), 233–243. doi:10.2105/AJPH.2005.065409.

Bloom, D. E., & Canning, D. (2008). *Population health and economic growth*. Washington D.C.: The International Bank for Reconstruction and Development/The World Bank On behalf of the Commission on Growth and Development.

Bornemeier, J. (2009). The Robert Wood Johnson Foundation's efforts to combat drug addiction. In S. L. Isaacs & D. C. Colby (Eds.), *To improve health and health care* (Vol. XIII, pp. 1–17). San Francisco: Jossey-Bass.

Bosworth, K., & Judkins, M. (2011). *Teachers and counselors teaming to teach a NIH neuroscience curriculum for drug prevention*. Presented at the 2011 AERA Annual Meeting, New Orleans, LA.

Bosworth, K., & Sailes, J. (1993). Content and teaching strategies in 10 selected drug abuse prevention curricula. *Journal of School Health, 63*(6), 247–253. doi:10.111/j.1746–1561.1993.tb06134.x.

Bosworth, K., Espelage, D. L., DuBay, T., Daytner, G., & Karageorge, K. (2000). A preliminary evaluation of a multimedia violence prevention program for early adolescence. *American Journal of Health Behavior, 24*(4), 268–280.

Bradshaw, C. P., Goldweber, A., Fishbein, D., & Greenberg, M. T. (2012). Infusing developmental neuroscience into school-based preventive interventions: Implications and future directions. *Journal of Adolescent Health, 51*(2), S41–S47. doi:10.1016/j.jadohealth.2012.04.020.

Bradshaw, C. P., Bottiani, J. H., Osher, D., & Sugai, G. (2014). Integrating positive behavioral interventions and supports (PBIS) and social and emotional learning (SEL) In M. D. Weist, N. A. Lever, C. P. Bradshaw, & J. Owens (Eds.), *Handbook of school mental health: Advancing practice and research* (2nd ed., pp. 101–118). New York: Springer US. doi:10.1007/978-1-4614-7624-58.

Brown, B. S. (1975). Drugs and public health: Issues and answers. *The ANNALS of the American Academy of Political and Social Science, 417*, 110–119. doi:10.1177/000271627541700111.

Bukoski, W. J. (1986). School-based substance abuse prevention: A review of program research. *Journal of Children in Contemporary Society, 18*(1–2), 95–115. doi:10.1300/J274v18n01_06.

Bukoski, W. J. (1990). The federal approach to primary drug abuse prevention and education. In J. A. Iniciardi (Ed.), *Handbook of drug control in the United States* (pp. 93–114). California: Greenwood Publishing Group.

Calear, A. L., & Christensen, H. (2010). Systematic review of school-based prevention and early intervention programs for depression. *Journal of Adolescence, 33*(3), 429–438. doi:0.1016/j.adolescence.2009.07.004.

Chaparro, E. A., Smolkowski, K., Baker, S. K., Hanson, N., & Ryan-Jackson, K. (2012). A model for system-wide collaboration to support integrated social behavior and literacy evidence-based practices. *Psychology in the Schools, 49*(5), 465–482. doi:10.1002/pits.21607.

Cho, H., Hallfors, D. D., Iritani, B. J., & Hartman, S. (2009). The influence of "no child left behind" legislation on drug prevention in US schools. *Evaluation Review, 33*(5), 446–463.doi:1 0.1177/0193841X09335050.

Coie, J. D., & Watt, N. F., West, S. G., Hawkins, J. D., Asarnow, J. R., Markman, H. J., Ramey, S. L., Shure, M. B., Long, B. (1993). The science of prevention: A conceptual framework and some directions for a national research program. *American Psychologist, 48*(10),1013–1022. http://dx.doi.org/10.1037/0003-066X.48.10.

Dills, A. K., & Miron, J. A. (2004). Alcohol prohibition and cirrhosis. *American Law and Economics Review, 6*(2), 285–318. doi:10.1093/aler/ahh003.

Doll, R., & Hill, A. B. (1954). The mortality of doctors in relation to their smoking habits. *British Medical Journal, 1*(4877), 1451.

Domitrovich, C. E., Bradshaw, C. P., Greenberg, M. T., Embry, D., Poduska, J. M., & Ialongo, N. S. (2010). Integrated models of school-based prevention: Logic and theory. *Psychology in the Schools, 47*(1), 71–88. doi:10.1002/pits.20452.

Durlak, J. A., & Wells, A. M. (1997). Primary prevention mental health programs for children and adolescents: A meta-analytic review. *American Journal of Community Psychology, 25*(2), 115–152.

Durlak, J. A., Rubin, L. A., & Kahng, R. D. (2001). Cognitive behavioral therapy for children and adolescents with externalizing problems. *Journal of Cognitive Psychotherapy, 15*(3), 183–194. 2001100000015/00000003/art00003.

Dusenbury, L., & Falco, M. (1995). Eleven components of effective drug abuse prevention curricula. *The Journal of School Health, 65*(10), 420–425. doi:10.1111/j.1746–1561.1995.tb08205.x.

Dusenbury, L., Falco, M., Lake, A., Brannigan, R., & Bosworth, K. (1997). Nine critical elements of promising violence prevention programs. *The Journal of School Health, 67*(10), 409–414. doi:10.1111/j.1746–1561.1997.tb01286.x.

Elias, M. J., Zins, J. E., Graczyk, P. A., & Weissberg, R. P. (2003). Implementation, sustainability, and scaling up of social-emotional and academic innovations in public schools. *School Psychology Review, 32*(3), 303–319.

Elliott, D. S., & Mihalic, S. (2004). Issues in disseminating and replicating effective prevention programs. *Prevention Science, 5*(1), 47–53. /10.1023/B:PREV.0000013981.28071.52.

Ennett, S. T., Tobler, N. S., Ringwalt, C. L., & Flewelling, R. L. (1994). How effective is drug abuse resistance education? A meta-analysis of Project DARE outcome evaluations. *American Journal of Public Health, 84*(9), 1394–1401. doi:10.2105/AJPH.84.9.1394.

Evans, R. I. (1976). Smoking in children: Developing a social psychological strategy of deterrence. *Preventive Medicine, 5*(1), 122–127. doi:10.1016/0091-7435(76)90015-3.

Evans, R. I. (1998). An historical perspective on effective prevention. In W. J. Bukoski & R. I. Evans (Eds.), *National Institute on Drug Abuse Research Monograph Series No. 176, Cost-Benefit/Cost-Effectiveness Research on Drug.Abuse Prevention: Implications for Programming and Policy*. NIH Publication No. 98-4021 (pp. 37–58). Washington DC: U. S. Department of Health and Human Services, National Institutes of Health, Superintendent of Documents, U. S. Government Printing Office.

Evans, R. I., Rozelle, R. M., Mittelmark, M., Hansen, W. B., Bane, A., & Havis, J. (1978). Deterring the onset of smoking in children: Knowledge of immediate psychological effects and coping with peer pressure, media pressure, and parent modeling. *Journal of Applied Social Psychology, 8*, 126–135.

Fagan, A. A., & Catalano, R. F. (2013). What works in youth violence prevention: A review of the literature. *Research on Social Work Practice, 23*(2), 141–156. doi:10.1177/1049731512465899.

Flay, B. R. (2009). School-based smoking prevention programs with the promise of long-term effects. *Tobacco Induced Diseases, 5*(6), 1–18.

Fonagy, P. (2012). The neuroscience of prevention. *Journal of the Royal Society of Medicine, 105*(3), 97–100. doi:10.1258/jrsm.2012.12k008.

Gandhi, A. G., Murphy-Graham, E., Petrosino, A., Chrismer, S. S., & Weiss, C. H. (2007). The devil is in the details: Examining the evidence for "proven" school-based drug abuse prevention programs. *Evaluation Review, 31*(1), 43–74. doi:10.1177/0193841X06287188.

Garfinkel, L. (1997). Trends in cigarette smoking in the United States. *Preventive Medicine, 26*(4), 447–450. doi:10.1006/pmed.1997.0191.

Glantz MD, Sloboda Z. (1999). Analysis and reconceptualization of resilience. In M. D. Glantz & J. L. Johnson (Eds.), *Resilience and Development: Positive Life Adaptations* (pp. 109–126). Dordrecht: Kluwer Academic Publishers.

Goodstadt, M. S., & Sheppard, M. A. (1983). Three approaches to alcohol education. *Journal of Studies on Alcohol and Drugs, 44*(2), 362–380.

Gorman, D. M. (1998). The irrelevance of evidence in the development of school-based drug prevention policy, 1986–1996. *Evaluation Review, 22*(1), 118–146. doi:10.1177/019384 1X9802200106.

Gottfredson, D. C., & Wilson, D. B. (2003). Characteristics of effective school-based substance abuse prevention. *Prevention Science, 4*(1), 27–38. doi:10.1023/A:1021782710278.

Greenberg, M. T., Weissberg, R. P., O'Brien, M. D., Zins, J. E., Fredericks, L., Resnik, H., & Elias, M. J. (2003). Enhancing school-based prevention and youth development through coordinated social, emotional, and academic learning. *American psychologist, 58*(6–7), 466. DOi: 10.1037/0003-066X.58.6-7.466.

Greenberg, M. T. (2010). School-based prevention: Current status and future challenges. *Effective Education, 2*(1), 27–52. doi:10.1080/19415531003616862.

Garmezy, N. (1985). Stress-resistant children: The search for protective factors. *Recent Research in Developmental Psychopathology, 4*, 213–233.

Hale, D. R., Fitzgerald-Yau, N., & Viner, R. M. (2014). A systematic review of effective interventions for reducing multiple health risk behaviors in adolescence. *American Journal of Public Health, 104*(5), e19–e41. doi:10.2105/AJPH.2014.301874.

Hallfors, D., & Godette, D. (2002). Will the principles of effectiveness' improve prevention practice? Early findings from a diffusion study. *Health Education Research, 17*(4), 461–470.

Hansen, W. B. (1992). School-based substance abuse prevention: A review of the state of the art in curriculum, 1980–1990. *Health Education Research, 7*(3), 403–430. doi:10.1093/her/7.3.403.

Hantman, I., & Crosse, S. (2000). Progress in prevention: Report on the National Study of Local Education Agency Activities under the Safe and Drug Free Schools and Communities Act. http://files.eric.ed.gov/fulltext/ED466014.pdf.

Harmon, M. A. (1993). Reducing the risk of drug involvement among early adolescents an evaluation of drug abuse resistance education (DARE). *Evaluation Review, 17*(2), 221–239. doi:10.1177/0193841×9301700206.

Hawkins, J. D., Catalano, R. F., & Miller, J. Y. (1992). Risk and protective factors for alcohol and other drug problems in adolescence and early adulthood: Implications for substance abuse prevention. *Psychological Bulletin, 112*(1), 64. doi:10.1037/0033-2909.112.1.64.

Hirayama, T. (2000). Non-smoking wives of heavy smokers have a higher risk of lung cancer: A study from Japan. *Bulletin of the World Health Organization, 78*(7), 940–942. doi:10.1590/S0042-96862000000700013.

Hoagwood, K. E., Olin, S. S., Kerker, B. D., Kratochwill, T. R., Crowe, M., & Saka, N. (2007). Empirically based school interventions target at academic and mental health functioning. *Journal of Emotional and Behavioral Disorders, 15*(2), 66–92.

Hogan, J. A., Gabrielsen, K. R., Luna, N., & Grothaus, D. (2003). *Substance abuse prevention: The intersection of science and practice.* Boston: Pearson Education, Inc.

Holder, H. (2009). Prevention programs in the 21st century: What we do not discuss in public, *105*, 578–581. doi:10.1111/j.1360-443.2009.02725.x.

Housman, M. (2001). Smoking and health: 1964 U.S. surgeon general's report as a turning point in the anti-smoking movement. *Harvard Health Policy Review, 2*, 119–127.

Institute of Medicine. (1993). *Emergency medical services for children.* Washington, DC: National Academy Press.

Institute of Medicine. (2001). *Crossing the quality chasm: A new health system for the 21st Century.* Washington, DC: National Academy Press; 2001.

Institute of Medicine. (2007). *Ending the tobacco problem: A blueprint for the nation,* are available from the National Academies Press, 500 Fifth Street, N.W., Lockbox 285, Washington, DC.

Institute of Medicine of the National Academies. (2003, September). Reducing underage drinking: A collective responsibility. [Report Brief]. http://www.iom.edu/~/media/Files/Report%20Files/2003/Reducing-Underage-Drinking-A-CollectiveResponsibility/ReducingUnderage-Drinking.pdf.

Institute of Medicine of the National Academies. (2007, May). Ending the tobacco problem: A blueprint for the nation. [Report Brief]. https://www.iom.edu/~/media/Files/Report%20Files/2007/Ending-the-Tobacco-Problem-A-Blueprint-for-theNation/Tobaccoreportbriefgeneral.pdf.

Jessor, R., & Jessor, S. L. (1977). *Problem behavior and psychosocial development: A longitudinal study of youth.* New York: Academic Press.

Johnston, L. D., Bachman, J. G., & O'Malley, P. M. (1979). *Monitoring the future: Questionnaire responses from the nation's high school seniors.* Ann Arbor: Institute for Social Research, University of Michigan.

Kohn, P. M., Goodstadt, M. S., Cook, G. M., Sheppard, M., & Chan, G. (1982). Ineffectiveness of threat appeals about drinking and driving. *Accident Analysis & Prevention, 14*(6), 457–464. doi:10.1016/0001-4575(82)90059-8.

Lynam, D. R., Milich, R., Zimmerman, R., Novak, S. P., Logan, T. K., Martin, C., Clayton, R., et al. (1999). Project DARE: No effects at 10-year follow-up. *Journal of Consulting and Clinical Psychology, 67*(4), 590. doi:10.1037/0022-006X.67.4.590.

MacKinnon, D. P., & Lockwood, C. M. (2003). Advances in statistical methods for substance abuse prevention research. *Prevention Science, 4*(3), 155–171. doi:10.1023/A:1024649822872.

McClellan, J., & Perera, R. (2013). School-based programmes for preventing smoking (review). *Cochrane Database of Systemic Review, 2013*(4) Art No.: CD001293. doi:10.1002/14651858.CD001293.pub3.

Mezvinsky, N. (1961). Scientific temperance instruction in the schools. *History of Education Quarterly, 1*(1), 48–56. doi:10.2307/367201.

Mosher, J. F., & Yanagisako, K. L. (1991). Public health, not social warfare: A public health approach to illegal drug policy. *Journal of Public Health Policy, 12*(3), 278–323. doi:10.2307/3342844.

Moskowitz, J. M. (1983). Preventing adolescent substance abuse through drug education. In T. J. Glynn, C. G. Leukefeld, & J. P. Ludford (Eds.), *NIDA Research Monograph Series, 47,* (pp. 233–249). Washington, D.C.: U.S. Government Printing Office.

Mrazek, P. J., & Haggerty, R. J. (1994). *Reducing risks for mental disorders: Frontiers for preventive intervention research.* Washington, D.C.: National Academy Press.

Muñoz, R. F., Mrazek, P. J., & Haggeliy, R. J. (1996). Institute of medicine report on prevention of mental disorders: summary and commentary. *American Psychologist, 51*(11), 1116.

National Institute on Drug Abuse. (1997). *Preventing drug use among children and adolescents: A research-based guide.* Rockville: U.S. Department of Health and Human Services.

Orcutt, J. D., & Turner, J. B. (1993). Shocking numbers and graphic accounts: Quantified images of drug problems in the print media. *Society for the Study of Social Problems, 40*(2), 190–206. doi:10.2307/3096921.

Padget, A., Bell, M. L., Shamblen, S. R., & Ringwalt, C. L. (2006). Does learning about the effects of alcohol on the developing brain affect children's alcohol use? *Prevention Science, 7*(3), 293–302. doi:10.1007/s11121-006-0030-9.

Pentz, M., Johnson, C. A., Dwyer, J. H., MacKinnon, D. M., Hansen, W. B., & Flay, B. R. (1989). A comprehensive community approach to adolescent drug abuse prevention: Effects on cardiovascular disease risk behaviors. *Annals of Medicine, 21,* 219–222. doi:10.3109/07853898909149937.

Perry, C. L., & Kelder, S. H. (1992). Models for effective prevention. *Journal of Adolescent Health, 13,* 355–363. doi:10.1016/1054–139X(92)90028-A.

Reinke, W. M., Stormont, M., Herman, K. C., Puri, R., & Goel, N. (2011). Supporting children's mental health in schools: Teacher perceptions of needs, roles, and barriers. *School Psychology Quarterly, 26*(1). 1–13. doi:10.1037/a0022714.

Rutter, M. (1985). Resilience in the face of adversity. Protective factors and resistance to psychiatric disorder. *The British Journal of Psychiatry, 147*(6), 598–611. Doi:10.1192/bjp.147.6.598.

Rutter, M. (1993). Resilience: Some conceptual considerations. *Journal of Adolescent Health 14*(8), 626–631. doi:10.1016/1054-139X(93)901196-V.

Sanson, A. V., Havinghurst, S. S., & Zubrick, S. R. (2011). The science of prevention for children and youth. *Australian Review of Public Affairs, 10*(1), 79–83.

Shepard, S., Armstrong, L. M., Silver, R. B, Berger, R., & Seifer, R. (2012). Embedding the family check up and evidence-based parenting programs in Head Start to increase parent engagement and reduce conduct problems in young children. *Advances in School Mental Health Promotion, 5*(3), 194–207. Published online 2012 Aug 7. doi: 10.1 080/1754730X.2012.707432.

Sigelman, C. K., Rinehart, C. S., Sorongon, A. G., Bridges, L. J., & Wirtz, P. W. (2004). Teaching a coherent theory of drug action to elementary school children. *Health Education Research, 19*(5), 501–513. doi:10.1093/her/cyg058.

Sloboda, Z. (2012). In celebration of prevention science. [PowerPoint slides].

Sloboda, Z. (2014). Reconceptualizing drug use prevention processes. *Adicciones: Revista de socidrogalcohol, 26*(1), 3–9.

Sloboda, Z., & Petras, H. (2014). *Defining prevention science.* New York: Springer.

Spoth, R., Rohrbach, L. A., Greenberg, M., Leaf, P., Brown, C. H., Fagan, A., Hawkins, J. D., et al. (2013). Addressing core challenges for the next generation of type 2 translation research and systems: The translation science to population impact (TSci Impact) framework. *Prevention Science, 14*(4), 319–351.

Swisher, J. D., & Hoffman, A. (1975). Information: The irrelevant variable in drug education. In W. C. Brown (Ed.), *Drug abuse prevention: Perspectives and approaches for educators.* Dubuque, IA: William C. Brown.

Tenant, R. Goens, C., Barlow, J., Day, C., & Stewart-Smith, S. (2007). A systematic review of interventions to promote mental health and prevent mental health problems in children and young people. *Journal of Public Mental Health, 6*, 25–34. Doi: 10.1108/17465729200700005.

Thompson, E. L. (1977). Smoking education program 1960–1976. *American Journal of Public Health, 68*(3), 250–257. doi:10.2105/AJPH.68.3.250.

Tobler, N. S. (1986). Meta-analysis of 143 adolescent drug prevention programs: Quantitative outcome results of program participants compared to a control or comparison group. *Journal of Drug Issues, 16*(4), 537–567.

Tobler, N. S. (1992). Drug prevention programs can work. *Journal of Addictive Diseases, 11(3)*, 1–28. doi:10.1300/J069v11n03_01.

Weiss, C. H., Murphy-Graham, E., Petrosino, A., & Gandhi, A. G. (2008). The fairy godmother—and her warts: Making the dream of evidence-based policy come true. *American Journal of Evaluation, 29*(1), 29. doi:10.1177/1098214007313742.

Werner, E. E., & Smith, R. S. (1989). *Vulnerable, but invincible.* Brewster, NY: Adams, Bannister, Cox.

Wilson, D. B., Gottfredson, D. C., & Najaka, S. S. (2001). School-based prevention of problem behaviors: A meta-analysis. *Journal of Quantitative Criminology, 17*(3), 247–272.

Wynder, E. L., & Graham, E. A. (1950). Tobacco smoking as a possible etiologic factor in bronchiogenic carcinoma: A study of six hundred and eighty-four proved cases. *Journal of the American Medical Association, 143*(4), 329–336. doi:10.1001/jama.1950.02910390001001.

Zimmerman, J. (1999). *Distilling democracy: Alcohol education in America's public schools* (pp. 1880–1925). Lawrence: University Press of Kansas.

Chapter 8
Developing School-Based Prevention Curricula

Jonathan Pettigrew and Michael L. Hecht

8.1 A Recent History of U.S. Prevention Efforts

School-based prevention likely emerged because of both political and practical concerns. Although one could go back as far as the Prohibition era to cite an early intervention, we start with the emergence of school-based interventions. This period likely begins in earnest during the 1960s, when a new drug culture centered on marijuana and other illicit substances emerged alongside the mainstream use of tobacco and alcohol. Since that time, the "drug of choice" has varied, being at different times marijuana, cocaine/crack, methamphetamines, or prescription drugs. Overall youth use rates also have fluctuated since the 1960s, though showing a general increase through the 1980s with a leveling off and decrease since that time (Johnston et al. 2013). Prevention interventions, as we know them, emerged during this period, with mandated attendance making schools an ideal context for their delivery (Chap. 7).

In the early days of school-based prevention during the 1970s and 1980s, curricula were based almost exclusively on a cognitive educational approach, which proved ineffective (Swisher et al. 1971; Tobler 1986). The false assumption was that if students were given enough information about substances' physiological effects and mortality outcomes, they would choose to avoid use. The concurrent assumption was that health outcomes would motivate youth to avoid or cease use through

J. Pettigrew (✉)
University of Tennessee, 37996 Knoxville, TN, USA

Hugh Downs School of Human Communication, P.O.Box 871205, 85287, Tempe, AZ, USA
e-mail: jonathan.pettigrew@asu.edu

M. L. Hecht
The Pennsylvania State University, State College, PA 16801, USA

REAL Prevention 765 Long Hill Road, 07933 Gillette, NJ, USA
e-mail: hechtpsu@gmail.com

© Springer Science+Business Media New York 2015   151
K. Bosworth (ed.), *Prevention Science in School Settings*,
Advances in Prevention Science, DOI 10.1007/978-1-4939-3155-2_8

fear and rational decision-making. Prevention curricula proliferated based on this premise. The iconic public service announcement of the late 1980s—"This is your brain. (Show egg.) This is your brain on drugs. (Drop egg into frying pan). Any questions?"—captures this ideology. This claim alone, sans evidence, was expected to thwart unwanted behaviors.

Criticisms of this approach can be summarized in two primary categories: curriculum content and delivery processes (Tobler and Stratton 1997). First, the premise that people make exclusively rational choices based on information (e.g., health consequences) and fear of negative outcomes proved naive. The approach failed to take into account the complexities of behavioral motivation. Factors such as social forces (e.g., behavioral norms, peer pressure, popularity, and friendship), past experiences (e.g., parental use and attitudes toward substances), biological mechanisms (e.g., puberty, adolescent cognitive development, and nervous system myelination), and alternative persuasive messaging (e.g., advertisements and substance offers) all factor into substance use decisions. In a landmark meta-analysis of 120 prevention programs, Tobler and Stratton (1997) concluded that knowledge- or attitude-only programs are not as effective as programs that teach social skills along with knowledge about substances. In fact, presenting detailed information about substances—including their street names, potential side effects, and average costs—may have provided some youth with a cafeteria offering of drugs and their potential highs. Tobler's work (e.g., Tobler et al. 2000) also highlighted the importance of considering substance use as a social process. Adolescents' substance use decisions are based on an array of interdependent social influences (e.g., parents, peers, and teachers), thus underscoring the need to teach adolescents general social competence and refusal skills.

Second, the delivery of cognitive educational programs failed to account for the way students learn (Tobler and Stratton 1997). Based on prevailing teaching practices of the 1950s, programs used didactic delivery of information in a one-way, noninteractive fashion. This teaching method proved to be inadequate. Tobler and Stratton (1997) pointed instead to the importance of interactive delivery mechanisms. Their analysis categorized programs as noninteractive (i.e., knowledge only, affective only, and knowledge plus affective interventions) versus interactive (i.e., social influence and comprehensive life skills). Findings showed that interactive programs outperformed noninteractive ones. A more recent meta-analysis confirms this finding for after-school programs and, similar to the previous review, suggests that interactive delivery is paramount to program success (Durlak et al. 2010); specifically, the researchers advocate for a SAFE model of program delivery: sequenced, active, focused, and explicit. These meta-analytic studies demonstrate that better implemented programs have stronger effects, which draws attention to issues of fidelity and implementation quality.

Marking a clear break from cognitive educational approaches, the next paradigm relied on theories of social influence and identification of risk and resiliency factors using the emerging technology of group randomized trials. Such trials were typified by the Adolescent Alcohol Prevention Trial (AAPT) conducted at the University of Southern California (Hansen and Graham 1991). The AAPT curriculum moved beyond simply trying to inform adolescents about the effects of various substances. Instead it used social cognitive theory to modify known risk and protective factors associated with substance use by, for example, attempting to teach the skills needed to resist substances. AAPT also considered how program content would be delivered (Rohrbach et al. 1993). This transition ushered in an era of theory-based curriculum development and evaluation during which evidence-based interventions proliferated.

Despite rather clear-cut research conclusions leading to the emergence of evidence-based curricula, practice still lags behind science. Studies clearly demonstrate a gap between knowledge of what works and actual practice (Ennett et al. 2003; Ringwalt et al. 2011). A 1999 nationally representative survey of teachers and school administrators in public and private schools with middle grades found that only 62 % of the schools used content identified as effective by Tobler's meta-analyses (Ennett et al. 2003). Almost 80 % of the teachers privileged noninteractive teaching methods, and only 17 % met the criteria for effective, highly interactive delivery; even fewer (14 %) met the criteria for teaching effective content through effective delivery methods (Ennett et al. 2003). Finally, Ennett and colleagues (2003) found that schools using evidence-based programs were about 1.5 times more likely to teach effective content through effective delivery methods than schools that did not use evidence-based programs. As dismal as these findings are, more recent research shows little improvement. In 2011 Ringwalt and colleagues reported that only 47 % of middle schools used evidence-based programming. We turn next to what is known about developing effective prevention curricula.

8.2 Considerations for Creating Effective Curricula

Research points to several considerations program developers should take into account when designing prevention curricula. These considerations are not mutually exclusive. Sometimes developers emphasize one consideration over others and many program developers account for several of these issues in their curricula.

8.2.1 Practical Considerations

Schools face a number of challenges in fulfilling their charge to educate the nation's children, which, quite simply, makes it difficult to convince them to spend time on prevention, including substance use prevention. As Miller-Day and colleagues (2013) point out, "delivery of prevention programs is a negotiation among the curriculum, teachers' classroom management and interests, students' behavior and needs, and administrative influence" (p. 325). Gaining access to schools, for example, can be difficult because local school officials (e.g., principals, teachers) often are required to coordinate with district administrators and school boards before implementing programs. To compensate for this challenge, curriculum writers might consider linking their curriculum to core standards (e.g., showing how teaching about drug risks develops critical thinking) or research demonstrating effects on school performance. Lessons that are modularized and can be taught in short segments also may generate less resistance. Developers do well to consider logistical challenges involved in administering prevention curricula in the public school context.

8.2.2 Logic Model

Curriculum design begins with a theoretical model that articulates causal factors and then designs a curriculum to address each factor. The model also anticipates the types of outcomes or effects that can be achieved. A theory of behavior change guides the process by articulating the mechanisms of change and the strategies for obtaining effects. Causal factors, curriculum components, and expected outcomes are linked through theories of behavior change in what is often termed a logic model, which depicts how the program works. Although research testing the active ingredients of interventions is still needed (Chakraborty et al. 2009; Embry and Biglan 2008), extant prevention research that identifies specific mediators and moderators of program effects provides the best evidence for what to incorporate into intervention programs to modify specific outcomes. Julian et al. (1995) state that a "major strength" of the logic model is that it encourages curriculum developers to "consider linkages between problems/conditions, activities, outcomes and impacts" (p. 334). Thus, successful drug prevention programs link specific lesson content to mediators of outcomes so that program content influences participants' beliefs and behaviors (e.g., Hansen 1996).

8.2.3 Risk and Resiliency/Protection

One of the most common models for curriculum development builds on empirically identified risk and resiliency/protective factors. Curricula based on this model seek to bolster protective factors and reduce risk factors (Hawkins et al. 1992). The National Institute on Drug Abuse (NIDA 2003) states, "An important goal of prevention is to change the balance between risk and protective factors so that protective factors outweigh risk factors" (p. 7).

Risk factors are generally defined as social or individual conditions that enhance the likelihood of substance use, whereas resiliency, or protective, factors do the opposite. Curriculum developers do not seek to alter all known or existing risk and protective factors, but focus on modifiable factors. For example, parental psychopathology is a known risk factor for drug abuse (Durlak 1998), but it is not considered malleable through a brief school-based intervention. In contrast, poor social skills, academic underperformance, perceptions that drug use is acceptable, and association with drug-abusing peers are more malleable risk factors, whereas association with academically successful peers is considered a modifiable protective factor (NIDA 2003). A curriculum based on a resiliency model seeks to enhance participants' social skills, alter their perceptions of the acceptability of use, and promote positive peer associations.

In an article summarizing and critiquing the risk/resiliency perspective, Sloboda et al. (2012) advocate a vulnerability model that differs from the risk/resiliency perspective by taking cumulative biosocial development into account. They critique as over simplistic the assumption that "risks" cause substance use; in fact, the manifestation of problematic substance use is dependent on a complex, longitudinal interplay of risk, and protective factors that are aspects of both the individual and the environment. Genetics, neurobiology, and psychopathology can indeed predispose an individual to substance use. Predisposition, however, does not determine behavior and these researchers point out that early behavior becomes part of the milieu of factors that affect later outcomes. For example, early experimentation with drugs becomes part of the cascade of behaviors and experiences that predispose certain individuals to later abuse.

Both risk/resiliency and vulnerability models help direct curriculum developers to consider predictors of substance use and how and when to intervene in significant ways to alter the individual or environment to reduce problematic substance use. The vulnerability model in particular warns curriculum writers to incorporate developmentally appropriate intervention components to prevent a negative cascade of behaviors leading to substance use.

8.2.4 Developmental Appropriateness

Another consideration is the developmental appropriateness of curriculum content and delivery. Whether conceptualized as risks/resiliencies or vulnerabilities, most of these factors typically change with age. For example, only 11 % of the 8th graders report drinking alcohol in the last 30 days, whereas 42 % of the high school seniors report doing so (Johnston et al. 2013). Thus the differential exposure to and accessibility of substances influences perceptions of acceptability and social norms.

One of the main theoretical advances in developing age-appropriate curricula emerges out of socio-emotional learning theory (SEL; Chap. 13). SEL argues that developmentally appropriate social and emotional competencies are the key to healthy and successful lives. The Collaborative for Academic, Social, and Emotional Learning (CASEL) group has identified socio-emotional learning as self-awareness, self-management, social awareness, relationship skills, and responsible decision-making (see CASEL.org, n.d.). These broad concepts take different forms as a person matures from childhood to adolescence to adulthood. What counts as socially competent for a 5th grader is different than for a 12th grader. So too, the competencies that require mastery differ across the lifespan. Late elementary schoolchildren may be actively working on engaging in socially competent conversation whereas middle school students need training in resistance skills. Research supports this view, showing, for example, that when youth control their emotional reactions to events they do better in life (see Chap. 13).

Matching curriculum content with developmental goals is an important consideration. Figure 8.1 offers a hypothetical example of how a school district might target particular individual competencies across different ages and what existing evidence-based programs incorporate these skills in age-appropriate ways.

8.2.5 Culture

Culture is another important consideration for developing prevention curricula. Culture has been broadly defined by demographics such as nationality, ethnicity, or geographic location. Income, parental education, or socioeconomic status may also be important markers of culture. This demographic approach to culture, however, has been criticized as an "ethnic gloss" that ignores large within-group variation and focuses curriculum on simplistic, perhaps even stereotypic, representations.

A more complex, sophisticated approach to culture has been suggested by a number of researchers (e.g., Castro et al. 2010; Hecht and Krieger 2006; Kreuter and McClure 2004; Resnicow et al. 1999). This work conceptualizes culture as a "social construction" rather than an a priori variable. In other words, culture is more a group's perspective or a way of making sense of experience than a static structure. In addition, people have multiple cultural group memberships and, as a result, identity or membership is crucial for intervention design.

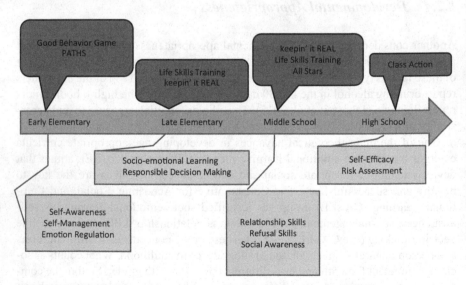

Fig. 8.1 Matching curriculum and competencies with evidence-based programs

Hecht and colleagues have incorporated this approach to culture in curriculum development. In their work they used community-based participatory research methods to develop culture-specific and multicultural versions of a curriculum (see Miller et al. 2000). Hecht and Krieger (2006) articulate the model for cultural grounding that was used. The model begins with the voices of the target population and integrates their perspectives, attitudes, beliefs, and practices into an intervention. Miller et al. (2000) describe this perspective as "from kids, through kids, to kids," or "kid-centric," because youth are involved in all stages of message development. The narrative form involved in describing youth practices and presenting the curriculum are keys to capturing the richness of culture.

Barrera et al. (2011) offer a typology that spans interventions ranging from researcher-driven to community-driven. They begin with prevention research cycle interventions, which are least culturally adapted, and move to cultural adaptation of evidence-based interventions and investigator-initiated culturally grounded interventions, both of which account for culture in curriculum design. They suggest that community-initiated indigenous interventions are the most culturally adapted.

Integrating culture into a curriculum is important because outcomes may lessen when target groups do not identify with curriculum material (Castro et al. 2010; Dusenbury and Falco 1995). In a study that compared three cultural versions of a curriculum—a Latino version, a white/black version, and a multicultural version—the multicultural version demonstrated the best effects, even among the majority Latino youth in the schools involved (Hecht et al. 2006; Hecht et al. 2003; Kulis et al. 2005). This is a promising finding given the diversity in most schools.

8.3 Exemplars

Several evidence-based programs are being delivered in schools. The "evidence-based" label shares a scientific as well as sociopolitical origin. To be evidence-based, essentially, means there is reasonable scientific evidence that the program affects its targeted outcomes. The Society for Prevention Research published a set of criteria for defining evidence-based curricula from a research perspective, which defines three hierarchical levels of interventions (Flay et al. 2005). These range from efficacy, the most basic level, to effectiveness, to dissemination-ready. *Efficacy* is demonstrated by experimental studies which show a given intervention causes positive outcomes under tightly controlled research conditions, whereas *effectiveness* requires that the intervention be scrutinized under natural or real-world implementation conditions, which tend to be suboptimal. Efficacy is typically established by the program designers, whereas effectiveness requires evidence from an unbiased source. A program is considered ready for dissemination when it has proven effectiveness and has established a support structure adequate to cover adoption- and implementation-related concerns. In addition, dissemination-ready programs provide information about program costs and tools for ongoing program evaluation.

The complexity of these issues has given rise to various "lists" of evidence-based practices that have become essential in providing the sociopolitical definition of "evidence-based" programming. Developers often are asked to prove that their programs qualify as "evidence-based," typically through inclusion on lists such as the National Registry of Evidence-based Programs and Practices (NREPP), Office of Juvenile Justice and Delinquency Prevention Model programs, and Blueprints for Violence Prevention. Being added to these "lists" has become the practical marker of a successful program. Funding often is necessary to conduct the rigorous research required to establish sufficient evidence to meet the inclusion criteria. Federal dollars for outcome research has primarily come from NIDA or the National Institute on Alcohol Abuse and Alcoholism. In this section, we briefly describe the three evidence-based school programs rated most cost-effective according to a recent Substance Abuse and Mental Health Services Administration (SAMHSA) study (Miller and Hendrie 2008) and outline a promising model for curriculum delivery and sustainability. We restrict our discussion to school-based programs designed to intervene with youth, not families. Unfortunately, that means we do not discuss evidence-based interventions with a broader focus, such as the Good Behavior Game (Poduska et al. 2008), Project ALERT (Ringwalt et al. 2010), Project Northland (Stigler et al. 2006), Project STAR (Brown et al. 2011), and Project TND (Rohrbach et al. 2010) as well as programs without a firm evidence base, such as Too Good for Drugs (Bacon 2003) and AlcoholEdu (Outside the Classroom, Inc. 2006).

8.3.1 All Stars (www.allstarsprevention.com)

All Stars was developed by William Hansen in the 1980s based on the social influence model. All Stars seeks to produce positive norms, strong personal commitments, parental attentiveness, positive future orientation and aspirations, and school and community bonding. These five protective factors have been shown to mediate program outcomes and are integrated into the All Stars logic model (Hansen 1996). All Stars incorporates developmentally appropriate material to reach youth during the time frame when they are most vulnerable to problematic risk behaviors. The core program is designed for 11- to 14-year-olds and contains 13 sessions of 45 min with eight additional booster sessions. There are additional All Stars Jr. sessions for elementary students and All Start Sr. sessions for high school students. A series of evaluation studies demonstrate effects on both theoretically derived mediators and substance use (e.g., Harrington et al. 2001; McNeal et al. 2004). The independent cost-benefit analysis commissioned by the SAMHSA reports that All Stars returns US$32 for every dollar spent, the highest return for any school-based program (Miller and Hendrie 2008). The following provides an excerpt from an interview with William Hansen.

Interview with William Hansen

1. How did you develop curriculum activities that teach the concepts and develop the skills identified by your logic model?

The first step I followed was to have a clear understanding of what needed to be addressed, the "targeted mediating variable." To be worth addressing in a curriculum, the targeted mediator (a) must be strongly statistically related to the outcome of interest, and (b) must be capable of modification. Once identified, I gained an understanding of the targeted mediator's developmental characteristics. For example, in All Stars, the three primary targeted mediating variables all have a similar characteristic; they each "erode" as young people grow older. So, the goal of intervention became one of trying to capitalize on positive qualities to either forestall or reverse the normal course of erosion. So, activities typically focused on providing opportunities for preexisting positive qualities to be reinforced. To do this, the curriculum has the teacher lead a lot of guided discussions using questions that naturally prompt positive responses from students. Activity development focused on starting with things known to be of interest to the target population and gradually moving toward revealing underlying positive conclusions that naturally strengthen the targeted mediator.

2. Any advice for someone just getting started in curriculum development? What resources do you recommend for this?

My first suggestion is to get used to disappointment. No intervention goes very far without field trials, and most field trials result in less than spectacular results. For every ten bright ideas, one will work once it is fully developed. There needs to be a very good understanding about how to try out an intervention. Also, a curriculum developer needs to observe how the intervention is interpreted by both teacher and student to identify weak spots that can be corrected. Finally, gain as much practical theoretical insight as possible. Kurt Lewin said, "There is nothing as practical as a good theory. If you want to know how something works, try to change it." You need an understanding that surpasses the kind of theory that you typically find among research publications. Curriculum development requires extensive psychological, sociological, and developmental understanding. The best resource for gaining these insights is a knowledgeable mentor.

8.3.2 keepin' it REAL (kiR) (www.real-prevention.com)

keepin' it REAL (kiR), created by Michael Hecht and Michelle Miller-Day, was the first evidence-based multicultural curriculum. The original middle school curriculum was based on narrative engagement and social-cognitive theories (Hecht and Miller-Day 2009), although the current elementary and middle school curricula are based on SEL theory. The research underlying kiR began more than 20 years ago to explain the social pressures youth feel when they are offered substances and to develop new ways to prevent use (Miller et al. 2000). This narrative research was among the first to describe the social processes of substance use offers and the role of race, ethnicity, and gender. A new approach to prevention curriculum development, cultural grounding, was created so that youth would identify with the lessons (Hecht and Krieger 2006). The elementary curriculum focuses on understanding risks and consequences, and making safe and responsible choices while learning the five SEL competencies. The multicultural middle school curriculum extends this focus on choices and places further emphasis on communication competence in social influence processes. The middle school curriculum reduced alcohol, marijuana, and tobacco use in a group randomized trial (Hecht et al. 2006; Hecht et al. 2003), with two at least partially successful replications (Kulis et al. 2005; Marsiglia et al. 2010; Pettigrew et al. 2015).

The independent cost-benefit analysis of the middle school curriculum commissioned by the SAMHSA reports that kiR returns US$27 for every dollar spent, the second best return for any school-based program (Miller and Hendrie 2008). kiR is now believed to be the most widely disseminated school-based program. Since its adoption by Drug Abuse Resistance Education (D.A.R.E.) for elementary and middle schools, it reaches approximately 2 million US students as well as students in 47 countries around the world.

Interview with Michelle Miller-Day

1. How did you develop curriculum activities that teach the concepts and develop the skills identified by your logic model?

keepin' It REAL is promoted as "From kids, through kids, to kids." In our curricula, adolescent drug use and drug offer-resistance episodes are considered within a cultural context to ensure the motivations, knowledge, and skills promoted and practiced in the curriculum are both effective and appropriate in a variety of social situations. We do this by culturally grounding the content (e.g., examples, role-play situations, illustrative scenarios, and curriculum media) in youth culture by collecting copious personal narratives from youth as the basis of curriculum development. Youth experience provides a basis for content and activities in these curricula, with youth serving as advisers on curriculum content, as creators of curriculum media (e.g., videos), and with students' stories as an integral element of implementation. Taking a communication competence approach, our curricula provide youth with the motivation to resist offers of drugs, the knowledge about substances and norms to make informed decisions about substance use, the decision-making and resistance skills, and skills practice to both effectively and appropriately resist direct and indirect offers of substances.

2. Any advice for someone just getting started in curriculum development? What resources do you recommend for this?

Curriculum development is both fun and challenging. You can receive formal training in curriculum development, but many scholars learn this process by "doing." Some questions to ask include, Is there a template I can use? What content needs to be addressed in each lesson to accomplish curriculum goals? How is content reinforced with learning that uses multiple senses and serves different learning styles? What are creative ways to engage the learner? Efforts may be guided by the "who, what, where, when, why, and how" approach: Who is needed for each component of the lesson? What is needed (e.g., resources)? Where will the lesson activities occur (e.g., a computer lab)? When in the curriculum should particular information be conveyed? Why is each lesson component needed? and How is each component best implemented? No one is expected to be an expert at everything, and effective teamwork goes a long way. Partnering with a group that has diverse and complementary skills and knowledge can help. Finally, there are some practical guides, such as our book (Miller et al. 2000), which includes an appendix that outlines the procedures for developing a customized narrative-based prevention program.

8.3.3 LifeSkills Training (LST) (www.lifeskillstraining.com)

Gilbert Botvin and colleagues developed LST in the late 1980s. Using a risk/resiliency model the LST program targets factors associated with adolescent substance use and other risky behaviors. The curriculum aims to enhance students' resistance skills, self-esteem, anxiety coping skills, and decision-making abilities. LST has elementary, middle, and high school modules, each teaching developmentally appropriate skills in the aforementioned domains. A long-term follow-up study tracking participants from 7th through 12th grades demonstrated efficacy (Botvin et al. 1995). The program has been subjected to numerous other randomized trials, most of which have confirmed positive outcomes (e.g., Spoth et al. 2006). In addition, the independent cost-benefit analysis commissioned by SAMHSA reports that the LST returns US$19 for every dollar spent (Miller and Hendrie 2008).

8.4 Current Trends

In addition to describing various considerations involved in curriculum development and providing exemplars of school-based prevention curricula, we also identify trends that loom on the horizon of curriculum development. Some of these trends are in their infancy, just being proposed and debated. Others are being actively researched.

8.4.1 Develop Interventions with Implementation/End User in Mind

One emerging direction is evolving from the recognition that for maximum effect curricula should be developed with the end users in mind. Prevention curricula have different audiences or consumers, each with its own organizational culture, contingencies, needs, and opportunities that must be addressed. This is an important direction for the field because no matter how effective an intervention, if it does not match users' needs or is not adopted and disseminated, it cannot fulfill its design. Early prevention scientists sought to create interventions that reduced substance use, but once they accomplished this they quickly recognized that it was not enough—schools had to use the curricula appropriately to continue producing beneficial effects. This realization led some prevention scientists to argue that designers should consider how an intervention can be disseminated during the development phase, rather than figuring that out later. This strategy holds the potential for aligning intervention design with participants' preferences to maximize chances for dissemination.

Alignment can be accomplished in a number of ways. Rotheram-Borus and Duan (2003) recommended integrating business and marketing plans into intervention development models. Sandler et al. (2005) built on this idea to incorporate a consumer-driven model from the business field in proposing the Prevention Service Development Model (PSDM). Equating prevention curricula to a new service good, these authors articulated several steps for developing, testing, marketing, and disseminating interventions. As they point out, adequately marketing and disseminating research-based curricula require skills that often fall outside of traditional research training. Thus, a partnership between a marketing organization and a research institution is advisable as long as there is a close relationship between the two (Harris et al. 2012).

There also are opportunities for collaboration between curriculum developers and disseminators. A relatively recent example of such a partnership is that between D.A.R.E. America (the disseminator) and keepin' it REAL (now distributed by REAL Prevention). Since 2008, D.A.R.E. America has licensed keepin' it REAL curriculum for their middle school program, and in 2011 collaborated with the founders of REAL Prevention to develop an elementary version of keepin' it REAL for D.A.R.E. Recognizing the different skill sets of curriculum developers and dissemination agencies can help maximize the effectiveness of partnerships. In particular, Harris and colleagues (2012) suggest that researchers can shape dissemination efforts through such practices as conducting formative research, balancing fidelity and adaptation, monitoring and evaluating outcomes, and testing dissemination approaches.

8.4.2   Universal–Targeted–Tailored Interventions

A looming question on the horizon of prevention curriculum development is: To what level of specificity should an intervention be developed and administered? Three levels of intervention have been identified: universal, targeted, and tailored.

The first school-based interventions were universal, that is, designed to affect everyone in a population. This seemed logical because the easiest way to implement school-based curriculum is in class units. Researchers recognized, however, that the overall population was made up of different cultural units, and research demonstrated that interventions targeted toward a specific subgroup (identified by race, ethnicity, gender, risk level, etc.) were more effective than universal interventions at reaching some segments of the population (e.g., Berkley-Patton et al. 2009). These targeted interventions customized some aspects of the intervention to the target population. For example, interventions designed for particular ethnicities might incorporate common phrases or idioms from each group. This approach, however, raises the issue of how to separate the targeted groups for implementation.

A relatively new approach on the horizon of curriculum development is to tailor interventions to individuals. A tailored intervention can be defined as, "Any combination of information or change strategies *intended to reach one specific person*, based on characteristics that are unique to that person, related to the outcome of interest, and have been *derived from an individual assessment*" (Kreuter and Skinner 2000, p. 1, emphasis in original). Tailored messages customize material for an individual based on that individual's responses to various pre-intervention measures. Whereas targeted interventions select content based on demographic (overt, objective) characteristics, tailored interventions customize content based on individuals' subjective preferences, responses, or needs. Research has not yet made clear what elements of an intervention require tailoring as opposed to simply being targeted.

Another variant of tailoring is to adjust the intervention content based on risk level. Called "unified interventions" (Brown and Liao 1999) or "adaptive interventions" (Collins et al. 2004), such programs incorporate a system of planned flexibility that seeks to adjust the dosage of intervention to the needs of each participant. The goal, according to Brown and Liao (1999) is "to apply the right amount of intervention to each subject" (p. 689). Unified interventions can be administered sequentially or concurrently. For example, if some participants show no difference after receiving a universal intervention, they might be enrolled in a selected intervention. Alternatively, given a priori knowledge of risk in a population, those individuals identified as high risk might be enrolled in both universal and selected interventions simultaneously.

Similarly, the adaptive intervention framework seeks to customize an intervention or intervention components to the needs of participants (Collins et al. 2004). Within this framework, targeting variables are measured and dosages, or treatment components are then customized based on an explicit set of decision rules. Importantly, a targeting variable is not necessarily risk level. For example, for a curriculum designed with multiple components, a set of screening questions answered by a school principal, counselor, or teacher might determine which components should be implemented in that setting. Important to adaptive interventions is a periodic recalibration of the intervention system through reassessment of targeting variables. Retesting the targeting variable after 6 months of intervention, for example, might indicate some components should be repeated while some new components should be incorporated. Adaptation is not based on race, gender, or risk level per se, but on measurement of specific indicators that adhere to an explicit set of decision rules. Adaptive interventions hold promise for optimizing prevention programs for varied settings but end users need more ongoing training and technical support compared to universal programs. Further research is needed to learn how to manage these needs.

The advent of Internet technology clearly facilitates targeted and tailored approaches. Students can gain access through websites and be presented with messages adapted by group (targeted) or individual (tailored) characteristics. Two recent meta-analyses (Baker et al. 2010; Noar et al. 2007) show tailoring does accrue statistically significant advantages in effecting behavior change over control conditions (i.e., targeted, generic, or no-message groups); however, the overall effect size is quite small (e.g., $d = 0.074$; Noar et al. 2007). When isolating studies that compared tailored messages against either generic or targeted messages, the effect size was $d = 0.058$. Because these analyses did not explicitly compare tailored versus targeted messages, it is unclear what value tailoring adds. One experiment examining these relationships with regard to disease prevention shows improvements for tailored over targeted and generic messages for perceived susceptibility to disease, but no differences among these conditions for intentions to ask a doctor about the disease (Roberto et al. 2009). Baker and colleagues (2010) caution that there is insufficient evidence regarding the cost-effectiveness of tailoring over generic or targeted messages and that there is little empirical evidence that could inform developers about the most effective approaches to tailoring messages. These areas are ripe for research and results will be directly applicable to curriculum developers, especially as communication technologies continue to innovate and proliferate.

8.4.3   Adaptation in Dissemination

Finally, adaptation becomes a crucial issue as interventions are widely implemented. We argue that interventions should be developed with adaptation in mind. Clearly, some degree of fidelity is needed or one cannot say the intervention is being used. However, adaptation appears inevitable (for a review, see Durlak and DuPre 2008). Facing this reality means developing interventions with the expectation they will be adapted. Planning for adaptation can involve utilizing adaptive intervention frameworks, identifying core components, and noting what should be included and may be omitted given limitations such as time, or considering how interventions might be adapted at various moments in the delivery system. We encourage intervention developers to assume that adaptation is a normal part of intervention development

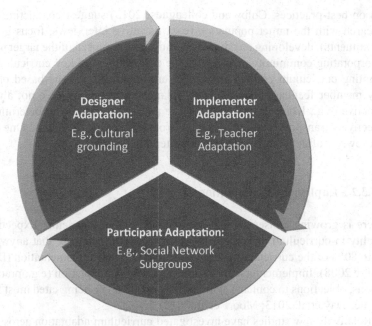

Fig. 8.2 Adaptation cycle

and implementation. Figure 8.2 summarizes what we term the adaptation cycle. In our view, adaptation occurs in at least three interrelated phases. Designers can adapt a curriculum, much like targeting an intervention to a population segment. Implementers also can adapt a curriculum for various practical and philosophical reasons. Finally, participants can adapt prevention messages.

8.4.3.1 Designer Adaptation

Designer adaptation involves undergoing a systematic process to adjust a curriculum in order to best meet the needs of a target population that may have different traits from the population for/with whom the curriculum was originally developed. Designer adaptation may follow systematic steps for altering the intervention or may entail cultural regrounding. Lee et al. (2008) proposed that planned adaptation of a curriculum involves four steps: developers must (a) examine the theory of change or core components, (b) identify differences between the original and target populations, (c) adapt program content for the target population, and (d) adapt the evaluation strategy. Although these steps are logical, they are relatively abstract. In the article, the researchers flesh out these general steps, offering suggestions for how each might be completed.

Another approach to designer adaptation involves regrounding a curriculum in a new target culture. Colby and colleagues (2013) detail a model of cultural regrounding and provide an exemplar of these processes. Following a call from Trickett and colleagues (2011), regrounding provides a set of best-processes rather than focus on best-practices, Colby and colleagues (2013) suggest conducting formative research with the target population (e.g., narrative interviews, focus groups with constituents), developing an advisory committee composed of the target population, incorporating community members in the development of key curriculum content, adapting curriculum content as needed, and making revisions based on community member feedback. Unfortunately, planned adaptations have not always been effective (e.g., Komro et al. 2008). More research is needed to determine how to effectively transport curriculum content from one setting to another. One factor that is known to affect outcomes is implementer adaptation.

8.4.3.2 Implementer Adaptation

There is growing consensus that implementers adapt curricula. Expecting 100% fidelity in curriculum delivery is unreasonable. Estimates are that anywhere from 20 to 80% of the curricular material is adapted during implementation (Durlak and DuPre 2008). Implementers cite various reasons for adaptation (e.g., practical limitations, objections to content), with logistics of delivery being cited most frequently (Miller-Day et al. 2013; Moore et al. 2013).

Relatively few studies have investigated curriculum adaptation across time, but those that have suggest that teachers (a) change how they teach from year to year, and (b) adapt curricula to fit their own teaching style. One study shows that teachers tend to decrease the amount of material covered from year to year (McCormick et al. 1995), whereas another demonstrates that teachers approach an average level of adaptation over a 3-year period (Ringwalt et al. 2009). Some research also has shown that a particular implementer tends to adapt multiple curricula in similar ways across time, suggesting an individual adaptation style (Hansen et al. 2013). In their analysis of teachers delivering the same curriculum to different classes of students during the same year, Pettigrew and colleagues (2013) conclude that teachers tend to adapt curricula in "practical, systematic ways to accommodate their delivery pattern" (p. 53). These tentative findings about the ways teachers adapt school-based curricula underscores the need to understand when and how adaptations enhance versus detract from program effects. For evidence-based programs that incorporate active learning techniques and theoretically informed content, adaptation may be inappropriate and measures assessing lack of fidelity may serve as a proxy for departure from empirically validated delivery and content. Thus, it is important to understand adaptation valence (e.g., positive, neutral, and negative), or the degree to which an adaptation is consistent with the underlying logic model of a program (Hansen et al. 2013; Miller-Day et al. 2013; Moore et al. 2013; Pettigrew et al. 2013). Curriculum developers, too, should be aware that adaptations will occur and potentially should account for these when writing curricula.

8.4.3.3 Participant Adaptation

Students are not passive recipients of prevention curricula but active agents who sort and filter material. Thus, even after delivery, curricula remain subject to adaptation. There is very little research on how students interpret material or construe the prevention messages; however, there are at least two ways participants adapt prevention messages. First, they filter the messages through their own interpretive processes. Their experiences, attitudes, and perspectives all can affect how they receive, interpret, and act on a prevention message. For example, studies of prevention outcomes tend to find that programming is most effective with students who are at high risk at pretest (Brown and Liao 1999). For high-risk youth, prevention messages are likely novel or diverge from their typical behaviors; thus, these messages have an observable effect. For youth at normal or low risk, messages may be redundant or may already align with their typical behaviors, and therefore less effect is observable. Future research might investigate how prevention messages are interpreted among groups with different risk levels.

Another aspect of participant adaptation is the social proliferation (Larkey and Hecht 2010; Miller-Day and Hecht 2013) of prevention messages. Narrative engagement theory (NET), for example, argues that effective interventions will stimulate conversations outside the classroom (Miller-Day and Hecht 2013). Whereas previous research might have considered this contamination, especially if it occurred across treatment and control groups, NET argues that engaging narratives will become the topic of ongoing conversations. Emerging research involving network analysis is particularly suited to illuminate how messages proliferate through a social network and how these messages are altered through multiple interactions with peers, family members, and others. It is expected that students would interpret and reinterpret prevention messages in light of interactions they have about prevention programs and messages as well as their social networks.

8.4.4 Integration of New Media

As technology and the way society uses technology develop, so too must interventions. Early in the 1980s, as computers were introduced into public schools, Body Awareness Resource Network (BARN)—a computer-based system—confidentially taught teens about the risks of alcohol, tobacco, and stress while using interactive lessons to teach refusal and other prosocial skills (Bosworth et al. 1983). Currently, some existing interventions incorporate available technologies. For example, the keepin' it REAL middle school program includes videos developed by high school students to illustrate resistance skills. Project ALERT also uses video vignettes to present prevention material. An online intervention called PEERx, developed by NIDA, offers a "choose your path" video-based activity hosted on youtube.com. Participants watch a short vignette from the first person perspective in which they are presented with a choice of using or not using a prescription drug. Based on the choice, different consequences play out in a second video that completes the vignette. Although the consequences may seem extreme or unrealistic, the intervention aptly illustrates how available technology might be used to intervention effect. Another example is a creative integration of video gaming and intervention messaging. Norris developed an interactive video game intervention designed to reduce risky sexual behavior among Latinas by teaching keepin' it REAL skills (Norris et al. 2013). The intervention involves participants entering a virtual space as an avatar and interacting with avatars controlled by a trained confederate (interactant or puppeteer), one of whom makes sexual advances. The experience is organized as a game, with the participants scored for their resistance behaviors.

Interventions that incorporate new technologies should build on the existing body of knowledge about what works in changing behavior. For example, the preceding examples seek to maintain the SAFE model (Durlak et al. 2010) of sequenced, active, focused, and explicit content while incorporating technologies that engage new audiences. In this way, technology is not the intervention per se, but a modality for intervention delivery that resonates with participants' daily experiences with these technologies. Technology offers exciting opportunities for future interventions. For example, St. Andrew Development, a Pennsylvania-based company, created a patented smartphone kiosk system for health information. A kiosk presents short messages, usually via video, then provides a QR (Quick Response) or bar code that can be swiped to receive text messages that provide additional information and links to websites. Others are developing cross-media-platform approaches. The MacCauley Honors College of the City University of New York, for example, hired Albie Hecht to start a "transmedia" lab to educate the next generation of information technologists trained to create content that transcends individual spaces. Clearly, the integration of technology has just begun.

8.4.5   Quality Control, Continuous Improvement

With any prevention programming, there is a need to continually improve and renew material. Although the core components of curricula (e.g., how to change individual behaviors) may remain relatively stable across time, other aspects will need to be updated to remain relevant for new generations of adolescents. The clothing actors wear in videos can become dated as fashions change. In addition, technology changes quickly, which may make curriculum examples humorously outdated. To illustrate, prior to the proliferation of mobile telephones, pagers were common among adolescents. References to pagers, however, are now laughable. Use of mobile phones for voice conversations also is not as common among adolescents as text messaging. Curricula should be continually updated to maintain current examples and scenarios congruent with adolescents' experiences.

At the level of implementation, there is also a need for continued quality improvement. Initial training coupled with continued technical support is a promising direction for enhancing delivery and program outcomes. For example, Dusenbury and colleagues developed a model for online technical support for school-based implementers; her work seeks to "bridge the gap" between prevention research and implementation practice. These online and DVD video training tools address (a) classroom management and teaching skills, (b) interactive teaching strategies, (c) basics related to effective program delivery, (d) evidence-based mechanisms to increase student engagement, and (e) teaching techniques for engaging high-risk youth and peer leaders, and for adapting programs (Dusenbury et al. 2010). Another avenue for continued implementation support is the use of learning communities or communities of practice. Some evidence suggests that participation in these communities can enhance implementation outcomes (Bumbarger 2010). Support and training in interactive delivery methods is especially needed (Ennett et al. 2011; Pettigrew et al. 2015).

8.4.6 Capacity Building

A final trend on the horizon of curriculum development is developing interventions that are sustainable through capacity building (Hawkins et al. 2008; Spoth et al. 2004). Considering the community context and capacity is important because interventions are situated within an ecological context. This implies that reducing the demand for cigarettes may in fact increase demand for alcohol. Conversely, administering multiple interventions may either reinforce or possibly compete with existing intervention efforts. School-based interventions may also overlap with community- or family-based interventions. On the horizon of prevention, then, is coordination among multiple interventions targeting several youth outcomes.

8.5 Conclusion

Curriculum development is a daunting but ultimately rewarding task. It requires simultaneous consideration of multiple components (e.g., culture, developmental appropriateness, and logic model), an ability to appease multiple audiences and users (e.g., teachers, students, dissemination agencies, and prevention scientists), creativity to develop effective instructional activities, persistence as many pilot testing and initial trials can prove unsuccessful, continual forward-thinking to stay abreast of developments in the fields of prevention science and education as well as legislative changes affecting schools and school-based interventions, and dedication to engage in rigorous science and report unbiased results for pilot, efficacy, and effectiveness trials, not to mention an ability to work well in a team as quality interventions owe their effectiveness to the contributions of many talented researchers, teachers, and developers. The promise of effectively developed school-based curricula, however, is the opportunity to positively influence the future of our nation's youth and our society.

References

Bacon, T. P. (2003). *Technical report: Evaluation of the too good for drugs–elementary school prevention program.* Report produced for a project funded by the Florida Department of Education, Department of Safe and Drug-Free Schools, Tallahassee, FL.

Baker, R., Camosso-Stefinovic, J., Gillies, C., Shaw, E. J., Cheater, F., Flottorp, S., & Robertson, N. (2010). Tailored interventions to overcome identified barriers to change: Effects on professional practice and health care outcomes. *Cochrane Database of Systematic Reviews 17*(3), CD005470. doi:10.1002/14651858.CD005470.pub2.

Barrera, M., Castro, F., & Steiker, L. (2011). A critical analysis of approaches to the development of preventive interventions for subcultural groups. *American Journal of Community Psychology, 48*, 439–454. doi:10.1007/s10464-010-9422-x.

Berkley-Patton, J., Goggin, K., Liston, R., Bradley-Ewing, A., & Neville, S. (2009). Adapting effective narrative-based HIV-prevention interventions to increase minorities' engagement in HIV/AIDS services. *Health Communication, 24*, 199–209. doi:10.1080/10410230902804091.

Bosworth, K., Gustafson, D. H., Hawkins, R. P., Chewning, B., & Day, T. (1983). Adolescents, health education, and computers: The Body Awareness Resource Network (BARN). *Health Education, 14*, 58–60.

Botvin, G. J., Baker, E., Dusenbury, L., Botvin, E. M., & Diaz, T. (1995). Long-term follow-up results of a randomized drug abuse prevention trial in a white middle-class population. *Journal of the American Medical Association, 273*, 1106–1112.

Brown, C. H., & Liao, J. (1999). Principles for designing randomized preventive trials in mental health: An emerging developmental epidemiology paradigm. *American Journal of Community Psychology, 27*, 673–710.

Brown, L. K., Nugent, N. R., Houck, C. D., Lescano, C. M., Whiteley, L. B., Barker, D., Viau, L., Zlotnick, C. (2011). Safe thinking and affect regulation (STAR): Human immunodeficiency virus prevention in alternative/therapeutic schools. *Journal of the American Academy of Child & Adolescent Psychiatry, 50*, 1065–1074. doi:10.1016/j.jaac.2011.06.018.

Bumbarger, B. K. (2010). *A low-cost model for improving implementation quality of evidence-based programs: A pilot efficacy trial.* (Final project report from the prevention research center for the promotion of human health, the Pennsylvania State University). www.revenue.state. pa.us/portal/server.pt/gateway/PTARGS_0_2_1045908_0_0_18/Bedford%20Implementation%20Study%20Final%20report%20to%20PCCD%201292010.pdf

CASEL. (n.d.). Website of the collaborative for academic, social, and emotional learning at www. casel.org

Castro, F. G., Barrera, M., & Holleran Steiker, L. K. (2010). Issues and challenges in the design of culturally adapted evidence-based interventions. *Annual Review of Clinical Psychology, 6*, 213–239. doi:10.1146/annurev-clinpsy-033109-132032.

Chakraborty, B., Collins, L. M., Strecher, V., & Murphy, S. A. (2009). Developing multicomponent interventions using fractional factorial designs. *Statistics in Medicine, 28*, 2687–2708.

Colby, M., Hecht, M. L., Miller-Day, M., Krieger, J. L., Syvertsen, A. K., Graham, J. W., & Pettigrew, J. (2013). Adapting school-based substance use prevention curriculum through cultural grounding: A review and exemplar of adaptation processes for rural schools. *American Journal of Community Psychology, 51*, 190–205. doi:10.1007/s10464-012-9524-8.

Collins, L. M., Murphy, S. A., & Bierman, K. L. (2004). A conceptual framework for adaptive preventive interventions. *Prevention Science, 5*, 185–196.

Durlak, J. A. (1998). Common risk and protective factors in successful prevention programs. *American Journal of Orthopsychiatry, 68*, 512–520. doi:10.1037/h0080360.

Durlak, J., & DuPre, E. (2008). Implementation matters: A review of research on the influence of implementation on program outcomes and the factors affecting implementation. *American Journal of Community Psychology, 41*, 327–350. doi:10.1007/s10464-008-9165-0.

Durlak, J., Weissberg, R., & Pachan, M. (2010). A meta-analysis of after-school programs that seek to promote personal and social skills in children and adolescents. *American Journal of Community Psychology, 45,* 294–309. doi:10.1007/s10464-010-9300-6.

Dusenbury, L., & Falco, M. (1995). Eleven components of effective drug abuse prevention curricula. *Journal of School Health, 65,* 420–425. doi:10.1111/j.1746-1561.1995.tb08205.x.

Dusenbury, L., Hansen, W. B., Jackson-Newsom, J., Pittman, D., Wilson, C., Simley, K., Ringwalt, C., Pankratz, M., & Giles, S. (2010). Coaching to enhance quality of implementation in prevention. *Health Education, 110,* 43–60.

Embry, D. D., & Biglan, A. (2008). Evidence-based kernels: Fundamental units of behavioral influence. *Clinical Child and Family Psychology Review, 11,* 75–113. doi:10.1007/s10567-008-0036-x.

Ennett, S. T., Ringwalt, C. L., Thorne, J., Rohrbach, L. A., Vincus, A., Simons-Rudolph, A., & Jones, S. (2003). A comparison of current practice in school-based substance use prevention programs with meta-analysis findings. *Prevention Science, 4,* 1–14. doi:10.1023/A:1021777109369.

Ennett, S. T., Haws, S., Ringwalt, C. L., Vincus, A. A., Hanley, S., Bowling, J. M., & Rohrbach, L. A. (2011). Evidence-based practicein school substance use prevention: Fidelity of implementation under real-world conditions. *Health Education Research, 26,* 361–371. doi:10.1093/her/cyr013.

Flay, B. R., Biglan, A., Boruch, R. F., Castro, F. G., Gottfredson, D., Kellam, S., & Ji, P. (2005). Standards of evidence: Criteria for efficacy, effectiveness and dissemination. *Prevention Science, 6,* 151–175. doi:10.1007/s11121-005-5553-y

Hansen, W. B. (1996). Pilot test results comparing the all stars program with seventh-grade D.A.R.E.: Program integrity and mediating variable analysis. *Substance Use & Misuse, 31,* 1359–1377.

Hansen, W. B., & Graham, J. W. (1991). Preventing alcohol, marijuana, and cigarette use among adolescents: Peer pressure resistance training versus establishing conservative norms. *Preventive Medicine, 20,* 414–430. doi:10.1016/0091-7435(91)90039-7.

Hansen, W. B., Pankratz, M. M., Dusenbury, L., Giles, S. M., Bishop, D. C., Albritton, J., & Strack, J. (2013). Styles of adaptation: The impact of frequency and valence of adaptation on preventing substance use. *Health Education, 113,* 345–363. doi:10.1108/09654281311329268.

Harrington, N. G., Giles, S. M., Hoyle, R. H., Feeney, G. J., & Yungbluth, S. C. (2001). Evaluation of the all stars character education and problem behavior prevention program: Effects on mediator and outcome variables for middle school students. *Health Education & Behavior, 28,* 533–546.

Harris, J., Cheadle, A., Hannon, P., Forehand, M., Lichiello, P., Mahoney, E., Snyder, S., Yarrow, J. (2012). A framework for disseminating evidence-based health promotion practices. *Preventing Chronic Disease, 9,* E22. doi:10.5888/pcd9.110081.

Hawkins, J. D., Catalano, R. F., & Miller, J. Y. (1992). Risk and protective factors for alcohol and other drug problems in adolescence and early adulthood: Implications for substance abuse prevention. *Psychological Bulletin, 112,* 64–105. doi:10.1037/0033-2909.112.1.64.

Hawkins, J. D., Brown, E. C., Oesterle, S., Arthur, M. W., Abbott, R. D., & Catalano, R. F. (2008). Early effects of Communities That Care on targeted risks and initiation of delinquent behavior and substance use. *Journal of Adolescent Health, 53,* 15–22.

Hecht, M. L., & Krieger, J. L. R. (2006). The principle of cultural grounding in school-based substance abuse prevention. *Journal of Language and Social Psychology, 25,* 301–319. doi:10.1177/0261927X06289476.

Hecht, M. L., & Miller-Day, M. (2009). The drug resistance strategies project: Using narrative theory to enhance adolescents' communication competence. In L. Frey & K. Cissna (Eds.), *Routledge handbook of applied communication* (pp. 535–557). New York: Routledge.

Hecht, M. L., Marsiglia, F. F., Elek, E., Wagstaff, D. A, Kulis, S., Dustman, P., & Miller-Day, M. (2003). Culturally-grounded substance use prevention: An evaluation of the *keepin' it R.E.A.L.* curriculum. *Prevention Science, 4,* 233–248.

Hecht, M. L., Graham, J. W., & Elek, E. (2006). The drug resistance strategies intervention: Program effects on substance use. *Health Communication, 20,* 267–276.

Johnston, L. D., O'Malley, P. M., Bachman, J. G., & Schulenberg, J. E. (2013). *Monitoring the Future national results on drug use: 2012 overview, key findings on adolescent drug use*. Ann Arbor: Institute for Social Research, University of Michigan.

Julian, D. A., Jones, A., & Deyo, D. (1995). Open systems evaluation and the logic model: Program planning and evaluation tools. *Evaluation and Program Planning, 18,* 333–341. doi:10.1016/0149-7189(95)00034-8.

Komro, K. A., Perry, C. L., Veblen-Mortenson, S., Farbakhsh, K., Toomey, T. L., Stigler, M. H., & Williams, C. L. (2008). Outcomes from a randomized controlled trial of a multi-component alcohol use preventive intervention for urban youth: Project Northland Chicago. *Addiction, 103,* 606–618. doi:10.1111/j.1360-0443.2007.02110.x.

Kreuter, M. W., & Skinner, C. S. (2000). Tailoring: What's in a name? *Health Education Research, 15,* 1–4. doi:10.1093/her/15.1.1.

Kreuter, M. W., & McClure, S. M. (2004). The role of culture in health communication. *Annual Review of Public Health, 25,* 439–455. doi:10.1146/annurev.publhealth.25.101802.123000.

Kulis, S., Marsiglia, F. F., Elek-Fisk, E., Dustman, P., Wagstaff, D., & Hecht, M. L. (2005). Mexican/Mexican American adolescents and keepin' It REAL: An evidence-based, substance abuse prevention program. *Children and Schools, 27,* 133–145.

Larkey, L. K., & Hecht, M. (2010). A model of effects of narrative as culture-centric health promotion. *Journal of Health Communication, 15,* 114–135. doi:10.1080/10810730903528017.

Lee, S. J., Altschul, I., & Mowbray, C. T. (2008). Using planned adaptation to implement evidence-based programs with new populations. *American Journal of Community Psychology, 41,* 290–303. doi:10.1007/s10464-008-9160-5.

Marsiglia, F. F., Kulis, S., Yabiku, S. T., Nieri, T. A., & Coleman, E. (2010). When to intervene: Elementary school, middle school or both? Effects of keepin' it REAL on substance use trajectories of Mexican heritage youth. *Prevention Science, 12,* 48–62.

McCormick, L. K., Steckler, A. B., & McLeroy, K. R. (1995). Diffusion of innovations in schools: A study of adoption and implementation of school-based tobacco prevention curricula. *American Journal of Health Promotion, 9,* 210–219.

McNeal, R. B. Jr., Hansen, W. B., Harrington, N. G., & Giles, S. M. (2004). How all stars works: An examination of program effects on mediating variables. *Health Education & Behavior, 31,* 165–178. doi:10.1177/1090198103259852.

Miller, T., & Hendrie, D. (2008). *Substance abuse prevention dollars and cents: A cost-benefit analysis. (DHHS Pub. No. [SMA] 07-4298)*. Rockville: Center for Substance Abuse Prevention, SAMHSA.

Miller, M. A., Alberts, J. K., Hecht, M. L., Trost, M., & Krizek, R. L. (2000). *Adolescent relationships and drug use*. Mahwah: Lawrence Erlbaum.

Miller-Day, M., & Hecht, M. L. (2013). Narrative means to preventative ends: A narrative engagement approach to adolescent substance use prevention. *Health Communication, 28,* 657–670. doi:10.1080/10410236.2012.762861.

Miller-Day, M., Pettigrew, J., Hecht, M. L., Shin, Y., Graham, J., & Krieger, J. (2013). How prevention curricula are taught under real-world conditions: Types of and reasons for teacher curriculum adaptations. *Health Education, 113,* 324–344. doi:10.1108/09654281311329259.

Moore, J. E., Bumbarger, B. K., & Rhoades, B. L. (2013). Examining adaptations of evidence based programs in natural contexts. *Journal of Primary Prevention, 34,* 147–161. doi:10.1007/s10935-013-0303-6.

National Institute on Drug Abuse (NIDA). (2003). *Preventing drug abuse among children and adolescents* (2nd ed.) (NIH Publication No. 04-4212(A)). Bethesda: National Institutes of Health.

Noar, S. M., Benac, C. N., & Harris, M. S. (2007). Does tailoring matter? Meta-analytic review of tailored print health behavior change interventions. *Psychological Bulletin, 133,* 673–693. doi:10.1037/0033-2909.133.4.673.

Norris, A. E., Hughes, C., Hecht, M., Peragallo, N., & Nickerson, D. (2013). Randomized trial of a peer resistance skill-building game for Hispanic early adolescent girls. *Nursing Research, 62,* 25–35. doi:10.1097/NNR.0b013e318276138f.

Outside the Classroom, Inc. (2006). *NREPP application summary for alcoholedu for high school*. Needham: Author.

Pettigrew, J., Miller-Day, M., Shin, Y., Hecht, M. L., Krieger, J. L., & Graham, J. W. (2013). Describing teacher–student interactions: A qualitative assessment of teacher implementation of the 7th-grade keepin' it REAL substance use intervention. *American Journal of Community Psychology, 51*, 43–56. doi:10.1007/s10464-012-9539-1.

Pettigrew, J., Graham, J. W., Miller-Day, M., Hecht, M. L., Krieger, J. L., & Shin, Y (2015). Adherence and delivery quality: Implementation quality and outcomes of 7th grade keepin' it REAL program. *Prevention Science, 16*, 90–99. doi: 10.1007/s11121-014-0459-1.

Poduska, J. M., Kellam, S. G., Wang, W., Brown, C. H., Ialongo, N. S., & Toyinbo, P. (2008). Impact of the good behavior game, a universal classroom-based behavior intervention, on young adult service use for problems with emotions, behavior, or drugs or alcohol. *Drug and Alcohol Dependence, 95*, S29–S44.

Resnicow, K., Baranowski, T., Ahluwalia, J. S., & Braithwaite, R. L. (1999). Cultural sensitivity in public health: Defined and demystified. *Ethnicity and Disease, 9*, 10–21.

Ringwalt, C. L., Pankratz, M. M., Jackson-Newsom, J., Gottfredson, N. C., Hansen, W. B., Giles, S. M., & Dusenbury, L. (2009). Three-year trajectory of teachers' fidelity to a drug prevention curriculum. *Prevention Science, 11*, 67–76. doi:10.1007/s11121-009-0150-0

Ringwalt, C. L., Clark, H. K., Hanley, S., Shamblen, S. R., & Flewelling, R. L. (2010). The effects of project ALERT one year past curriculum completion. *Prevention Science, 11*, 172–184. doi:10.1007/s11121-009-0163-8.

Ringwalt, C. L., Vincus, A., Hanley, S., Ennett, S., Bowling, J., & Haws, S. (2011). The prevalence of evidence-based drug use prevention curricula in U.S. middle schools in 2008. *Prevention Science, 12*, 63–69. doi:10.1007/s11121-010-0184-3.

Roberto, A. J., Krieger, J. L., & Beam, M. A. (2009). Enhancing web-based kidney disease prevention messages for Hispanics using targeting and tailoring. *Journal of Health Communication, 14*, 525–540. doi:10.1080/10810730903089606.

Rohrbach, L. A., Graham, J. W., & Hansen, W. B. (1993). Diffusion of a school-based substance abuse prevention program: Predictors of program implementation. *Preventive Medicine, 22*, 237–260. doi:10.1006/pmed.1993.1020.

Rohrbach, L. A., Gunning, M., Sun, P., & Sussman, S. (2010). The project towards no drug abuse (TND) dissemination trial: Implementation fidelity and immediate outcomes. *Prevention Science, 11*, 77–88. doi:10.1007/s11121-009-0151-z.

Rotheram-Borus, M. J., & Duan, N. (2003). Next generation of preventive interventions. *Journal of the American Academy of Child & Adolescent Psychiatry, 42*, 518–526. doi:10.1097/01. CHI.0000046836.90931.E9.

Sandler, I., Ostrom, A., Bitner, M. J., Ayers, T. S., Wolchik, S., & Daniels, V.-S. (2005). Developing effective prevention services for the real world: A prevention service development model. *American Journal of Community Psychology, 35*, 127–142. doi:10.1007/s10464-005-3389-z.

Sloboda, Z., Glantz, M. D., & Tarter, R. E. (2012). Revisiting the concepts of risk and protective factors for understanding the etiology and development of substance use and substance use disorders: Implications for prevention. *Substance Use & Misuse, 47*, 944–962. doi:10.3109/1 0826084.2012.663280.

Spoth, R. L., Greenberg, M., Bierman, K., & Redmond, C. (2004). PROSPER community–university partnership model for public education systems: Capacity-building for evidence-based, competence-building prevention. *Prevention Science, 5*, 31–39. doi:10.1023/ B:PREV.0000013979.52796.8b.

Spoth, R. L., Clair, S., Shin, C., & Redmond, C. (2006). Long-term effects of universal preventive interventions on methamphetamine use among adolescents. *Archives of Pediatrics & Adolescent Medicine, 160*, 876–882. doi:10.1001/archpedi.160.9.876.

Stigler, M. H., Perry, C. L., Komro, K. A., Cudeck, R., & Williams, C. L. (2006). Teasing apart a multiple component approach to adolescent alcohol prevention: What worked in Project Northland? *Prevention Science, 7*, 269–280. doi:10.1007/s11121-006-0040-7.

Swisher, J. D., Crawford, J., Goldstein, R., & Yura, M. (1971). Drug education: Pushing or preventing? *Peabody Journal of Education, 49*, 68–75.

Tobler, N. S. (1986). Meta-analysis of 143 adolescent drug prevention programs: Quantitative outcome results of program participants compared to a control or comparison group. *Journal of Drug Issues, 16*, 537–567.

Tobler, N. S., & Stratton, H. H. (1997). Effectiveness of school-based drug prevention programs: A meta-analysis of the research. *Journal of Primary Prevention, 18*, 71–128. doi:10.1023/A:1024630205999.

Tobler, N. S., Roona, M. R., Ochshorn, P., Marshall, D. G., Streke, A. V., & Stackpole, K. M. (2000). School-based adolescent drug prevention programs: 1998 meta-analysis. *Journal of Primary Prevention, 20*, 275–336. doi:10.1023/A:1021314704811.

Trickett, E. J., Beehler, S., Deutsch, C., Green, L. W., Hawe, P., McLeroy, K., Miller, R. L., Rapkin, B. D., Schensul, J. J., Schulz, A. J., Trimble, J. E. (2011). Advancing the science of community-level interventions. *American Journal of Public Health, 101*(8), 1410. doi:10.1007/s10464-012-9524-8.

Chapter 9
Scaling Up Evidence-Based Preventive Interventions

Louise A. Rohrbach and Stephanie R. Dyal

Schools offer enormous opportunity to reach large numbers of adolescents for the promotion of health and prevention of disease. There is now substantial empirical evidence that a number of school-based interventions, programs, and policies are effective in preventing a broad range of social, emotional, behavioral, and health problems among youth, such as unhealthy eating, physical inactivity, substance abuse, teen pregnancy, school failure, delinquent behavior, and violence (National Research Council & Institute of Medicine 2009). These evidence-based interventions utilize a broad range of approaches, including universal education (e.g., curricula that discourage risk-taking behaviors and promote healthy lifestyles), provision of selected preventive services (e.g., mental health assessments), and environmental strategies (e.g., school-wide programs to prevent bullying and policies that promote consumption of healthy beverages). When implemented with fidelity (as intended by the original design) on a large scale, evidence-based preventive interventions (EBIs) have the potential to achieve significant public health impact (Spoth et al. 2013).

Despite this potential, there are unique contextual factors embedded within school systems that are likely to impede large-scale implementation of prevention programs (Chen 1998; Domitrovich et al. 2008). For example, the complexity of school organizational structures, which often require approval and buy-in for new strategies from multiple levels of decision makers (e.g., superintendents, principals, teachers, school boards, and community partners), can be a barrier to program implementation (Greenberg 2010). Furthermore, school system decision makers

L. A. Rohrbach (✉) · S. R. Dyal
Department of Preventive Medicine, University of Southern California, 2001 N. Soto Street, MC 9239, Los Angeles, CA 90032, USA
e-mail: rohrbach@usc.edu

S. R. Dyal
e-mail: stepharp@usc.edu

© Springer Science+Business Media New York 2015   175
K. Bosworth (ed.), *Prevention Science in School Settings*,
Advances in Prevention Science, DOI 10.1007/978-1-4939-3155-2_9

may believe that implementing prevention programs interferes with their primary mission to promote learning through reading, writing, math, and other academic subjects. Another contextual factor that may impede program adoption is that many school systems are facing significant reductions in public funds; thus, some are more focused on experimenting with broad school reform measures in an effort to cope with these crises than adoption of new programs and curricula.

A large gap exists between the programs, policies, and services suggested as best practices for school-based health promotion and disease prevention, and those that are currently being implemented in schools (Lee and Gortmaker 2013). In 2006, the School Health Programs and Policies Study estimated that only 61 % of schools nationwide required health education in at least one specific grade, less than 10 % of schools required daily physical education, and less than 5 % of schools made condoms available to students (Kann et al. 2007). Furthermore, a number of studies have shown that only a small percentage of health promotion programming in schools is evidence-based (Gottfredson and Gottfredson 2002; Ringwalt et al. 2009a). For example, in a national longitudinal survey of middle schools, Ringwalt and colleagues (Ringwalt et al. 2009a) found that only 34.4 and 42.6 % of schools were implementing evidence-based substance abuse prevention programs in 1999 and 2005, respectively. This is despite years of government policies (e.g., Safe and Drug Free Schools Act of 1999 and the No Child Left Behind Act of 2001) mandating the use of evidence-based programs (Hallfors and Godette 2002).

9.1 What Is Scaling Up?

The goal of disseminating and implementing EBIs on a large scale has been called the "new frontier" for the twenty-first century (National Research Council & Institute of Medicine, 2009). *Scaling up* or *going to scale* refers to the process by which evidence-based preventive interventions become disseminated, implemented, and institutionalized widely throughout a program, organization, or geographic area (Elmore 1996). The process of scaling up is guided by a body of research known as *translation research,* which investigates the complex processes and mechanisms through which tested and proven interventions are integrated into policy and practice on a large scale, in a sustainable way, and across various targeted populations and settings (Rohrbach et al. 2006).

The typical life cycle for an intervention starts with an investigation of the determinants of the health or behavioral problem, which is applied to the development of programs and strategies that are tested in rigorous experimental trials to determine *proof of concept* or *efficacy.* Interventions with proven efficacy are then tested among a wider range of population groups and settings to evaluate effectiveness when they are implemented under less well-controlled or "real-world" conditions. At this point in the cycle, effective interventions may be made available to schools and other community organizations for adoption. In the next phase, researchers may begin to investigate the best strategies for disseminating and implementing them on a wide scale (Mrazek and Haggerty 1994). An implicit expectation exists in this approach that schools will adopt and implement evidence-based preventive interventions with a high degree of fidelity to what was intended by the program developers and described in the original protocol (Pas and Bradshaw 2012). However, a growing body of research shows that there are many challenges involved in transporting preventive interventions that produced favorable outcomes during research trials to real-world school settings, and often, fidelity is lower when interventions are implemented under real-world conditions (Dusenbury et al. 2003; Durlak and DuPre 2008).

Scaling up of EBIs is generally recognized as a multifaceted and multilayered activity that requires building considerable resources, infrastructures, and capacities for high-quality, sustained program implementation (Spoth et al. 2013). To achieve a stronger impact of preventive interventions on the health of young people, scaling up also requires greater discovery and advances in the field of translation research. In this chapter, we will address the key challenges in scaling up evidence-based preventive interventions (EBIs) for the prevention of social, emotional, behavioral, and health problems among youth in school settings. We will summarize findings from studies on the multilevel factors that contribute to successful adoption and implementation, discuss some challenges of scaling up that are unique to the school setting, and present a case study that demonstrates one approach to addressing these challenges and issues.

9.2 Conceptual Frameworks

At present, there are not explicit theories that guide the process of scaling up evidence-based prevention in schools, but conceptual frameworks such as social-ecological models (McLeroy et al. 1988), the Reach Effectiveness Adoption Implementation Maintenance (RE-AIM) framework (Glasgow, et al. 1999), and interactive systems models (e.g., Durlak and DuPre 2008; Wandersman 2008) have been applied to guide research and practice related to scaling up. Most of these frameworks are grounded in the diffusion of innovations theory (Rogers 1983), which describes how ideas or practices that are perceived as new, such as EBIs, are communicated through a variety of channels over time among members of a social system. One of the core concepts of the theory is that innovations diffuse through a series of nonlinear "stages" that broadly include adoption (the intention to try the innovation), implementation (putting it into use), and sustained implementation or maintenance. A multitude of factors can influence the likelihood of adoption and implementation of innovations, including characteristics of the innovation (e.g., relative advantage over current practices, compatibility with current values, trialability, and observability) and setting (e.g., culture and politics) (Rogers 1983). Applying and expanding upon these concepts, recent heuristic frameworks posit that dissemination and implementation of EBIs will be influenced by a complex interaction of factors related to the EBI, the prevention delivery system (e.g., features related to the capacity of the organization in which it is delivered), and the prevention support system (e.g., training) (Durlak and DuPre 2008; Spoth et al. 2013; Wandersman et al. 2008; Wilson et al. 2011). As applied to school settings, these frameworks suggest that multiple factors—such as perceptions of the value and "fit" of the intervention, the school climate and culture, the capacity of school personnel to implement the intervention, and delivery of training—will interact within the multilevel context provided by the school district, community, and state department of education to determine the success of scaling up the EBIs.

In the next section, we discuss key factors that influence the dissemination, adoption, and implementation stages in the scaling-up process.

9.3 Dissemination and Adoption

How Do Schools Access Information About Evidence-Based Preventive Interventions? Schools and school districts access information about educational innovations from a variety of sources. They may actively search for or passively receive this information. For example, in a national survey of school personnel, Rohrbach and colleagues (Rohrbach et al. 2005) found that professional conferences, state departments of education, and marketing brochures were the most commonly accessed sources of information about evidence-based substance abuse prevention programs. Even though current policies promote the use of prevention approaches that are science based (e.g., Philliber and Nolte 2009; Hallfors and Godette 2002), research in school settings has shown that data on the effectiveness of an innovative program or curriculum are only one of several criteria that administrators consider when making decisions about adoption. Typically, school personnel rely more on their own experiences, staff of neighboring schools, opinions of parents and other community members, and data collected from their own students to make these decisions (Honig and Coburn 2008). In addition, some decision makers in the school system may be skeptical about using a science-based approach. For example, in a study of barriers to adoption of evidence-based pregnancy prevention programs, Philliber and Nolte (2009) found that some school decision makers did not see any reason to give preference to well-evaluated programs and even questioned both the quality of the research and the motivations of the program developers.

Information received through personal experience and community sources may be highly influential, as it may increase community buy-in and support for innovations. Parents and community members may encourage administrators to pay attention to information disseminated by mass media (Honig and Coburn 2008). For example, when evaluations suggesting the Drug Abuse Resistance Education (DARE) program was ineffective were popularized in television and newspaper reports, administrators used this information to support removal of the DARE program locally (Weiss et al. 2005).

While articles in peer-reviewed scientific journals are the primary way that researchers disseminate information about effective preventive interventions, such sources are much less likely to reach school administrators than prevention scientists (Rohrbach et al. 2005). Furthermore, school personnel may be pressed for time or lack interest in reading published articles about EBI research, or they may not have the specialized skills necessary to interpret the findings. Addressing this problem, various governmental and nongovernmental organizations have developed registries, print materials, and websites of lists of "best practice," "research-validated," and "evidence-based" preventive interventions in an effort to facilitate effective decision-making. These materials address characteristics of EBIs, findings from evaluations, criteria for appropriate EBI selection, and other pertinent information (Powers et al. 2011). Examples of these sources of information include the Blueprints for Healthy Youth Development website, developed by University of Colorado Center for the Study and Prevention of Violence, which provides information about EBIs to reduce antisocial behavior and promote a healthy course of youth development (http://www.colorado.edu/cspv/blueprints); the List of Evidence-Based Teen Pregnancy Prevention Program Models, developed by the U.S. Department of Health and Human Services, that identifies programs with evidence of effectiveness for impacting rates of pregnancy, sexually transmitted infections (STIs), or sexual risk behaviors (e.g., sexual activity, contraceptive use, number of sexual partners, etc.) (http://www.hhs.gov/ash/oah/oah-initiatives/teen_pregnancy/db/); the National Registry of Evidence-Based Programs and Practices that was developed to help the public learn about evidence-based substance abuse and mental health interventions (http://nrepp.samhsa.gov/); and the Research-Tested Intervention Programs (RTIPs) website, developed by the National Cancer Institute, designed to provide program planners with information about interventions that address diet, nutrition, physical activity, sun safety, and tobacco control (http://rtips.cancer.gov/rtips/index.do).

Although these resources are designed to help decision makers select youth-related interventions that can work in school settings, they still do not address all of the information needs of school administrators (Powers et al. 2011). For example, they tend to provide very little information about *how* to successfully implement specific EBIs in a school setting. The ratings they provide tend to emphasize the quality of research that determined program effectiveness, rather than the process by which the program can be implemented in real-world settings and the quality of technical assistance available to support implementation. In addition, each information source has its own process and criteria for identifying programs that are worthy of recommendation, which may lead school decision makers to conclude that there is inconsistent evidence for a specific program's effectiveness.

In sum, schools receive information regarding EBIs from personal and professional contacts, community members, conferences, marketing publications, mass media, online resources, government agencies, local research, published journal articles, and reports that compile multiple sources of information. These varied sources differ in credibility, accessibility, (perceived) relevance, and perceived trustworthiness. Difficulty in balancing input from these sources contributes to the complexity of making decisions about adopting EBIs.

How Do Schools Make Decisions About Which Evidence-Based Programs to Adopt? School districts differ greatly in how decisions about new programs are made, and decision-making is a complex process involving many personnel with different rank, input, and information. Typically, decisions about new programs are made by administrators, with teachers as "opinion givers" but not the ultimate decision makers. However, usually it is individual teachers who decide *whether and how* new curricula are used (Rohrbach et al. 1996). Furthermore, community and school politics are important factors in the decision-making process.

In regard to EBIs, the decision-maker (principal or district coordinator) is influenced by the public and teachers' preference, both due to social influence and the need for buy-in and support of the chosen EBI. Administrators may decide to adopt an EBI to conform to decisions made by neighboring schools. Often, schools get the impetus to adopt an EBI because they apply for and are awarded grant funding that guides them, and sometimes mandates them, to implement EBIs. Thus, decision-makers are not independent in the choices they make about adoption of prevention interventions; rather, they aim to make choices that are accepted by school personnel, the public, other schools in the district, and their external funding sources.

Sometimes, the decision to adopt an EBI is related directly to the decision to apply for a grant that will fund implementation of the specific EBI. Educators may recognize the need for an intervention, apply for a grant, and be awarded funding within a government program that provides guidance (sometimes in the form of requirements) in selecting a specific intervention. For example, Little and colleagues (Little et al. 2014) found that schools in California that applied for and received competitive grant funds for tobacco prevention education from the state were significantly more likely to adopt evidence-based tobacco prevention programs than schools that did not apply for funds.

9.3.1 Partnerships

School decision makers may contact purveyor organizations to help them access and interpret information about prevention interventions (Fixsen et al. 2005). Some purveyors are private organizations that provide information about specific programs as well as program-related materials, research support, and training for evidence-based preventive interventions, such as National Health Promotion Associates, Inc. (http://www.lifeskillstraining.com), which disseminates the Life Skills Training Program (Botvin et al. 1995), and ETR Associates (http://www.etr.org), which disseminates Reducing the Risk (Kirby et al. 1991), and many other programs. Another type of purveyor organization is the Blueprints for Healthy Youth Development, initiated by the University of Colorado Center for the Study and Prevention of Violence (http://www.colorado.edu/cwpv/blueprints), which promotes the adoption of evidence-based programs and provides information that supports effective and sustainable implementation of a broad range of programs. Schools may find organizations such as these useful to guide their decisions about which EBIs might fit well in their particular setting.

Another structure that may aid schools in decision-making about prevention curricula is the development of partnerships with public health researchers or university faculty (Honig and Coburn 2008). School–researcher partnerships have the potential to overcome several of the challenges to program adoption, including enhancing the "fit" between the school and the newly adopted EBI, anticipating the school's capacity-building needs for program implementation, and increasing local support for prevention (Spoth et al. 2013). One mechanism that has led to successful partnerships between school personnel, public health professionals, and researchers for the dissemination and implementation of EBIs is the Prevention Research Center program funded by the Centers for Disease Control and Prevention (CDC) (Franks et al. 2007). Prevention research centers based in several academic institutions have created successful partnerships with local educational agencies for research and scaling up of the Coordinated Approach to Child Health (CATCH), Planet Health and Not-on-Tobacco (N-O-T) programs (Franks et al. 2007). Other examples of models for effective practitioner–scientist partnerships that have led to large-scale implementation of school-based EBIs for substance abuse prevention are the Promoting School-University-Partnerships to Enhance Resilience (PROSPER) model (Spoth et al. 2011) and Communities that Care (CTC) coalitions (Fagan et al. 2009).

9.3.2 Factors Related to School Readiness and Capacity for Implementing Evidence-Based Programs

Successful implementation of EBIs depends on more than appropriate selection. Schools' organizational capacity has an influence on quality of implementation. Many schools are not prepared to implement EBIs, and do not assess their capacity to do so, resulting in a lack of preparation for implementation (Bumbarger and Perkins 2008). Recently, greater attention has been paid to assessment of readiness as an initial step in developing the "delivery system" for EBIs (Durlak and DuPre 2008). Community readiness for EBIs may be measurable at multiple levels—organizational, individual, community, and school (Bumbarger and Perkins 2008). EBI implementation can be improved by assessing school readiness and improving organizational function at multiple levels prior to EBI adoption. In the next section, we provide examples of characteristics that have been shown to improve implementation. One might consider a school that is "ready for prevention" as one that has at least some, if not most, of these characteristics.

An example of a tool that may be useful in assessing school readiness for prevention is the Bridge-It system developed by Bosworth and colleagues (Bosworth et al. 1999; Gingiss et al. 2006). Bridge-It includes survey items that assess facilitation processes, resources, school-based leadership, implementers, external environment, compatibility, external leadership, and innovation characteristics, which are summarized in scales that schools can use to identify weaknesses or barriers to EBI implementation. As is discussed below, there are a variety of factors that characterize schools that are prepared for prevention program implementation, such as having norms that reflect an openness to change, a positive work climate, a willingness to integrate the new program into existing practices, a shared vision regarding the value and purpose of the program, a process for collaborative decision-making, effective communication mechanisms, a plan that contains clear roles and responsibilities for program implementation, strong leadership for the program (including support, encouragement, priority setting, and incentives), motivated staff who have received training to enhance skills and self-efficacy to implement the program, and a system for providing ongoing technical assistance to staff during program implementation (Durlak and DuPre 2008). Enhancement of the factors that facilitate implementation as well as reduction of barriers can improve implementation fidelity and program impact.

9.3.3 Factors Associated With Adoption and Implementation of EBIs

For more than 50 years, researchers have studied factors associated with adoption and successful implementation of a wide range of innovative practices, programs, and policies in school settings (Berman and Pauly 1975; Fullan 1992; Hall 1979; Huberman and Miles 1984). Currently, there is a growing body of research on factors that explain how prevention innovations, in particular, are put into use in schools. These studies suggest that a combination of factors at multiple levels are associated with the likelihood schools will adopt EBIs and implement them successfully, including factors related to program characteristics; the school, district, and community context in which the program will be implemented; and the individuals who implement the program (Chen 1998; Rohrbach et al. 1996; Durlak and DuPre 2008). Below, we summarize the key findings from this research literature.

9.3.4 Characteristics of the Intervention

Like any product, EBIs have to be marketed in an acceptable and appealing way for them to be adopted (Fixsen et al. 2005; Rotheram-Borus and Duan 2003; Sandler et al. 2005). Interventions that are perceived to be easy to use and compatible with the organization's policies, procedures, and curriculum standards are most likely to be adopted (Rohrbach et al. 1996, 2006; Spoth et al. 2013). For example, teachers are more likely to adopt programs that are well specified (e.g., have a clearly written teaching manual), use teaching methods with which they are familiar, and contain audiovisual materials. Also, adoption of a specific EBI is more likely if teachers perceive incentives for adopting it, and the program is viewed as having benefits over the curriculum they currently use (Rohrbach et al. 2005).

Financial factors are associated with program adoption, in particular, the cost of materials, other resources, and teacher training (Spoth et al. 2013). Information about program cost, student/staff time requirements, and training can be difficult for schools to access, creating a potential barrier to adoption (Powers et al. 2011). While they recognize the benefits of prevention programs, many school organizations perceive the costs as too high (Cho et al. 2009; Hallfors and Godette 2002; Roberts-Gray et al. 2007). Concerns about the financial costs of implementing prevention programs have become even stronger as school districts experience significant reductions in public funding for education in general. Some sources of funding for school-based prevention programming, such as the Safe and Drug-Free Communities Act of 1999, have been eliminated entirely. As a result, the districts that are more likely to implement evidence-based prevention approaches are both larger districts, which may have greater discretionary funding by virtue of their size, and those that can allocate sufficient resources to develop applications for external funding (Cho et al. 2009; Little et al. 2014; Rohrbach et al. 2005). These findings suggest a need for increased funding mechanisms as well as improvements in schools' ability to determine their funding needs to increase adoption and sustained implementation of evidence-based prevention (Bumbarger and Perkins 2008).

9.3.5   Organizational and Community Factors

Various factors related to the community and organizational context are associated with adoption and successful implementation of EBIs in schools. Prevention programs are more likely to be adopted in communities that are stable and where adults demonstrate less opposition to prevention (Gingiss et al. 2006; Roberts-Gray et al. 2007). The presence of an administrator or teacher who functions as the "program champion" increases the likelihood that evidence-based prevention programs will be adopted and implemented over time (Fagan et al. 2008; Fagan and Mihalic 2003; Little et al. 2014; Roberts-Gray et al. 2007; Rohrbach et al. 2005, 2006). Also, adoption of prevention programs is greater in school districts that have a clear or perceived mandate to implement these programs (Little et al. 2014; Rohrbach et al. 2005).

The effect of the climate of the workplace, or the shared perception of the work environment, has long been the subject of examination by researchers (e.g., Glisson and James 2002). School climate has been referred to as "the quality and character of school life" (Cohen et al. 2009, p. 180). It encompasses people's perceptions of the schools' norms, goals, values, interpersonal relationships, teaching and learning practices, and organizational structures (Cohen et al. 2009). For example, schools are seen as having a positive climate when both vertical (principal to teacher, teacher to student) and horizontal (teacher to teacher) relationships are open and supportive (Gregory et al. 2007). Furthermore, a positive school climate fosters youth development and learning necessary for a productive and satisfying life in our society (Cohen et al. 2009).

A consistent finding in the literature is that a positive school climate is associated with greater adoption and more successful implementation of prevention programs (Beets et al. 2008; Ennett et al. 2003; Gittelsohn et al. 2003; Kallestad and Olweus 2003; Rohrbach et al. 2005). Teachers and administrators in organizations with a positive climate, including high teacher morale, a high degree of teacher involvement in decision-making, open communication and collaboration among staff, and active support of administrators for innovations are more willing to try new programs (Rohrbach et al. 1996, 2005). Furthermore, school organizations with a positive climate have greater capacity to deal with problems that arise during implementation (Gingiss et al. 2006; Gittelsohn et al. 2003; Mihalic et al. 2008; Roberts-Gray et al. 2007; St. Pierre and Kaltreider 2004; Thaker et al. 2008). School principals play a critical role in that they can provide positive incentives to staff for implementation and help to promote positive attitudes toward the program among teachers and parents (Gregory et al. 2007; Kam et al. 2003).

9.3.6 Characteristics of Program Implementers

Several studies have examined whether specific characteristics of teachers are associated with a greater likelihood of adopting prevention programs and implementing them with integrity (Rohrbach et al. 2006). There is some evidence that younger teachers, female teachers, and those with a confident and non-authoritarian teaching style may be more likely to implement evidence-based prevention programs (Ennett et al. 2003; Rohrbach et al. 1993); however, other studies have failed to find an association between teachers' background characteristics and program implementation (Kallestad and Olweus 2003; McGraw et al. 1996). A more consistent finding is that teachers who have positive beliefs about the prevention program, such as the perception that it is effective and fits well with their student population, are more likely to try the program and implement it successfully (Beets et al. 2008; Kallestad and Olweus 2003; Klimes-Dougan et al. 2009). In addition, implementation is more likely to be successful when teachers have strong self-efficacy or confidence that implementation will work, as well as greater comfort with the interactive teaching techniques that are common to prevention programs (Rohrbach et al. 19931996; Ennett et al. 2003).

Increasing Capacity for Implementation: Training The most common strategy that has been used to help faculty schools prepare for prevention program implementation is teacher training. Some training is broad, providing an overview of prevention approaches, but in many cases it is program specific. Sometimes training is provided to all teachers in a particular subject area (e.g., health) or grade level (e.g., 9th); in other cases, the school administration invites to training sessions only those teachers who will be implementing the program. The typical approach to program-specific training is to conduct a pre-implementation in-service workshop, which provides information about the theoretical and empirical base for the program, demonstrates key program lessons and components, and provides opportunities to practice key program activities. For some EBIs, this training is provided by purveyor organizations on behalf of program developers (Fixsen et al. 2005). There is substantial evidence that teachers who participate in these types of training workshops deliver a greater proportion of health education program components and adhere more closely to program manuals than do teachers who have not been trained (Blake et al. 2005; Ennett et al. 2003; Fagan et al. 2008; Gingiss et al. 2006; Hallfors and Godette 2002; Roberts-Gray et al. 2007; Rohrbach et al. 2006). Training workshops can provide the skills needed to implement the program as well as help to generate enthusiasm and commitment for implementation (Gottfredson and Gottfredson 2002; Rohrbach et al. 2006). Recent studies have suggested that other modalities for providing pre-implementation training, such as online education, may be a promising, less expensive alternative to in-person workshop training (Bishop et al. 2005).

In light of the many challenges that organizations encounter in implementing evidence-based prevention programs in school settings (e.g., Fagan and Mihalic 2003; Mihalic et al. 2008), successful implementation may require teacher training that goes beyond workshops and extends throughout the implementation period (Fixsen et al. 2005; Mihalic and Irwin 2003). Ongoing training, often referred to as *technical assistance,* may take the form of coaching, "just-in-time" reminders and suggestions, access to online resources, and/or access to training staff for problem solving and general support. Mihalic and Irwin (2003) conducted an evaluation of 42 communities that implemented evidence-based prevention programs identified by the Blueprints for Violence Prevention initiative (currently known as Blueprints for Healthy Youth Development; see http://www.colorado.edu/cspv/blueprints/), and found that teachers' perceptions that the quality of technical assistance they received was high (e.g., informative, supportive, etc.) were positively related to program fidelity and sustainability (Mihalic and Irwin 2003). While research supports the value of teacher coaching to enhance implementation of innovative curricula (Joyce and Showers 2002), in two recent trials of coaching interventions for evidence-based substance abuse prevention programs, teachers who were coached were no more likely to attain better program outcomes than teachers who were not coached (Ringwalt et al. 2009b; Rohrbach et al. 2010c). Overall, the literature suggests that a multicomponent approach to teacher training, which combines pre-implementation workshops with ongoing technical assistance (via coaching, telephone, and/or online support) will improve program implementation relative to pre-implementation training alone (Spoth et al. 2013).

Implementation Fidelity and Adaptation One of the major issues in scaling up of evidence-based prevention approaches has been the tension between fidelity of implementation to the original intervention design and adaptation of interventions to meet local needs and preferences. On one side of the debate, prevention program developers emphasize the importance of implementing with fidelity to the program design that was tested in evaluation research. Some prevention scientists (e.g., Elliott and Miahlic 2004) argue that the field does not have adequate research data to guide decisions about adapting or removing specific components. That is, we may know that certain interventions in their entirety are effective, but we have not conducted studies that enable us to identify which parts, or components, of interventions are critical to their success. Thus, many program developers push for close adherence to the intervention design. This approach is supported by evidence demonstrating that implementation fidelity matters; that is, school-based preventive interventions implemented with higher fidelity have produced stronger outcomes than those implemented with lower fidelity (Durlak and DuPre 2008; Domitrovich and Greenberg 2000).

On the other side of the debate, it is argued that adaptations of interventions are acceptable as long as they fall short of a "zone of drastic mutation" (Hall 1979). Hall (1979) suggested that program developers place changes (mutations) to their interventions along a continuum of zones, ranging a zone in which mutations are minimal and acceptable, to a zone in which mutations are so drastic, the intervention does not resemble what was originally developed. Thus, proponents of adaptation side of the fidelity-adaptation debate suggest that users of the intervention have the greatest knowledge about how it needs to be adapted to address local needs and capabilities, and making adaptations does not jeopardize program effectiveness as long as the adaptations are not "drastic," but consistent with the program design. Furthermore, it is argued that the process of adapting an intervention may increase local buy-in for it, as well as increase the likelihood that program implementation will be sustained (Berman and Pauly 1975).

Thus, at the center of the fidelity-adaptation debate is the question of whether program adaptations reduce or improve program effectiveness. Evaluations of prevention programs implemented in real-world school settings have shown both considerable variability in the quality of implementation and a fairly high prevalence of adaptation (Ringwalt et al. 2003; Rohrbach et al. 2006). For example, teachers have reported eliminating some of the key content of prevention programs, changing modules that involve using interactive teaching techniques (e.g., role playing and small group exercises) to the use of methods that are less interactive (e.g., lectures), and generally deviating from the program as written (Rohrbach et al. 1996 2006).

The challenge to the prevention field is that although adaptation of evidence-based programs appears to be ubiquitous, we know very little about how it affects program outcomes. In one study of adaptations that teachers made to the Life Skills Training program (Botvin et al. 1995), researchers observed program delivery and coded the valence of teachers' adaptations, concluding the majority were negative (i.e., inconsistent with or detracting from the program's objectives) (Dusenbury et al. 2005). In another study, teachers and students were interviewed and asked to generate suggestions for adaptations to two prevention programs, Project Towards No Drug Abuse (TND) (Sussman et al. 2004b) and Too Good for Drugs and Violence (Mendez Foundation 2000). About three quarters of the adaptations that respondents suggested were judged independently by the program developers as acceptable and consistent with the program theory (Ozer et al. 2010). In the future, more research is needed to understand the relationship between program outcomes and adaptations that are observed by outside staff or self-reported by teachers.

With the assumption that it is inevitable that teachers will make adaptations to evidence-based prevention programs as they put them into use in the real world (e.g., Ringwalt et al. 2003), one approach that may improve program outcomes is *guided adaptation*, in which school personnel work with program developers to plan adaptations carefully. For example, to guide practitioners in their potential adaptation of school-based programs for prevention of pregnancy and sexually transmitted diseases, the CDC established a framework that distinguishes between core content and pedagogical methods that can and cannot be modified, and uses a stoplight metaphor to apply the framework (Rolleri et al. 2014). In addition, in the future it is important that prevention researchers conduct rigorous evaluations of different approaches to adaptation and how they are related to program outcomes. One example of this type of research is a current study by Hecht and his colleagues (Colby et al. 2013; Hecht, et al. 2006; Miller-Day et al. 2013), in which an adapted version of the *keepin' it REAL* drug abuse prevention program, customized by the program developers for rural students, is being compared to the original version of the program and a control group. Another example of adaptation research compared two approaches of the delivery of the evidence-based Life Skills Training Program (Botvin et al. 1995)—the standard approach, in which curriculum lessons were taught as a stand-alone program, and the infused method, in which lesson material was integrated into the existing grade-level subject curricula (Vicary et al. 2006). The findings indicated that neither version of the program was found effective for the entire sample, although the standard approach showed some promising effects among females (Vicary et al. 2006).

9.4 Case Study: Project Towards No Drug Abuse Background

Below, we present a case study that describes the scaling up of Project TND (Sussman et al. 2002, 2004b). Project TND is a 12-session school-based prevention program developed to deter youth from smoking cigarettes, drinking alcohol, and using illicit substances including marijuana and hard drugs. The program was developed for older teens, particularly those at relatively high risk for drug abuse (e.g., alternative high school youth). Based on theories in psychology (clinical, cognitive, and social) and sociology, as well as recovery or chemical dependency treatment-related approaches, the TND model incorporates (a) pro-social motivation enhancement, (b) life and social skills, and (c) decision-making components to decrease youths' vulnerability to a wide range of problem behaviors that can interfere with learning and be personally destructive (Sussman et al. 2004a).

The effectiveness of Project TND has been evaluated in seven randomized control trials, each of which has involved experimental manipulation of different aspects of the program. In all seven studies, a favorable program effect on "hard" drug use (e.g., cocaine, stimulants, tranquilizers, etc.) has been demonstrated at 1-year follow-up (Rohrbach et al 2010c; Sun et al. 2006, 2008; Sussman et al. 2002, 2012; Valente et al. 2007). The effect of the program on youths' tobacco and alcohol use has been less consistent across the trials. In addition, two of the early evaluation studies suggested that the program can have a preventive effect on violence-related behaviors (Sussman et al. 2002).

9.4.1 Going to Scale

The research team that developed and evaluated Project TND began dissemination of the program in 2001, 8 years after the start of the first evaluation study. Two specific events created the initial demand for the program and provided the impetus for taking it to scale. The first was the designation of Project TND as a "model" program by the federal Substance Abuse and Mental Health Services Administration (SAMSHA).[1] The second event was the passage of Title V of the No Child Left Behind Act of 2001, which included a requirement that states use research-based programs to reduce drug use (as well as to improve school safety). As school districts sought information about evidence-based substance abuse prevention programs that were appropriate for implementation at the high school level, many were referred to Project TND.

Our research team needed to complete several tasks to get Project TND ready for wider dissemination and implementation. First, we needed to decide whether we would distribute the program ourselves, in our university setting, or identify a purveyor organization that would publish the program materials and provide teacher training and other technical support. After carefully weighing our options, we decided to maintain full control of the program and established resources, both internal and external, to facilitate its distribution. Second, we modified the Project TND manual to make it more user-friendly to teachers, for example, clarifying and reordering some of the lesson steps and reformatting the manual to make it more appealing. Third, because we planned to strongly recommend teacher training for organizations that adopted Project TND, we needed to create a system for providing training on a large scale. We established cadre of health education specialists who became certified Project TND trainers available to conduct teacher training workshops at the site of organizations that requested it. Fourth, we created a website that provided detailed information about the program theory, components, evaluation results, training, and costs.

9.4.2 Evidence for Successful Scaling Up

The Project TND curriculum is designed for implementation in a classroom setting over a 4- to 6-week period. Across the studies that established the evidence base for Project TND, we found that program delivery by both prevention specialists from outside of the school system and regular classroom teachers was effective in

---

[1] Since their initial efforts to provide information that practitioners could use to guide decision-making about evidence-based substance abuse prevention programs, SAMHSA has revised its approach and eliminated the distinction between "model" programs and others that have been evaluated (see the National Registry of Evidence-based Programs and Practices, http://nrepp.samsha.gov).

reducing substance use among youth (Rohrbach et al. 2007). As the program was scaled up, we suggested that it could be delivered in schools as well as other types of community settings, by implementers with various professional backgrounds (e.g., classroom teacher, health educator, counselor, nurse, mental health professional, etc.) who had participated in TND-certified training. In a survey of 120 early adopters of TND, we found that the majority of organizations implemented the program in high schools (57 %), but a substantial minority (28–38 %) reported they delivered it in nonschool settings (e.g., community centers), suggesting that the program generalizes to a variety of settings (Rohrbach et al. 2010a).

In 2003, we initiated the Project TND Dissemination Trial, funded by the National Institute on Drug Abuse, which focused on two primary research questions: (1) Is TND effective when implemented under real-world conditions? and (2) Is a comprehensive teacher training approach that combines a pre-implementation training workshop with coaching and technical assistance more effective than a training workshop alone? (Rohrbach et al. 2010b, c). A total of 65 high schools from 14 districts across the USA that had contacted us for information about Project TND were recruited and randomly assigned to one of three groups: (1) comprehensive training, (2) workshop training only, or (3) non-intervention control. With regard to our first research question, we found that program delivery in the real-world context of high schools produced reductions in marijuana use and hard drug use (the latter for baseline nonusers only); however, overall the effects were weaker than those demonstrated in the more controlled evaluations of the program (Rohrbach et al. 2010c). With regard to training approaches, our comparison showed that teachers who received the comprehensive training delivered the program with greater implementation fidelity that did teachers who received the workshop only (Rohrbach et al. 2010b); however, we found no evidence for improved student outcomes in the comprehensive training condition (Rohrbach et al. 2010c).

Self-reported process evaluation data showed that acceptance of the program was moderate-to-high among both teachers and students; for example, students' average rating of the program was 2.28 (± 0.04) on 4-point scale, and 70 % of teachers planned to continue teaching the program in the next year (Rohrbach et al. 2010b). Furthermore, written comments from teachers and notes from trainers' observations provided a wide variety of suggestions for revisions to TND that could make the program more acceptable to teachers and more feasible to deliver. Based on these suggestions, as well as input from an additional group of teachers included in the qualitative study conducted by Ozer and colleagues (Ozer et al. 2010), we revised the curriculum. In particular, the format was improved (e.g., adding text boxes of teaching tips to lesson plans), options were added (e.g., conducting a program activity as a group rather than individual exercise), and program examples were updated.

9.4.3   Lessons Learned

Below we summarize the lessons we have learned from the research described above, as well as from more than one decade of experience in scaling up Project TND.

1. **Implementation.** We have learned that implementation of TND is feasible in both school and community (i.e., nonschool) settings. In schools, successful implementation of TND requires careful planning and a supportive climate. In the high schools that participated in our dissemination study, two of the greatest challenges were finding a "home" for program delivery (i.e., a subject area or specific class in which the curriculum would be delivered) and adequate time for delivery. While administrators may want to maximize the number of students reached by the program by mandating that all relevant teachers be provided with training and program materials, a more cost-efficient delivery model may be to incentivize and train only those teachers who have positive attitudes toward the program, report they are comfortable with its approach, and are willing to commit the time it takes to implement all of the program lessons. Another model that we have found facilitates implementation involves establishing partnerships between schools and local social service agencies, in which external funding for the program is obtained and agency staff are trained to deliver TND in the participating high schools.

2. **Training.** Building on our evaluation results that show the program is effective when it is implemented by trained teachers (Rohrbach et al. 2007, 2010b), the information that we disseminate to potential program adopters emphasizes the importance of providing a face-to-face workshop to prepare teachers for implementation. Previous research suggests that once implementation is initiated, ongoing training and technical assistance can improve implementation fidelity (e.g., Mihalic et al. 2008). Our dissemination study was one of the first experimental tests of the "value added" in providing ongoing teacher training (i.e., coaching and technical assistance) for prevention program delivery in schools (Rohrbach et al. 2010b). We found that comprehensive training produced greater implementation fidelity and stronger short-term student outcomes compared to workshop training alone; however, these short-term benefits did not translate into more positive student behavioral changes (Rohrbach et al. 2010b, c). Despite declining resources available for prevention programming, it is important to provide program-specific training to those who will deliver the program. In addition, future research in the prevention field should focus on the ideal amount and best modalities for providing training to those who will implement prevention programs in school settings.

3. **Evaluation.** Similar to other prevention programs that have been scaled up in schools, we have limited data on the outcomes of Project TND when it is implemented in real-world school contexts. There are enormous challenges in conducting evaluation research in school settings, such as the costs involved, the difficulty of tracking changes over time, and competition with school's primary mission. Nevertheless, to increase the scale-up of Project TND and its potential impact on public health, rigorous evaluations of implementation of TND in everyday schools settings are needed. One way in which this can be accomplished is to increase partnerships between universities and school organizations, particularly if external funding that "braids" research and practice is available to support the research.

9.5 Summary

Research conducted during the past several decades has established the effectiveness of a number of interventions for the prevention of social, emotional, behavioral, and health problems among youth, such as unhealthy eating, physical inactivity, substance abuse, teen pregnancy, school failure, delinquent behavior, and violence. However, current implementation of these evidence-based interventions (EBIs) in the school setting is low, despite national and state policies requiring their use. To maximize their potential impact on public health, EBIs need to be delivered on a large scale. *Scaling up* or *going-to-scale* refers to the process by which EBIs become disseminated, implemented, and institutionalized widely throughout a program, organization, or geographic area. In this chapter, we addressed the key challenges in scaling up evidence-based prevention programming in school settings.

Multiple factors will interact within the multilevel context provided by the school, school district, community, and state department of education to explain success in scale-up of EBIs. The current focus on academic achievement in the nation's schools, coupled with school reform efforts, reductions in funding, complex decision-making mechanisms, and limited time and resources for prevention programming have impeded large-scale implementation of prevention programs.

Schools receive information regarding effective prevention interventions from a variety of sources, such as personal and professional contacts, conferences, marketing publications, mass media, and online resources. While there are several registries and websites available to help schools select specific programs, they tend to emphasize providing information about program effectiveness rather than best practices for program implementation.

The decision to adopt and implement an EBI is influenced by a number of factors related to the school and district organizational context (e.g., leadership, administrative support, school climate, etc.), characteristics of the personnel who will deliver the program (e.g., attitudes toward the program, self-efficacy to implement it), and characteristics of the intervention itself (e.g., perceived ease of use, flexibility, fit with organizational goals, etc.). Recent evidence suggests that it is important for schools to assess their level of readiness to implement EBIs and apply that information to improve organizational capacity, prior to initiating EBI adoption and implementation. Some educational organizations have found it useful to establish partnerships with community organizations, coalitions, or local universities to build capacity for prevention program implementation. Another critical element of capacity building is the provision of program-specific teacher training and technical assistance, both before the intervention begins and throughout the implementation process.

While policy makers and developers of EBIs have emphasized the importance of implementing interventions as intended by the original design (fidelity) to achieve positive program outcomes, evaluations of EBI delivery in real-world settings have documented considerable variability in implementation fidelity and a high prevalence of program adaptations. Currently, we know very little about the effects of most adaptations on program outcomes. One approach that may be promising is to encourage guided adaptation, in which teachers receive input from the program developer and/or published materials to plan careful adaptations to meet local needs that are consistent with the program approach and theoretical framework.

Finally, we presented a case study of the successful scaling up of TND, an evidence-based drug abuse prevention curriculum that targets high school-aged youth. We discussed our process of revising the curriculum to make it better suited for wide-scale use, the development of a training system, and research we have conducted to evaluate program effectiveness when the program is implemented in real-world school settings.

References

Beets, M. W., Flay, B. R., Vuchinich, S., Acock, A. C., Li, K.-K., & Allred, C. (2008). School climate and teachers' beliefs and attitudes associated with implementation of the positive action program: A diffusion of innovations model. *Prevention Science, 9*, 264–275. doi:10.1007/s11121-008-0102-2.

Berman, P., & Pauly, E. W. (1975). Federal programs supporting educational change. Vol. II, Factors affecting change agent projects. (Document No: R-1589/2-HEW). Santa Monica: RAND Corporation.

Bishop, D. C., Giles, S. M., & Bryant, K. S. (2005). Teacher receptiveness toward web-based training and support. *Teaching and Teacher Education, 21*(1), 3–14. doi:10.1016/j.tate.2004.11.002.

Blake, S. M., Ledsky, R. A., Sawyer, R. J., Goodenow, C., Banspach, S., Lohrmann, D. K., & Hack, T. (2005). Local school district adoption of state-recommended policies on HIV prevention education. *Preventive Medicine: An International Journal Devoted to Practice and Theory, 40*(2), 239–248. http://www.sciencedirect.com/science/article/pii/S0091743504002993.

Bosworth, K., Gingiss, P. M., Potthoff, S., & Roberts-Gray, C. (1999). A Bayesian model to predict the success of the implementation of health and education innovations in school-centered programs. *Evaluation and Program Planning, 22*, 1–11. doi:10.1016/S0149-7189(98)00035-4.

Botvin, G. J., Baker, E., Dusenbury, L., Botvin, E. M., & Diaz, T. (1995). Long-term follow-up results of a randomized drug abuse prevention trial in a white middle-class population. *Journal of the American Medical Association, 273*(14), 1106–1112. doi:10.1001/jama.1995.03520380042033.

Bumbarger, B. K., & Perkins, D. F. (2008). After randomized trials: Issues related to dissemination of evidence-based interventions. *Journal of Children's Services, 3*, 53–61. doi:10.1108/17466660200800012.

Chen, H. T. (1998). Theory-driven evaluations. *Advances in Educational Productivity, 7*, 15–34.

Cho, H., Hallfors, D. D., Iritani, B. J., & Hartman, S. (2009). The influence of "No Child Left Behind" legislation on drug prevention in U.S. schools. *Evaluation Review, 33*(5), 446–463. doi:10.1177/0193841×09335050.

Cohen, J., McCabe, E. M., Michelli, N. M., & Pickeral, T. (2009). School climate: Research, policy, practice, and teacher education. *Teachers College Record, 111*(1), 180–213.

Colby, M., Hecht, M. L., Miller-Day, M., Krieger, J. R., Syvertsen, A. K., Graham, J. W., & Pettigrew, J. (2013). Adapting school-based substance use prevention curriculum through cultural grounding: A review and exemplar of adaptation processes for rural schools. *American Journal of Community Psychology, 51*(1–2), 190–205. doi:10.1007/s10464-012-9524-8.

Domitrovich, C. E., & Greenberg, M. T. (2000). The study of implementation: Current findings from effective programs that prevent mental disorders in school-aged children. *Journal of Educational and Psychological Consultation, 11*(2), 193–221. doi:10.1207/S1532768XJ-EPC1102_04.

Domitrovich, C. E., Bradshaw, C. P., Poduska, J. M., Hoagwood, K., Buckley, J. A., Olin, S., Ro-
manelli, L. H., & Ialongo, N. S. (2008). Maximizing the implementation quality of evidence-
based preventive interventions in schools: A conceptual framework. *Advances in School Mental Health Promotion, 1*(3), 6–28. doi:10.1080/1754730X.2008.9715730.

Durlak, J. A., & DuPre, E. P. (2008). Implementation matters: A review of research on the influence of implementation on program outcomes and the factors affecting implementation. *American Journal of Community Psychology, 41*(3–4), 327–350. doi:10.1007/s10464-008-9165-0.

Dusenbury, L., Brannigan, R., Falco, M., & Hansen, W. B. (2003). A review of research on fidelity
of implementation: Implications for drug abuse prevention in school settings. *Health Education Research, 18*(2), 237–256. doi:10.1093/her/18.2.237.

Dusenbury, L., Brannigan, R., Hansen, W. B., Walsh, J., & Falco, M. (2005). Quality of implementation: Developing measures crucial to understanding the diffusion of preventive interventions.
Health Education Research, 20(3), 308–313. doi:10.1093/her/cyg134.

Elliott, D. S., & Mihalic, S. (2004). Issues in disseminating and replicating effective prevention
programs. *Prevention Science, 5*(1), 47–53. doi:10.1023/B:PREV.0000013981.28071.52.

Elmore, R. F. (1996). Getting to scale with good educational practices. *Harvard Educational Review, 66,* 1–26. http://her.hepg.org/content/g73266758j348t33/.

Ennett, S. T., Ringwalt, C. L., Thorne, J., Rohrbach, L. A., Vincus, A., Simons-Rudolph, A., & Jones,
S. (2003). A comparison of current practice in school-based substance use prevention programs
with meta-analysis findings. *Prevention Science, 4*(1), 1–14. doi:10.1023/A:1021777109369.

Fagan, A. A., & Mihalic, S. (2003). Strategies for enhancing the adoption of school-based prevention programs: Lessons learned from the Blueprints for Violence Prevention replications of the
Life Skills Training program. *Journal of Community Psychology, 31*(3), 235–253. doi:10.1002/
jcop.10045.

Fagan, A. A., Hanson, K., Hawkins, J. D., & Arthur, M. W. (2008). Bridging science to practice:
Achieving prevention program implementation fidelity in the community youth development
study. *American Journal of Community Psychology, 41*(3–4), 235–249. doi:10.1007/s10464-
008-9176-x.

Fagan, A. A., Hanson, K., Hawkins, J. D., & Arthur, M. W. (2009). Translation research in action:
Implementation of the communities that care prevention system in 12 communities. *Journal of
Community Psychology, 37,* 809–829. doi:10.1002/jcop.20332.

Fixsen, D., Naoom, S. F., Blase, D. A., Friedman, R. M., & Wallace, F. (2005). *Implementation
research: A synthesis of the literature (FMHI Publication #231)*. Tampa: University of South
Florida, Louis de la Parte Florida Mental Health Institute, The National Implementation Research Network.

Franks, A. L., Kelder, S. H., Dino, G. A., Horn, K. A., Gortmaker, S. L., Wiecha, J. L., & Simoes,
E. J. (2007). School-based programs: Lessons learned from CATCH, Planet Health, and Not-
On-Tobacco. *Preventing Chronic Disease: Public Health Research, Practice, and Policy, 4*(2),
1–9. http://www.cdc.gov/pcd/issues/2007/apr/pdf/06_0105.pdf.

Fullan, M. G. (1992). *Successful school improvement: The implementation perspective and beyond*. Philadelphia: Open University Press.

Gingiss, P. M., Roberts-Gray, C., & Boerm, M. (2006). Bridge-It: A system for predicting implementation fidelity for school-based tobacco prevention programs. *Prevention Science, 7*(2),
197–207. doi:10.1007/s11121-006-0038-1.

Gittelsohn, J., Merkle, S., Story, M., Stone, E. J., Steckler, A., Noel, J., & Ethelbah, B. (2003).
School climate and implementation of the pathways study. *Preventive Medicine, 37*(Supplement 1), S97–S106. doi:10.1016/j.ypmed.2003.08.010.

Glasgow, R. E., Vogt, T. M., & Boles, S. M. (1999). Evaluating the public health impact of health
promotion interventions: The RE-AIM framework. *American Journal of Public Health, 89,*
1323–1327. doi:10.2105/AJPH.89.9.1322.

Glisson, C., & James, L. R. (2002). The cross-level effects of culture and climate in human service
teams. *Journal of Organizational Behavior, 23*(6), 767–794. doi:10.1002/job.162.

Gottfredson, D. C., & Gottfredson, G. D. (2002). Quality of school-based prevention programs: Results from a national survey. *Journal of Research in Crime and Delinquency, 39*(1), 3–35. doi:10.1177/002242780203900101.

Greenberg, M. T. (2010). School-based prevention: Current status and future challenges. *Effective Education, 2*(1), 27–52. doi:10.1080/19415531003616862.

Gregory, A., Henry, D. B., & Schoeny, M. E. (2007). School climate and implementation of a preventive intervention. *American Journal of Community Psychology, 40*(3–4), 250–260. doi:10.1007/s10464-007-9142-z.

Hall, G. E. (1979). The concern-based approach to facilitating change. *Educational Horizons, 57*, 202–208.

Hallfors, D., & Godette, D. (2002). Will the "Principles of Effectiveness" improve prevention practice? Early findings from a diffusion study. *Health Education Research, 17*(4), 461–470. doi:10.1093/her/17.4.461.

Hecht, M. L., Graham, J. W., & Elek, E. (2006). The drug resistance strategies intervention: Program effects on substance use. *Health Communication, 20*, 267–276. doi:10.1207/s15327027hc2003_6.

Honig, M. I., & Coburn, C. (2008). Evidence-based decision making in school district central offices: Toward a policy and research agenda. *Educational Policy, 22*(4), 578–608. doi:10.1177/0895904807307067.

Huberman, A. M., & Miles, M. B. (1984). *Innovation up close: How school improvement works*. New York: Plenum Press.

Joyce, B., & Showers, B. (2002). *Student achievement through staff development* (3rd edn.). Alexandria: Association for Supervision and Curriculum Development.

Kallestad, J. H., & Olweus, D. (2003). Predicting teachers' and schools' implementation of the Olweus Bullying Prevention Program: A multilevel study. *Prevention & Treatment, 6*(1). doi:10.1037/1522-3736.6.1.621a.

Kam, C.-M., Greenberg, M. T., & Walls, C. T. (2003). Examining the role of implementation quality in school-based prevention using the PATHS curriculum. *Prevention Science, 4*(1), 55–63. doi:10.1023/A:1021786811186.

Kann, L., Telljohann, S. K., & Wooley, S. F. (2007). Health education: Results from the School Health Policies and Programs Study 2006. *Journal of School Health, 77*(8), 408–434. doi:10.1111/j.1746-1561.2007.00228.x.

Kirby, D., Barth, R. P., Leland, N., & Fetro, J. V. (1991). Reducing the risk: Impact of a new curriculum on sexual risk-taking. *Family Planning Perspectives, 23*(6), 253–263.

Klimes-Dougan, B., August, G. J., Lee, C.-Y. S., Realmuto, G. M., Bloomquist, M. L., Horowitz, J. L., & Eisenberg, T. L. (2009). Practitioner and site characteristics that relate to fidelity of implementation: The early risers prevention program in a going-to-scale intervention trial. *Professional Psychology: Research and Practice, 40*(5), 467–475. doi:10.1037/a0014623.

Lee, R., & Gortmaker, S. (2013). Health dissemination and implementation within schools. In R. C. Brownson, G. A. Colditz, & E. K. Proctor (Eds.), *Dissemination and implementation research in health* (pp. 419–436). Oxford: Oxford University Press.

Little, M. A., Pokhrel, P., Sussman, S., & Rohrbach, L. A. (2014). The process of adoption of evidence-based tobacco use prevention programs in California Schools. *Prevention Science*. doi:10.1007/s11121-013-0457-8.

McGraw, S. A., Sellers, D. E., Johnson, C. C., Stone, E. J., Bachman, K. J., Bebchuk, J., et al. (1996). Using process data to explain outcomes: An illustration from the Child and Adolescent Trial for Cardiovascular Health (CATCH). *Evaluation Review, 20*(3), 291–312.

McLeroy, K. R., Bibeau, D., Steckler, A., & Glanz, K. (1988). An ecological perspective on health promotion programs. *Health Education & Behavior, 15*, 351–377. doi:10.1177/109019818801500401.

Mendez Foundation. (2000). *Too good for drugs and violence—High school*. Tampa: Mendez Foundation.

Mihalic, S. F., & Irwin, K. (2003). Blueprints for violence prevention: From research to real-world settings—factors influencing the successful replication of model programs. *Youth Violence and Juvenile Justice, 1*(4), 307–329. doi:10.1177/1541204003255841.

Mihalic, S. F., Fagan, A. A., & Argamaso, S. (2008). Implementing the life skills training drug prevention program: Factors related to implementation fidelity. *Implementation Science, 3*(1), 5. doi:10.1186/1748-5908-3-5.

Miller-Day, M., Pettigrew, J., Hecht, M. L., Shin, Y., Graham, J., & Krieger, J. (2013). How prevention curricula are taught under real-world conditions: Types of and reasons for teacher curriculum adaptations in 7th grade drug prevention curriculum. *Health Education, 113*(4), 324–344. doi:10.1108/09654281311329259.

Mrazek, P., & Haggerty, R. (1994). *Reducing risks for mental disorders: Frontiers for preventive intervention research.* Washington: National Academy Press.

National Research Council & Institute of Medicine, Committee on the Prevention of Mental Disorders and Substance Abuse Among Children, Youth, and Young Adults: Research Advances and Promising Interventions. (2009). *Preventing mental, emotional, and behavioral disorders among young people: Progress and possibilities.* Washington: The National Academies Press.

Ozer, E. J., Wanis, M. G., & Bazell, N. (2010). Diffusion of school-based prevention programs in two urban districts: Adaptations, rationales, and suggestions for change. *Prevention Science, 11,* 42–55. doi:10.1007/s11121-009-0148-7.

Pas, E. T., & Bradshaw, C. P. (2012). Examining the association between implementation and outcomes: State-wide scale-up of school-wide positive behavior intervention and supports. *Journal of Behavioral Health Services & Research, 39*(4), 417–433. doi:0.1007/s11414-012-9290-2.

Philliber, S., & Nolte, K. (2009). Implementation science: Promoting science-based approaches to teen pregnancy. *Prevention Science, 9*(3), 166–177. doi:10.1007/s11121-008-0094-9.

Pierre, St. T. L., & Kaltreider, D. L. (2004). Tales of refusal, adoption, and maintenance: Evidence-based substance abuse prevention via school-extension collaborations. *American Journal of Evaluation, 25*(4), 479–491. doi:10.1016/j.ameval.2004.09.006.

Powers, J. D., Bowen, N. K., & Bowen, G. L. (2011). Supporting evidence-based practice in schools with an online database of best practices. *Children & Schools, 33*(2), 119–128. doi:10.1093/cs/33.2.119.

Ringwalt, C. L., Ennett, S., Johnson, R., Rohrbach, L. A., Simons-Rudolph, A., Vincus, A., & Thorne, J. (2003). Factors associated with fidelity to substance use prevention curriculum guides in the nation's middle schools. *Health Education & Behavior, 30*(3), 375–391. doi:10.1177/1090198103030003010.

Ringwalt, C., Vincus, A. A., Hanley, S., Ennett, S. T., Bowling, J. M., & Rohrbach, L. A. (2009a). The prevalence of evidence-based drug use prevention curricula in U.S. middle schools in 2005. *Prevention Science, 10*(1), 33–40. doi:10.1007/s11121-008-0112-y.

Ringwalt, C. L., Pankratz, M. M., Hansen, W. B., Dusenbury, L., Jackson-Newsom, J., Giles, S. M., et al. (2009b). The potential of coaching as a strategy to improve the effectiveness of school-based substance use prevention curricula. *Health Education & Behavior, 36*(4), 696–710. doi:10.1177/1090198107303311.

Roberts-Gray, C., Gingiss, P. M., & Boerm, M. (2007). Evaluating school capacity to implement new programs. *Evaluation and Program Planning, 30*(3), 247–257. doi:10.1016/j.evalprogplan.2007.04.002.

Rogers, E. M. (1983). *Diffusion of innovations* (2nd ed.). New York: The Free Press.

Rohrbach, L. A., Graham, J. W., & Hansen, W. B. (1993). Diffusion of a school-based substance abuse prevention program: Predictors of program implementation. *Preventive Medicine, 22,* 237–260. doi:10.1006/pmed.1993.1020.

Rohrbach, L. A., D'Onofrio, C. N., Backer, T. E., & Montgomery, S. B. (1996). Diffusion of school-based substance abuse prevention programs. *American Behavioral Scientist, 39*(7), 919–934. doi:10.1177/0002764296039007012.

Rohrbach, L. A., Ringwalt, C. L., Ennett, S. T., & Vincus, A. A. (2005). Factors associated with adoption of evidence-based substance use prevention curricula in U.S. school districts. *Health Education Research, 20*(5), 514–526. doi:10.1093/her/cyh008.

Rohrbach, L. A., Grana, R., Sussman, S., & Valente, T. W. (2006). Type II translation: Transporting prevention interventions from research to real-world settings. *Evaluation & the Health Professions, 29*(3), 302–333. doi:10.1177/0163278706290408.

Rohrbach, L. A., Dent, C. W., Skara, S., Sun, P., & Sussman, S. (2007). Fidelity of implementation in Project Towards No Drug Abuse (TND): A comparison of classroom teachers and program specialists. *Prevention Science, 8,* 125–132. doi:10.1007/s11121-006-0056-z.

Rohrbach, L. A., Gunning, M., Sun, P., & Sussman, S. (2010a). The Project Towards No Drug Abuse (TND) dissemination trial: Implementation fidelity and immediate outcomes. *Prevention Science, 11,* 77–88. doi:10.1007/s11121-009-0151-z.

Rohrbach, L. A., Gunning, M., Grana, R., Gunning, G., & Sussman, S. (2010b). Dissemination of Project Towards No Drug Abuse (TND): Findings from a survey of program adopters. *Substance Use & Misuse, 45,* 2551–2566. doi:10.3109/10826081003725278.

Rohrbach, L. A., Sun, P., & Sussman, S. (2010c). One-year follow-up evaluation of the Project Towards No Drug Abuse (TND) dissemination Trial. *Preventive Medicine, 51,* 313–319. doi:10.1016/j.ypmed.2008.07.003.

Rolleri, L. A., Fuller, T. R., Firpo-Triplett, R., Lesesne, C. A., Moore, C., & Leeks, K. D. (2014). Adaptation guidance for evidence-based teen pregnancy and STI/HIV prevention curricula: From development to practice. *American Journal of Sex Education, 9*(2), 135–154. doi: 10.1080/15546128.2014.900467.

Rotheram-Borus, M. J., & Duan, N. (2003). Next generation of preventive interventions. *American Academy of Child & Adolescent Psychiatry, 42*(5), 518–526. doi:10.1097/01.CHI.0000046836.90931.E9.

Sandler, I., Ostrom, A., Birner, M. J., Ayers, T. S., Wolchik, S. A., & Daniels, V.-S. (2005). Developing effective prevention services for the real world: A prevention service development model. *American Journal of Community Psychology, 35*(3–4), 127–142. doi:0.1007/s10464-005-3389-z.

Spoth, R., Redmond, C., Clair, S., Shin, C., Greenberg, M., & Feinberg, M. (2011). Preventing substance misuse through community-university partnerships and evidence-based interventions: PROSPER outcomes 4½ years past baseline. *American Journal of Preventive Medicine, 40,* 440–447. doi:10.1016/j.amepre.2010.12.012.

Spoth, R., Rohrbach, L. A., Greenberg, M., Leaf, P., Brown, C. H., Fagan, A., Catalano, R. F., Society for Prevention Research Type 2 Translational Task Force Members and Contributing Authors. (2013). Addressing core challenges for the next generation of type 2 translation research and systems: The translation science to population impact (TSci Impact) framework. *Prevention Science, 14*(4), 319–351. doi:10.1007/s11121-012-0362-6.

Sun, W., Skara, S., Sun, P., Dent, C. W., & Sussman, S. (2006). Project Towards No Drug Abuse: Long-term substance use outcomes evaluation. *Preventive Medicine, 42*(3), 188–192. doi:10.1016/j.ypmed.2005.11.011.

Sun, P., Dent, C. W., Sussman, S., & Rohrbach, L. A. (2008). One-year follow-up evaluation of Project Towards No Drug Abuse (TND4). *Preventive Medicine, 47,* 438–442. doi:10.1016/j.ypmed.2008.07.003.

Sussman, S., Dent, C. W., & Stacy, A. W. (2002). Project Towards No Drug Abuse: A review of the findings and future directions. *American Journal of Health Behavior, 26*(5), 354–365. doi:10.5993/AJHB.26.5.4.

Sussman, S., Earleywine, M., Wills, T., Cody, C., Biglan, T., Dent, C. W., & Newcomb, M. D. (2004a). The motivation, skills, and decision-making model of "drug abuse" prevention. *Substance Use & Misuse, 39,* 1971–2016. doi:10.1081/JA-200034769.

Sussman, S., Rohrbach, L., & Mihalic, S. (2004b). *Blueprints for violence prevention, book twelve: Project Towards No Drug Abuse.* Boulder: Center for the Study and Prevention of Violence.

Sussman, S., Sun, P., Rohrbach, L. A., & Spruijt-Metz, D. (2012). One-year outcomes of a drug abuse prevention program for older teens and emerging adults: Evaluating a motivational interviewing booster component. *Health Psychology, 31*(4), 476–485. doi:10.1037/a0025756.

Thaker, S., Steckler, A., Sánchez, V., Khatapoush, S., Rose, J., & Hallfors, D. D. (2008). Program characteristics and organizational factors affecting the implementation of a school-based indicated prevention program. *Health Education Research, 23*(2), 238–248. doi:10.1093/her/cym025.

Valente, T. W., Ritt-Olson, A., Stacy, A., Unger, J. B., Okamoto, J., & Sussman, S. (2007). Peer acceleration: Effects of a social network tailored substance abuse prevention program among high-risk adolescents. *Addiction, 102*(11), 1804–1815. doi:10.1111/j.1360–0443.2007.01992.x.

Vicary, J. R., Smith, E. A., Swisher, J. D., Hopkins, A. M., Elek, E., Bechtel, L. J., & Henry, K. L. (2006). Results of a 3-year study of two methods of delivery of life skills training. *Health Education and Behavior, 33,* 325–339. doi:10.1177/1090198105285020.

Wandersman, A., Duffy, J., Flaspohler, P., Noonan, R., Lubell, K., Stillman, L., & Saul, J. (2008). Bridging the gap between prevention research and practice: The interactive systems framework for dissemination and implementation. *American Journal of Community Psychology, 41*(3–4), 171–181. doi:10.1007/s10464-008-9174-z.

Weiss, C. H., Murphy-Graham, E., & Birkeland, S. (2005). An alternate route to policy influence: How evaluations affect D.A.R.E. *American Journal of Evaluation, 26*(1), 12–30. doi:10.1177/1098214004273337.

Wilson, K. M., Brady, T. J., Lesesne, C., & On Behalf of the NCCDPHP Work Group on Translation (2011). An organizing framework for translation in public health: The knowledge to action framework. *Preventing Chronic Disease, 8*(2), 1–7. doi:10.1089/jwh.2007.0699.

Part III
Research in and with Schools

Chapter 10
Schools as Venues for Prevention Programming

Terri N. Sullivan, Kevin S. Sutherland, Albert D. Farrell
and Katherine A. Taylor

Schools are frequently the setting for the implementation of programs focused on reducing the frequency of problem behaviors such as aggression, substance use, and truancy (Botvin et al. 2006; Espelage et al. 2013; MVPP 2009; Vo et al. 2012). The high prevalence rates and negative outcomes associated with risk behaviors among youths demonstrate the need for prevention programs. For example, annual prevalence rates for alcohol and marijuana use in a national survey of 8th, 10th, and 12th graders conducted in 2012 were 44 and 25%, respectively (Johnston et al. 2013). Results from a national survey of high school students conducted in 2011 indicated that in the past 12 months, 33% of students had been in a physical fight and 20% had been bullied on school grounds (Centers for Disease Control and Prevention 2011). Negative consequences of risk behaviors may include physical injury, substance abuse, poor academic performance, and early school leaving (Guerra and Bradshaw 2008). These statistics highlight the potential benefits of researchers and schools forming strong partnerships to effectively address risk behaviors.

Schools represent a particularly appropriate setting for implementing universal prevention programs. From a practical standpoint, they enable access to large numbers of students from early childhood to late adolescence and provide an opportunity to follow students over time (Farrell et al. 2001). Moreover, school staff members are trained to support youth development, and the public generally supports this

T. N. Sullivan (✉) · A. D. Farrell · K. A. Taylor
Department of Psychology, Virginia Commonwealth University, 810 West Franklin Street,
Richmond, VA 23284-9045, USA
e-mail: tnsulliv@vcu.edu

A. D. Farrell
e-mail: afarrell@vcu.edu

K. A. Taylor
e-mail: taylorka7@vcu.edu

K. S. Sutherland
Special Education and Disability Policy, School of Education, Virginia Commonwealth
University, 1015 West Main Street, Richmond, VA 23284-9045, USA
e-mail: kssuther@vcu.edu

© Springer Science+Business Media New York 2015
K. Bosworth (ed.), *Prevention Science in School Settings,*
Advances in Prevention Science, DOI 10.1007/978-1-4939-3155-2_10

focus (Gottfredson 2001). Although students spend only about 18% of their waking hours at school, the school context has a powerful influence on their development (Gottfredson and Gottfredson 2007). Peer groups typically form within the school context and often exert their influence during the school day. Schools may also place youths in contact with peers who have a variety of backgrounds and different values. Depending on the norms and attitudes of peers within various groups, peer influences may either encourage or discourage risk behaviors. Within the school environment, informal social norms may also support engagement in problem behaviors; for example, using aggression as a means to gain status and correct perceived injustices (Fagan and Wilkinson 1998). Other risk factors may also be present within the school environment. For example, although the most serious incidents of victimization (such as homicides) typically occur outside of school, youths are at elevated risk for experiencing a broader range of criminal victimization (e.g., theft, assault) when they are at school or on their way to and from school (Gottfredson and Gottfredson 2007). As Gottfredson (2001) noted, some of the likely causes of problem behavior at school are related, and many of these factors can be altered to reduce students' involvement in these behaviors.

10.1 The Focus of School-Based Prevention Efforts

School-based prevention programs have the potential to influence multiple levels of the social systems that influence students' behavior. Programs focused on individual students attempt to increase students' knowledge base and enhance skills such as communication, problem-solving, and emotion management that have been associated with specific risk behaviors (Botvin et al. 2006; Espelage et al. 2013; Farrell et al. 2001). For example, Second Step: Student Success Through Prevention is a violence prevention program for middle school students focused on enhancing empathy, communication, problem-solving, and anger management skills (Espelage et al. 2013). Another example of an individual-level skill-building program is the Life Skills Training Program, which addresses substance use prevention for elementary to high school students (Botvin et al. 2006). The Life Skills Training Program aims to improve youths' self-esteem and skills related to stress and coping, emotion management, resistance against peer and media pressure to use drugs, and social competence (Botvin and Tortu 1988). Implementing these types of programs in school settings provides students opportunities to learn, model, and apply targeted skills with peers on a day-to-day basis. Improvements in social and emotional learning may have broader benefits, as was documented by a recent meta-analysis showing that school-based interventions that concentrate on social and emotional learning significantly increased academic achievement (Durlak et al. 2011).

Programs that focus on the classroom level are designed to improve teachers' classroom management skills and effectiveness in dealing with students' disruptive or aggressive behavior, which can negatively affect academic success and classroom climate (van Lier et al. 2004; Vo et al. 2012). As an example, BEST in CLASS is a manualized program designed for preschool children at risk for emotional or behavioral disorders. This program uses a teacher training and coaching model to provide teachers direct assistance in learning and effectively implementing instructional and classroom management skills with the goal of fostering prosocial behavior and engagement in learning (Vo et al. 2012). The PAX Good Behavior Game focuses more generally on creating a positive and prosocial classroom, and thereby decreasing off-task and disruptive or aggressive behaviors. Students develop expectations for classroom behavior with their teacher, then the team of students who best meets these expectations wins the game and earns a reward. This program also incorporates evidence-based behavioral strategies designed to increase students' engagement in learning (Embry 2003). Prevention programs focused on the classroom level may not only improve students' behavior and academic achievement but also enhance positive relationships with peers and with teachers.

Prevention programs targeting the school environment often aim to create a warm and responsive school climate with high expectations for prosocial behavior and academic achievement (Embry et al. 1996; Olweus 2004). A key focus is on fostering positive relationships. Recognition of the transactional nature of social interactions among students and teachers, and of the effect of these interactions in supporting prosocial behavior, is central to achieving a positive school climate (Conroy et al. 2009). School environment programs may implement interventions at multiple levels of the school's social system. For example, the Olweus Bullying Prevention Program (Olweus 2004) includes a component to recognize individual students' prosocial behaviors and address individual bullying behaviors; a classroom-level component to foster positive student–student and student–teacher relationships; and a school-level component focused on adults' consistent implementation of school rules, an "on-the-spot" intervention to address bullying behaviors, and awareness and monitoring of "hot spots" where these behaviors are most likely to occur. A common thread woven through each of these components is parental involvement. Efforts to address broader influences through community outreach are also included. Ideally, such a comprehensive approach creates a protective environment that supports adaptive development and deters risk behaviors.

10.2 Complexities in Implementing Prevention Programs in Schools

Regardless of the specific focus of a school-based prevention program, schools present unique implementation challenges for researchers. Schools are complex systems containing youths with diverse needs, and school contexts are often changing and unpredictable (Forman et al. 2013). Researchers have found that the quality of implementation of prevention programs in schools is often low (Durlak 2010; Durlak and DuPre 2008; Forman et al. 2013; Gottfredson and Gottfredson 2002). This is unfortunate in that high-quality implementation (e.g., the implementer's skills and completeness of delivery) appears necessary for positive outcomes (Durlak and

DuPre 2008; Wilson et al. 2003). The replication and sustainability of research-based prevention programs in day-to-day practice also remain a concern. Variations in both the quality of implementation and in outcomes associated with evidence-based prevention programs have contributed to an increased focus on implementation science, which seeks to explore and explain how and why interventions work in real-world contexts (Kelly and Perkins 2012).

In the following sections, we use the health promotion intervention life cycle (Bopp et al. 2013) as the framework for addressing several aspects of partnering with schools as venues for prevention programs. This model is divided into three phases: (a) program development, adoption, and implementation; (b) sustainability, institutionalization, or termination; and (c) diffusion and dissemination. For this chapter, we focus primarily on the first and second phases, as diffusion and dissemination are addressed in Chap. 9. It is important to note that although we present phases of the model in a linear fashion, they are actually iterative in nature. For example, decisions made in the development and implementation of a school-based prevention program directly inform its sustainability, and factors that may enhance sustainability should be considered during development and implementation.

10.3   Program Development and Adoption

A key initial step for school staff and researchers is identifying the most appropriate prevention program for a particular school or set of schools. This involves consideration of characteristics of both the intervention and the setting where it will be implemented. The prevention program needs to be evidence-based, culturally and developmentally relevant, and focused on key risk and protective factors for the risk behavior being targeted within the student population. The capacity or readiness of the school to support the prevention program must also be considered. In this section, we discuss three issues that inform both program development and adoption: (a) identifying the needs of the schools, (b) selecting the most appropriate intervention, and (c) assessing the school's capacity or readiness for the program.

10.3.1   Identifying the Needs of the Schools

A key consideration in selecting a prevention program is how well it addresses the needs of the school. Interventions differ in their goals, the specific risk and protective factors they target, their intended population, the intervention strategies they use, and the resources they require for successful implementation (Farrell and Vulin-Reynolds 2007). Establishing a match between these features and the needs and characteristics of a particular school is critical to ensuring an intervention's success. School interventions are not likely to be successful without the support of teachers and other school staff, and such support is not likely to be present without a clear sense that the intervention addresses an important need. A logical starting point may involve conducting a needs assessment to identify the key concerns of teachers, school administrators, and other stakeholders, or collecting data that identify problems within the school (e.g., truancy rates, student reports of drug use). Specific goals might involve reducing a specific problem behavior (e.g., aggression, drug use, early school leaving), addressing a constellation of problem behaviors, or promoting positive development.

10.3.2 Selecting the Most Appropriate Intervention Approach

Interventions are not likely to have their desired impact if they do not address the factors responsible for the development or maintenance of the problem they are attempting to change (Coie et al. 1993). These factors are likely to vary across schools. Support for this notion was provided by a recent literature review that identified student (e.g., gender, initial level of aggression, parental monitoring), school (e.g., norms for aggression), and community (e.g., level of poverty and crime) characteristics that moderate the impact of school-based violence prevention programs (Farrell et al. 2013). Thus, the selection of appropriate prevention strategies must take into account the dynamics of the student population and the school and their specific profile of risk and protective factors (Farrell and Vulin-Reynolds 2007), as different risk factors may operate in different socio-ecological contexts. This reality underscores the need for assessing levels of risk and protective factors present within a given school and using this information to identify relevant intervention strategies. The Communities That Care model, which involves selecting interventions based on their match to data obtained from a community assessment of risk factors, provides an excellent example of this approach (Hawkins et al. 2012).

The comprehensiveness of an intervention approach is also important in that multiple interventions may be needed in the school setting, or across multiple settings, to address key risk and protective factors associated with a risk behavior and to provide adequate dosage to produce desired outcomes (Nation et al. 2003). Farrell and Camou (2006) provided a framework for comprehensive youth violence prevention programs based on a grid model that incorporated social setting (e.g., school, family, and community), developmental stage, and level of risk. Although many schools implement multiple programs, these do not necessarily represent a coordinated effort. Gottfredson and Gottfredson (2001), in their national survey of principals representing 635 schools, found that schools implemented a median of 14 different prevention activities. Although this level of activity may be of benefit, they suggested that such diverse efforts may reduce the impact of intervention by spreading resources too thin. Domitrovich et al. (2010) similarly noted that although schools often implement multiple prevention programs, these efforts are not always complementary. They discussed advantages of using theory and data to systematically integrate prevention programs (i.e., blending overlapping components and retaining unique elements) to address intervention targets. Integrated prevention efforts may cover a wider range of risk and protective factors (e.g., to systematically address a particular risk behavior or target multiple risk behaviors) and have both interactive and additive effects (Domitrovich et al. 2010). A comprehensive effort to address problem behaviors is more likely to be successful if it involves interventions that focus on multiple settings, both within and outside of the school context. According to this model, school-based prevention programs represent only one part of a larger effort.

10.3.3 Assessing School Capacity or Readiness for a Program

Another consideration for program adoption is the school's capacity or readiness for the program. Capacity represents "the skills, motivations, knowledge, and attitudes necessary to implement innovations, which exist at the individual, organization, and community levels," and is similar to the construct of readiness, which denotes the school's preparedness to begin and successfully complete program implementation (Flaspohler et al. 2008, p. 183). The literature on implementation science identifies numerous aspects of capacity (Bosworth et al. 1999), three of which appear particularly critical. First, it is important to differentiate between two implementation science frameworks. *Research-to-practice* models focus on the transfer of innovative, evidence-based programs that have been validated in controlled experimental settings into real-world settings, such as classrooms and schools (Aarons et al. 2010; Fixsen et al. 2005). In contrast, *community-centered* models begin by identifying community-based capacities and the ways in which novel prevention programs or innovations may be adapted to meet community needs, with the improvement of current practice superseding the introduction of innovations (Wandersman 2003).

Flaspohler et al. (2008) identified innovation-specific and general capacity factors that reflect a school's organizational capacity. Innovation-specific capacity, which is evaluated more often in research-to-practice models, encompasses program fit. *Fit* represents the degree to which the program (a) dovetails with the school's needs, goals, and day-to-day practice and (b) is socioculturally and developmentally relevant (Nation et al. 2003). For example, interventions need to address specific risk factors that emerge during specific stages of youth development (Farrell and Camou 2006). Programs that cover multiple grades may therefore require a different focus at each grade. For example, interventions focused on early grades may address factors such as impulse control, whereas those focused on secondary school students may address factors related to dating violence. Additional factors within innovation-specific capacity include school and, especially administrative, buy-in and support needed to supply sufficient time and resources and create a climate conducive to successful program implementation as well as the capability for ongoing training and program evaluation.

Compared to research-to-practice models, community-centered models may place more emphasis on an organization's general capacity, which consists of "leadership, organizational structure, management style, organizational climate, resource availability, staff capacity, and external relationships" with community members (Flaspohler et al. 2008, p. 191). In contrast to innovation-specific capacities (i.e., those needed to incorporate a specific innovation into the school setting), general capacities represent the broad-spectrum infrastructure, mission, and capabilities of the organization (Halgunseth et al. 2012). School personnel may experience tension between wanting to be receptive to prevention research innovations but at the same time needing to be confident that such innovations will fit within the school's general capacities. Flaspohler et al. (2008) also highlighted the need for researchers to more carefully consider general capacities prior to implementing research-to-practice models because general capacities influence implementation effectiveness.

Several researchers have developed measures to assess school capacity (e.g., Bosworth et al. 1999; Roberts-Gray et al. 2007). For example, Bosworth et al. (1999) created a model to assess the probability of successful implementation of school-based prevention efforts. In consultation with a panel knowledgeable about prevention programs and intervention theory, they identified several factors that may predict successful school-based implementation. Factors included the complexity of teaching and implementing the program, the plan for facilitating implementation (e.g., training, coaching, and fidelity monitoring), implementer characteristics (e.g., commitment and ability to implement the program based on other job duties), and the program's compatibility with school needs. They also listed broader factors related to leadership at the individual school and school district levels, external environment (e.g., policy and procedural support at the school district level and support from parents and the community), and availability of resources needed to deliver the program (Bosworth et al. 1999). Roberts-Gray et al. (2007) used these factors to assess the implementation success of the Texas Tobacco Prevention Initiative in 47 schools. Aggregated scores for the eight capacity factors predicted the quality of program adherence and the quantity of program activities implemented. Thus, this type of assessment may be helpful in evaluating the likelihood of program success in specific schools.

10.3.4   Collaborating with Schools on Intervention Selection and Development

Another issue related to selecting a specific intervention concerns how best to involve teachers, school administrators, and other key stakeholders in the decision-making process. Their active involvement is often key to obtaining support for program implementation. They may also have valuable insights into what may or may not meet the needs of their school, and the degree to which specific programs are feasible and acceptable to the community. Although actively involving teachers and administrators in intervention development and implementation planning can increase their buy-in, it can also pose some difficulties. There are numerous examples in the literature of well-intentioned, intuitively appealing prevention efforts that have ultimately been found to have limited effects, or in some cases negative effects

(Dishion et al. 1999). Many programs such as Drug Abuse Resistance Education (D.A.R.E.), Scared Straight, and boot camps continue to have widespread support despite evidence questioning their effectiveness (U.S. Surgeon General 2001). This underscores the need to involve key stakeholders in intervention selection where possible, but to limit choices to intervention strategies with research support for their effectiveness (Hawkins et al. 2012).

As this section illustrates, the process of program development and adoption requires considerable effort to ensure that it leads to a carefully developed intervention plan. This plan must begin with a careful consideration of the goals and characteristics of the settings where the intervention will be implemented, including information regarding the factors responsible for maintaining the problem being addressed. As we noted, the selection of an intervention requires identifying complementary components that have potential to accomplish these goals. Finally, the potential for success will also depend on the school's capacity to implement the program successfully. Case study 1 describes a collaborative adoption process whereby specific school needs were matched to evidence-based programming in order to maximize the likelihood of program effectiveness.

Case Study 1: Concept Mapping

This case study illustrates the use of a concept-mapping approach to involve key stakeholders in the identification of relevant issues related to youth violence prevention programs. The information gathered informed the intervention approach for a research project that focused on developing and testing the feasibility of a middle school violence prevention program for youth with and without disabilities (Sullivan et al. 2013). In the planning phase of this research project, concept mapping was used to identify the needs related to youth violence prevention at participating middle schools. Concept mapping, which has been promoted as a useful participatory research method for program planning, encompasses multiple steps: (a) brainstorming project-relevant ideas; (b) sorting and rating ideas based on similarity, importance, and feasibility; (c) visually representing stakeholders' ideas in the form of a concept map; (d) interpreting the map; and (e) utilizing the map for project planning (Trochim 1989).

The first component of the concept-mapping process involved a brainstorming activity where stakeholders were asked to generate goals for the project by listing statements in response to the open-ended prompt: "An important goal for school-based violence prevention programs for middle school students is...." A total of 57 adults participated, including middle school teachers, administrators, other school staff, researchers, community workers, parents, a school board member, and 16 middle school students with and without disabilities. Adult participants were given the option of completing brainstorming activities anonymously using a web-based concept-mapping program

(Concept Systems Incorporated) or completing a paper-and-pencil version of the activity. Students completed the paper-and-pencil version. This task generated 245 goals. Combining similar responses and eliminating redundant responses reduced the final number of goals to 85.

During the second stage of the project, 22 school staff, including some who had participated in the brainstorming activity, sorted the 85 goals into piles they thought were similar or related and rated each goal's importance and feasibility on a five-point scale where higher scores indicated greater importance or feasibility. A concept map was then generated based on participants' responses to the brainstorming and sorting and rating tasks. The concept map was a two-dimensional scatter plot of goals, where those that were closer together were considered more similar. Procedures described in previous research (e.g., Sutherland and Katz 2005; Trochim 1989) were then used to identify clusters that represented similar sets of goals. This led to the identification of eight discrete clusters of goals that related to (a) coping and conflict resolution skills, effective nonviolent alternatives, and problem recognition; (b) educating students about different forms of violence and teaching social skills/anger management; (c) safety, positive development, and specific aspects of violence prevention programs; (d) school policies and school climate and physical environment; (e) role models and mentors, outside influences on student behavior, and student engagement at school and in the community; (f) citizenship and relationships; (g) interdependence among the school, parents, and students, positive relationships between school staff and students, and strategies for teachers; and (h) community and parent involvement. Participants rated goals in the last cluster (community and parent involvement) as the most difficult to address.

Final clusters and cluster maps were then presented to the stakeholders involved in the concept-mapping process in order to facilitate the interpretation of the results and ensure their accuracy. Focus groups were also conducted to identify the potential supports and challenges to implementing program goals in the participating schools. Discussion centered on several topics that were useful in the assessment of each school's capacity and readiness for program implementation, including aspects of the school climate, resources, effective teaching methods, and parental support. Themes such as parent and community involvement, school climate, and students' social and emotional development echoed researchers' thoughts that prevention programs should address risk behaviors at multiple levels of the school ecology and in multiple settings (Nation et al. 2003).

This concept-mapping project was a first step toward engaging principal stakeholders in the selection of an intervention approach for middle school violence prevention. Ultimately, the ideas generated during this process were used to determine important and feasible areas for intervention. Taken together, the results suggested that the prevention program should address both the school environment and the individual student level related to skill building in areas such as problem-solving, emotion management, and communication. This resulted in the implementation of combined violence prevention programs that addressed multiple levels of the school environment (i.e., Olweus Bullying Prevention Program; Olweus 2004) and specific areas of individual-level skill building (i.e., Second Step: Student Success Through Prevention; Committee for Children 2008).

10.4   Implementation Phase

Having identified an appropriate intervention approach, the next step involves its implementation. *Implementation* is defined as the set of activities designed to put a program into practice in an organization such as a school (Forman et al. 2013). The goal of this phase is to have all components of an evidence-based program in place and integrated into practice, organizational and community structures, and policies. There are a myriad of interconnected aspects to implementing a new school-based prevention program, such as the capacity and culture of the school and the ongoing skill development of implementers (e.g., teachers; Fixsen et al. 2005). The unique interplay between practitioners' fear of change, their investment in the status quo, and the complexities of a particular environment create a tenuous context for implementation, particularly when implementing a new program.

Berkel et al. (2011) proposed a working model of prevention that highlights the relations between several dimensions of implementation and desirable outcomes among youths. To illustrate, they argued that the behaviors of program implementers (e.g., teachers) as they implement and adapt core components are associated with the behaviors of participants (e.g., students), such as attendance and engagement. From their perspective, a critical aspect of implementation research is how programs promote high levels of youth engagement, and how this engagement mediates program effectiveness. This model highlights the importance of both high-quality training and ongoing support for implementers (e.g., coaching of teachers, performance feedback), which can increase the likelihood of high-quality implementation as well as implementers using instructional behaviors associated with youth engagement (Aarons et al. 2010; Conroy et al. 2009; Domitrovich et al. 2012; Dunst and Trivette 2012; Fixsen et al. 2005; Vo et al. 2012).

One critical factor related to the successful implementation of a school-based intervention is getting the full support and cooperation of teachers and administrators. School staff members must perceive the need for the innovation before they will implement it (Gottfredson 2001). As previously noted, most schools have a history of implementing a variety of different prevention strategies (Gottfredson and Gottfredson 2001), which may not always have involved evidence-based interventions or been implemented with sufficient dosage or fidelity to produce their desired effects (Gottfredson and Gottfredson 2002). A long history of limited success may lead teachers and administrators to be quite skeptical that the next strategy they attempt will be any more successful. This may make it difficult to generate the degree of enthusiasm, support, and cooperation needed for successful implementation. It may also create negative expectations for success.

Efforts to obtain teacher and school administrator support for prevention programming are often hampered by the practice of having outside staff implement prevention programs. The use of outside interventionists under the direct control and supervision of researchers may increase the likelihood that an intervention will be conducted with fidelity. However, it also decreases the involvement of teachers and other key staff. Teachers play a critical role in the climate of a school, and their interactions with students and with each other provide opportunities for them to model the skills targeted by many intervention programs. Using outside interventionists may limit teachers' support for the intervention and the degree to which it is infused into the curriculum and other aspects of the school. One example of how interventions can increase the involvement of teachers and administrators is provided by the Olweus Bullying Prevention Program (Olweus 2004), which establishes a Bullying Prevention Coordinating Committee composed of teachers, administrators, and other school staff. In the research project discussed in case study 2, this committee receives performance-based feedback regarding teachers' adherence to and competence with intervention delivery, and based on this feedback they identify areas for improvement (and positive reinforcement for implementation successes).

Another factor related to successful implementation concerns the extent to which teachers and administrators feel that they "own" the intervention. Schools, particularly those located near a university, may have a history of researchers coming into the school to implement an intervention, collecting data, and disappearing when the project ends. Teachers may question the extent to which those outsiders, regardless of their academic credentials, have a clear understanding of their school and the issues students and teachers face. They may also feel disrespected if their opinions are not actively sought. Although their knowledge and insights may be of value in tailoring an intervention to meet the specific needs of a school, involving teachers and school staff in tailoring intervention strategies may be challenging. Adapting an intervention requires a clear understanding of which aspects must be implemented with fidelity and which can be modified to be more culturally or contextually appropriate to specific groups of students, or to meet practical constraints such as class schedules (Meyer et al. 2000). Whereas adaptations have historically been viewed as deviations from program core components that threaten internal validity, more recent work has focused upon how thoughtful adaptations may strengthen the effectiveness of prevention programs (Durlak and DuPre 2008; Fixsen et al. 2005; Forman et al. 2013). In their review of implementation research, Durlak and DuPre (2008) reported that of three studies assessing program adaptation, all found adaptation had a positive effect on outcomes. However, without strong measures of treatment fidelity, the core components of prevention programs cannot be measured, limiting our ability to identify effective versus harmful adaptations. Thus, an important focus in implementation research must be the monitoring of fidelity to the prevention program in order to assess adaptations in the school context (Bopp et al. 2013).

Providing quality training is critical to the success of a prevention program, regardless of whether researchers or school staff are responsible for implementation. High-quality training has been associated with better program implementation (Durlak and DuPre 2008). Research suggests that professional development in the form of one-time training does not result in proficient delivery of practices in authentic settings (Becker and Domitrovich 2011; Sholomskas et al. 2005), highlighting the need for implementers to receive ongoing coaching and performance feedback (Vo et al. 2012). A large literature suggests that coaching strategies such as collaborative decision-making, modeling, observation and performance feedback, and opportunities to problem solve enhance and sustain teacher delivery of prevention components (Han and Weiss 2005; Reinke et al. 2009; Reyes et al. 2012). Forman et al. (2013) noted that multiple models of implementation emphasize the importance of not only developing competent implementers (training and coaching) but also rewarding implementation and providing feedback to implementers on the process of implementation (e.g., fidelity) as well as program outcomes.

Ensuring that prevention programs are implemented as intended increases the likelihood that they will produce positive outcomes (Hulleman et al. 2013). *Treatment fidelity,* referring to the degree to which a program is delivered as intended, has three components—treatment adherence, treatment differentiation, and competence (McLeod et al. 2009). As it relates to prevention programs delivered in schools by teachers, *treatment adherence* refers to the extent to which the teacher delivers the program as designed (i.e., prescribed practices). *Treatment differentiation* refers to the extent to which treatments being implemented differ along appropriate lines defined by the treatment protocol (e.g., do not have protocol violations). Finally, *competence* refers to the level of skill and degree of responsiveness the teacher demonstrates when delivering the evidence-based instructional practices prescribed by the protocol. Each component captures a unique aspect of treatment fidelity that is important to assess in prevention research (Carroll and Nuro 2002).

A number of factors within schools can influence implementation fidelity, including the diverse training backgrounds of teachers (Kam et al. 2003), level of teacher training (Pianta and Rimm-Kaufman 2006), and resource restrictions (Domitrovich et al. 2010). More proximal factors associated with teacher and student behavior, such as teacher relationships with students and level of student involvement in classroom activities, may also influence outcomes. Indeed, prevention programs will not be effective if youths do not bond with teachers or actively participate in classroom activities (McLeod et al. 2009). It is plausible that such contextual factors may influence fidelity and thereby outcomes, so it is critical to assess implementation fidelity during the implementation phase.

Because a key part of implementation involves training and supervising teachers to deliver the instructional practices specified for a prevention program, ascertaining the extent to which these practices are delivered according to the treatment protocol is of critical importance (Sutherland et al. in press). Doing so requires assessing all three treatment fidelity components (McLeod et al. 2013). Indeed, it is necessary to assess implementation fidelity so that researchers can determine whether any "failure" to produce a desired outcome is due to the prevention program or its implementation. If it is due to the program (i.e., implementation is sufficient), this implies the need to adapt the program or select an alternative. In contrast, if the program was not appropriately implemented, this suggests the need for improvements in teacher training and support. Fidelity measurement of a prevention program may also assist researchers in identifying the components of an intervention that are most related to desirable outcomes, allowing for more efficient delivery. In addition, identifying the core components of a prevention program may assist in identifying those components that are amenable to adaptation, increasing the acceptability of the program. Unfortunately, the science and measurement of treatment fidelity is underdeveloped in school-based prevention (Sanetti and Kratochwill 2009). Most studies focus on adherence, which leaves competence of delivery and treatment differentiation largely unstudied (Sanetti and Fallon 2011).

The measurement of treatment fidelity is clearly important during implementation, and researchers and program purveyors strive for the highest levels of implementation fidelity possible. At the same time, full implementation is often not a realistic goal, and research has suggested that implementation fidelity ranging from 60 to 80% is associated with positive youth outcomes (Durlak and DuPre 2008). Thus, whereas new implementers can present challenges, particularly ones associated with the fidelity of implementation, they can also present unique opportunities to innovate and refine practices based upon school and programmatic needs (Fixsen et al. 2005). Several researchers (Dissemination Working Group 1999; Fixsen et al. 2005; Winter and Szulanski 2001) recommended innovation after full implementation with fidelity in order not to "escape the scrutiny of fidelity" (Fixsen et al. 2005, p. 17), noting that at some point if innovations to implementation are significant, they may warrant future scientific study. At the same time, the ability to innovate may enhance program acceptance, and if researchers have clearly identified the core components of their program that require implementation with fidelity, practitioners may feel some freedom to adapt a particular evidence-based program to their context without compromising the fidelity of implementation (Durlak 2010; Harn et al. 2013). In the next section, a case study of an ongoing research project is used to illustrate how adaptation and performance-based feedback provided to schools implementing the Olweus Bullying Prevention Program (Olweus 2004) are used to maintain and improve the fidelity of implementation of classroom meetings by teachers.

Case Study 2: Implementing the Olweus Bullying Prevention Program

The Olweus Bullying Prevention Program attempts to create a positive learning environment by addressing bullying behavior at the school-wide, classroom, and individual levels. Key components include staff development and the formation of a Bullying Prevention Coordinating Committee whose task it is to enhance school safety through monitoring and overseeing positive changes to the school environment and the application of school rules. The classroom component consists of weekly classroom meetings, where students and teachers engage in discussion and activities related to preventing bullying behavior.

The first six classroom meetings are scripted in order to provide structure around establishing school-wide rules and program expectations. Beyond these six meetings, teachers are expected to discuss bullying-related topics in the classroom meetings, but specific scripted meetings are not provided. A large number of teachers in the two middle schools in this case preferred more structured guides for classroom meetings, so we worked in partnership with teachers to identify relevant topics (e.g., problem-solving, emotional regulation, cyberbullying) then created meeting plans to address these. Teachers used their knowledge of their students and school culture to assist us in enhancing the cultural relevance of these meetings by adapting role plays, examples, and language. Such activities integrated the teachers as stakeholders in the adaptation process (Domenech-Rodriquez et al. 2011) and are in line with recommendations to make programs more culturally relevant (Bernal et al. 1995; Nation et al. 2003). Research also suggests that local adaptations may enhance the sustainability of intervention programs (Berkel et al. 2011; Rogers 2003).

Because teachers conduct the classroom meetings, measuring the extent to which these meetings are delivered according to the meeting plans is of critical importance for monitoring implementation fidelity. Thus, we assess both the adherence and competence of teacher delivery of classroom meetings as well as more general teacher instructional practices (e.g., providing youth with opportunities to respond, reinforcement procedures) and student engagement. Becker and Domitrovich (2011) have pointed out that although researchers collect data on treatment fidelity and program implementation, they typically do not share these data with the school where they are collected. We address this concern by collecting data on implementation fidelity on a weekly basis in at least 20 % of the classrooms implementing the Olweus program, and using these data to inform implementation procedures at the schools. Observational data are compiled and shared with each school's Bullying Prevention Coordinating Committee, which is made up of teachers, administrators, parents, and university partners. These presentations highlight both successes (e.g., improvements in teachers providing feedback to students) and areas for improvement (e.g., low rates of teacher reinforcement) while focusing on the links between teacher behaviors and youth engagement during the classroom meetings. In addition, twice a year these data are compiled and shared with the entire school faculty, again highlighting both strengths of program delivery and areas for improvement.

The work of the Bullying Prevention Coordinating Committee at each school, and the ongoing support and collaboration with university partners in this process, has promise for increasing the likelihood of both high-quality implementation and sustainability of the program.

The amount of time it takes to move from adoption to quality implementation of a major school-wide reform has not yet been established, with estimates ranging from a minimum of 1 year (e.g., Fixsen et al. 2005) to at least 3 years (e.g., Felner et al. 2001). Our use of a multiple baseline design provides a rare opportunity to examine changes in implementation fidelity over the course of the project. Our design involves implementing the intervention in three different schools but uses randomization to determine when intervention activities are initiated at each school. Following a year of baseline data collection, intervention implementation was started at school A in year 2 of the project and at school B in year 3; implementation will begin in school C at the end of the final year of the project. We are also engaged in efforts to sustain intervention activities at the conclusion of the project. This design allows us to examine changes related to implementation across school years. We are also able to benefit from our experience implementing the intervention at school A as we work with schools B then C.

Fidelity data from the first 2 years of our project provide some insight into the implementation of the Olweus program. At school A, adherence and competence both increased modestly from year 1 to year 2 and mean scores fell in the acceptable range. These data suggest that teachers are implementing the program in Year 2 at least as extensively and competently as they did in Year 1. Comparing competence data for the first year of implementation in school B with those for the second year of implementation in school A reveals that almost all time points for both schools were in the acceptable to excellent range. At school A, some increases in competence of delivery occurred over time, perhaps reflective of the teachers' experience in implementing the program the previous year, their approval of adaptations to classroom meetings made in the previous year, ongoing fidelity monitoring, or some combination thereof. Meanwhile, teachers in school B were energized about the program at the beginning of their first year of implementation. Interestingly, both schools have some fluctuations in competence that merit further examination to potentially link them with events and other activities going on in the schools. Our long-term goal is to use the ongoing data to plan for sustainability.

10.5   Sustainability

In the health promotion intervention life cycle, a critical point for many prevention programs is the time frame after implementation. At this point, the program may be sustained and move toward being institutionalized within a school or, as is more often the case, terminated and sometimes replaced by a new program (Bopp et al. 2013). Although the successful implementation of evidence-based prevention programs has great value, the ultimate goal is their sustainability in schools. *Sustain-*

ability is the ability to maintain and support the long-term survival and effectiveness of an evidence-based program at a particular intervention site (Fixsen et al. 2005). Ensuring that intervention activities will continue beyond the end of a research project requires that sustainability be considered from the onset through each phase of the project. Some of the issues we highlighted in the sections on program development and adoption (e.g., ensuring the program meets the school's needs and garnering program support) and implementation (e.g., providing ongoing training and coaching and tailoring the program as allowable to be more relevant for students and staff) enhance the likelihood of sustainability. Bopp et al. (2013) identified factors that promote sustainability, including characteristics of the prevention program, its implementers, and the implementation process, as well as the organization's general capacity and support for the program. In this section, we first present concerns related to difficulties in sustaining school-based prevention programs, then review factors that may promote sustainability in more detail.

The sustainability of prevention programs delivered in schools is a concern of prevention researchers and practitioners (Fixsen et al. 2009; Han and Weiss 2005; Reyes et al. 2012). Whereas there is substantial evidence that school-based prevention can have positive effects on students' academic and behavioral functioning (e.g., Durlak et al. 2011), the degree to which school-based implementers (e.g., teachers and other school personnel) can sustain high-quality implementation remains an open and vexing question. Fixsen et al. (2009) pointed out that efforts to implement evidence-based programs over the past two decades suggest that "research results are not being used with sufficient quantity and quality to impact human services and, therefore, have not provided the intended benefits to consumers and communities" (p. 531).

Several overarching factors influence the sustainability of school-based prevention programs. At the macro level, the availability of resources and the priorities and policies of the school district, which are influenced by resources and priorities at the state and federal levels, impact the agenda for prevention programs (Han and Weiss 2005). At the school level, some indicators of sustainability can be found by examining a school's general capacity (Halgunseth et al. 2012). The life span of a prevention program is influenced by the school's overall management, leadership, and organizational structure as well as administrative policies within the school that support the program and the availability of resources needed to sustain it (Flaspohler et al. 2008; Johnson et al. 2004). For grant-funded prevention programs, a resource gap often exists in that the resources available to initiate the program during the life cycle of the grant exceed those that remain after the grant ends. As Gottfredson (2001) noted, "Programs operated as part of research endeavors are generally implemented under unusual conditions" (p. 232).

A key concern for sustainability is ensuring that a program will continue to be implemented at the required level of fidelity, as in a national survey Gottfredson and Gottfredson (2002) found that the quality of school-based prevention practices implemented in the typical school was generally low. Their analysis of correlates of prevention quality suggested that implementation could be improved through better integration of prevention activities into school operations; more extensive local planning and involvement in selecting interventions; stronger organizational support in terms of high-quality training, supervision, and principal support; and use of more standardized program materials and methods.

Factors related to a particular school-based prevention program may also influence its sustainability. Universal programs aimed at changing the school environment generally have a framework that supports their integration into school operations, which can facilitate sustainability (Olweus 2004). Clearly, the degree to which the program is high quality, effective, and congruent with school needs and goals plays a role in sustainability. In addition, the presence of a school champion for the program and its perceived support by the principal are critical. In particular, school staff may use the principal's support as a gauge of the program's priority within the school; whether they will be held accountable for its implementation; and whether sufficient resources, time, and energy will be devoted to it both during the initial implementation and in the future (Han and Weiss 2005). One challenge is that interventions often must be in place for some time before they produce their intended effects. School climate is usually well established and somewhat resistant to change. Prevention programs targeted across multiple grade levels may need to be implemented for several years before effects on school climate are realized, allowing new students to enter a school in which the majority of students in older grades have participated in previous years of the intervention. Unfortunately, teachers and administrators may lose patience waiting to see signs of success and may be tempted to try something different. This has led to some school systems adopting a new program(s) in lieu of or in addition to existing programs.

Similar to the implementation phase, the extent to which the prevention program allows for adaptations can have implications for whether it is accepted by school staff and sustained by a school. Given that greater resources often exist when a prevention program is initially implemented than in subsequent years, adaptations that enhance the feasibility of continued implementation without damaging the integrity of the intervention are important. In fact, implementation research suggests that when programs are adapted locally, they may have a greater likelihood of being sustained (Berkel et al. 2011; Rogers 2003). Ensuring that program adaptations do not detract from the integrity of the intervention and monitoring program fidelity on an ongoing basis are critical if the prevention program is to maintain its evidence-based status as it is sustained in the school context (Aarons et al. 2010; Domitrovich et al. 2012). Moreover, researchers must have sustainability in mind as they develop and test prevention programs. The early identification of core components, development of fidelity measures that assess the adherence to and competence of delivery of core components, and assessment of adaptations (either through direct observations or via teacher focus groups) are all critically important to developing prevention programs that have a higher than average likelihood of sustainability.

Implementer characteristics—including attitudes toward the intervention, teaching ability, self-efficacy, commitment and motivation to change, and perceptions of program benefits—may also influence the sustainability of a prevention program. Initiating and maintaining ongoing collaborative work with teachers and other school personnel to ensure that prevention programs are feasible and acceptable can lead to greater implementation and sustainability. Prevention researchers have emphasized that if evidence-based prevention programs are to be delivered by teachers effectively, feedback from teachers should be used to address potential resistance to implementation. Such feedback can be incorporated into the design of program content as well as implementation of instructional practices (Becker et al. 2009; Greenberg et al. 2003). In addition, the ongoing measurement of treatment fidelity at multiple levels, such as training, delivery, coaching, and teacher implementation (adherence and competence of delivery) can assist in both planning for sustainability as well as making the program more flexible and adaptable. As Becker and Domitrovich (2011) note, researchers collect data on treatment fidelity and program implementation but typically do not share these data with the school in which they are collecting the data. By collecting fidelity data on a regular basis and using these data to inform implementation procedures, researchers can facilitate both the iterative development process and adaptations, with the ultimate goal of increasing program sustainability.

Johnson et al. (2004) emphasize that sustainability planning is an iterative process that continues over the life span of a prevention program. They identified two building blocks for sustainability; namely, ensuring that (a) the organization builds the infrastructure capacity to sustain the prevention program and (b) the program continues to meet shareholder needs, be implemented with fidelity, and maintain its effectiveness. They detailed five sustainability actions: assessing the organization's infrastructure capacity and readiness for the prevention program; developing a sustainability plan to target issues related to capacity and readiness; and executing, evaluating, and revising this plan as needed. These sustainability actions then lead to the proximal outcome of "sustainability readiness" and distal outcomes in terms of benefits for students and school staff when effective and relevant programs are well integrated within the organizational structure. Case study 3 describes efforts to increase the implementation fidelity, and subsequently the sustainability, of a program designed to prevent the development of emotional and behavioral disorders in young, high-risk children.

The last case study describes the BEST in CLASS project to exemplify issues of implementation and sustainability. Recall that BEST in CLASS is a secondary-level intervention that targets problem behaviors in preschool children at risk for emotional and behavioral disorders.

Case Study 3: Implementing BEST in CLASS for Sustainability

Teachers are trained to deliver BEST in CLASS through a 6-h professional development workshop and 14 weeks of performance-based coaching provided by trained coaches (see Vo et al. 2012, for a description of the program development process). Both training and coaching focus on eight learning modules: (a) Basics of Behavior and Development, (b) Rules, Expectations and Routines, (c) Behavior-Specific Praise, (d) Pre-correction and Active

Supervision, (e) Opportunities to Respond and Instructional Pacing, (f) Instructive and Corrective Feedback, (g) Home–School Communication, and (h) Linking and Mastery. The efficacy of BEST in CLASS is currently being investigated in a multisite randomized controlled trial, and preliminary data suggest that the program had an impact on observed teacher instructional and child behaviors (Conroy et al. 2013) and on standardized measures of child behavior (Vo et al. 2012).

BEST in CLASS was developed with an eye toward sustainability. Specifically, program administrators initially approached university researchers for assistance with an increasing number of young children arriving in preschool with high rates of problem behavior. Through a collaborative process, BEST in CLASS was developed with feasibility of implementation in mind. Accordingly, teachers deliver evidence-based instructional practices (i.e., core components) during their classroom instructional activities. Program development was guided by an iterative process (see Vo et al. 2012, for a description) wherein teachers implemented aspects of the program; direct observations of implementation were conducted focusing on adaptations, adherence, and competence of delivery; and focus groups were held to identify barriers and supports to program delivery.

In order to plan for implementation, BEST in CLASS was developed according to a consultation model. Existing literature and data collected during the development project (e.g., focus groups with teachers) guided development of a structured, practice-based coaching model whereby coaches provided teachers with weekly performance feedback on their implementation. In addition, observations and focus groups with teachers and coaches led to adaptations in both component delivery and coaching, adaptations which were integrated into training materials and procedures. These adaptations are in line with implementation literature which suggests that incorporating the knowledge program providers (e.g., teachers, program administrators) have about their particular context can lead to innovations that improve intervention (Durlak and DuPre 2008) and in turn increase the likelihood of sustainability (Berkel et al. 2011; Rogers 2003).

The identification of core program components also contributed to the development of a fidelity measure, the BEST in CLASS Adherence and Competence Scale (BiCACS; Sutherland et al. in press). This direct observational tool assesses the extensiveness (adherence) and quality (competence) of delivery of each of the eight core components of BEST in CLASS using a Likert-type scale. Two additional items (child responsiveness; engagement) assess children's responses to the program components. The BiCACS was found to have promising reliability and validity in an initial psychometric study (Sutherland et al. in press). This is important (and novel) as researchers have highlighted the need for reliable measures of integrity to advance the science of prevention (Durlak 2010; Sanetti and Kratochwill 2009; Wolery 2011).

The use of a rating scale rather than dichotomous checklists for the BiCACS allows for variation in fidelity measurement. As Durlak and DuPre (2008) noted, dichotomous designations of implementation (e.g., high vs low) are arbitrary and do not capture variations in implementation that may be useful in identifying the core components in a prevention program and measuring variations in competence and adherence over time, which can inform teacher training efforts.

In the efficacy trial, observers used the BiCACS to assess the use of the core components of BEST in CLASS in both treatment and comparison classrooms from baseline until maintenance (1 month after coaching ends). Posthoc analyses indicated no difference for adherence ratings between groups at pretreatment. In contrast, there were significant differences in adherence and competence ratings favoring the BEST in CLASS group at both posttreatment and maintenance. In addition, the comparison group showed no differences between phases across time for either adherence or competence.

In summary, the development and ongoing adaptation of BEST in CLASS, particularly during the project phase, resulted in a program designed in collaboration with teachers and program administrators that has promise for quality implementation and long-term sustainability. Initial data from the efficacy trial suggest that teachers implemented the program with increasing adherence and competence across time, and the use of an observational integrity tool, the BiCACS, with promising psychometrics to measure implementation fidelity has much potential for determining the core components of the program.

10.6   Conclusion

Schools represent a key context for youths' social, emotional, and academic development and are a natural fit for prevention programs that seek to strengthen these areas of development, thereby decreasing the incidence of problem behaviors. Strong partnerships between researchers and school staff are essential for the effective implementation of evidence-based programs. Prior to program implementation, it is important for researchers to identify the prevalence of the problem behavior in the target school population and the constellation of risk and protective factors that influence it. A thorough understanding of these risk and protective factors can then guide the selection of the evidence-based program or programs that most effectively target them. The school's readiness to implement the prevention program must also be considered. In this regard, the fit between the prevention program and the school's general capacity in terms of its organizational structure, mission, goals, and staff "buy-in" or support for the program should be addressed. Overall, it is essential that the prevention program meet the school's needs by (a) effectively targeting the risk behavior and (b) being feasible to implement.

During implementation, an understanding of which are the core components of the prevention program that must be implemented to preserve its integrity and which can be adapted to make the program more relevant and feasible to implement is needed. Program adaptations that maintain a program's integrity have been shown to enhance the likelihood of desired outcomes. However, the collection of fidelity data is necessary to ensure that these adaptations are well documented and do not alter the implementation of the program's core components. The benefits of prevention programs in mitigating serious negative outcomes for youth are well worth the trade-off in energy, time, and money spent on their implementation. However, unless researchers and school staff can improve the sustainability of these programs in schools, their true capacity to benefit youth over the course of development may remain unknown.

It is again worth emphasizing that schools are dynamic entities containing heterogeneous student populations embedded within diverse community contexts. Therefore, the process of implementing interventions within schools is necessarily iterative to meet the numerous needs extant in an individual school. Although many promising prevention programs have been developed (U.S. Surgeon General 2001), there is considerable room for improvement. The best of our current programs are based on an incomplete understanding of the myriad risk factors that influence and maintain problem behaviors in school-aged youth and of potential promotive and protective factors that could enhance their positive development (Farrell and Vulin-Reynolds 2007). Further progress in identifying these factors will guide the development of more effective prevention strategies. Further work is also needed to improve the effectiveness and efficiency of delivery of current interventions. There is growing evidence to suggest that the effectiveness of many school-based interventions varies across individuals, schools, and settings (Farrell et al. 2013). This implies a need to tailor interventions to best meet the needs of a target population. Unfortunately, we currently have limited information to determine which aspects of interventions can be adapted without reducing their impact. Finally, the dissemination of interventions and their sustainability continue to pose major challenges (Forman et al. 2013). Considerable efforts are needed to ensure that schools are able to devote their limited resources to programs that have the greatest likelihood of effectiveness, to implement these programs with sufficient integrity to ensure that they produce their intended effects, and to sustain quality implementation with their available resources. These efforts will require a sustained iterative effort whereby interventions are continuously (a) developed to address emerging information about the nature of the problem being targeted and the factors that maintain it, (b) evaluated to determine their impact and the conditions under which they are effective, and (c) disseminated to establish the factors that facilitate their widespread implementation (Gottfredson 1984).

References

Aarons, G. A., Glisson, C., Hoagwood, K., Kelleher, K., Landsverk, J., & Cafri, G. (2010). Psychometric properties and U.S. national norms of the Evidence-Based Practice Attitude Scale (EBPAS). *Psychological Assessment, 22*(2), 356–365. doi:10.1037/a0019188

Becker, K. D., & Domitrovich, C. E. (2011). The conceptualization, integration, and support of evidence-based interventions in the schools. *School Psychology Review, 40*(4), 582–589.

Becker, K. D., Nakamura, B., Young, J., & Chorpita, B. (2009). What better place than here? What better time than now? ABCT's burgeoning role in the dissemination and implementation of evidence-based practices. *Behavior Therapist, 32*(5), 89–96.

Berkel, C., Mauricio, A., Schoenfelder, E., & Sandler, I. (2011). Putting the pieces together: An integrated model of program implementation. *Prevention Sciences, 12*(1), 23–33. doi:10.1007/s11121-010-0186-1

Bernal, G., Bonilla, J., & Bellido, C. (1995). Ecological validity and cultural sensitivity for outcome research: Issues for the cultural adaptation and development of psychosocial treatments with Hispanics. *Journal of Abnormal Child Psychology, 23*(1), 67–82. doi:10.1007/BF01447045

Bopp, M., Saunders, R. P., & Lattimore, D. L. (2013). The tug-of-war: fidelity versus adaptation throughout the health promotion program life cycle. *Journal of Primary Prevention, 34*(3), 193–207. doi:10.1007/s10935-013-0299-y

Bosworth, K., Gingiss, P., Potthoff, S., & Roberts-Gray, C. (1999). A Bayesian model to predict the success of the implementation of a health education innovation. *Evaluation & Program Planning, 22*(1), 1–11.

Botvin, G. J., & Tortu, S. (1988). Preventing adolescent substance abuse through life skills training. In R. H. Price, E. L. Cowen, R. P. Lorion, & J. R. McKay (Eds.), *Fourteen ounces of prevention: A casebook for practitioners* (pp. 98–110). Washington, DC: American Psychological Association.

Botvin, G. J., Griffin, K. W., & Nichols, T. D. (2006). Preventing youth violence and delinquency through a universal school-based prevention approach. *Prevention Science, 7*(4), 403–408. doi:10.1007/s11121-006-0057-y

Carroll, K. M., & Nuro, K. F. (2002). One size cannot fit all: A stage model for psychotherapy manual development. *Clinical Psychology: Science & Practice, 9*(4), 396–406. doi:10.1093/clipsy.9.4.396

Centers for Disease Control and Prevention. (2011). *Web-based injury statistics query and reporting system (WISQARS)*. Atlanta: National Center for Injury Prevention and Control. http://www.cdc.gov/injury/wisqars/index.html.

Coie, J. D., Watt, N. F., West, S. G., Hawkins, J. D., Asarnow, J. R., Markman, H. J., Ramey, S. L., Shure, M. B., & Long, B. (1993). The science of prevention: A conceptual framework and some directions for a national research program. *American Psychologist, 48*(10), 1013–1022. doi:10.1037/0003-066X.48.10.1013

Committee for Children. (2008). *Second Step: Student success through prevention program*. Seattle: Author.

Conroy, M. A., Sutherland, K. S., Haydon, T., Stormont, M., & Harmon, J. (2009). Preventing and ameliorating young children's chronic problem behaviors: An ecological classroom-based approach. *Psychology in the Schools, 46*(1), 3–17. doi:10.1002/pits.20350

Conroy, M. A., Sutherland, K. S., Vo, A., Carr, S. E., & Ogston, P. (2013). Early childhood teachers' use of effective instructional practices and the collateral effects on young children's behavior. *Journal of Positive Behavioral Interventions*. doi:10.1177/1098300713478666

Dishion, T. J., McCord, J., & Poulin, F. (1999). When interventions harm: Peer groups and problem behavior. *American Psychologist, 54*(9), 755–764. doi:10.1037/0003-066X.54.9.755

Dissemination Working Group. (1999). *Common elements of developing and implementing program models*. Calgary: FYI Consulting, Ltd.

Domenech Rodriguez, M. M., Baumann, A., & Schwartz, A. (2011). Cultural adaptation of an empirically supported intervention: From theory to practice in a Latino/a community context. *American Journal of Community Psychology, 47*(1–2), 170–186. doi:10.1007/s10464-010-9371-4

Domitrovich, C. E., Bradshaw, C. P., Greenberg, M. T., Embry, D., Poduska, J. M., & Ialongo, N. S. (2010). Integrated models of school-based prevention: Logic and theory. *Psychology in the Schools, 47*(1), 71–88. doi:10.1002/pits.20452

Domitrovich, C. E., Moore, J. E., & Greenberg, M. T. (2012). Maximizing the effectiveness of social-emotional interventions for young children through high-quality implementation of evidence-based interventions. In B. Kelly & D. F. Perkins (Eds.), *Handbook of implementation science for psychology in education* (pp. 207–229). Cambridge: Cambridge University Press.

Dunst, C. J., & Trivette, C. M. (2012). Meta-analysis of implementation practice research. In B. Kelly & D. F. Perkins (Eds.), *Handbook of implementation science for psychology and education* (pp. 68–91). Cambridge: Cambridge University Press.

Durlak, J. (2010). The importance of doing well in whatever you do: A commentary on the special section: "Implementation research in early childhood education." *Early Childhood Research Quarterly, 25*(3), 348–357.

Durlak, J. A, & DuPre, E. P. (2008). Implementation matters: A review of research on the influence of implementation on program outcomes and the factors affecting implementation. *American Journal of Community Psychology, 41*(3–4), 327–350. doi:10.1007/s10464-008-9165-0

Durlak, J. A., Weissberg, R. P., Dymnicki, A. B., Taylor, R. D., & Schellinger, K. B. (2011). The impact of enhancing students' social and emotional learning: A meta-analysis of school-based universal interventions. *Child Development, 82*(1), 405–432. doi:10.1111/j.1467-8624.2010.01564.x

Embry, D. D. (2003). *PAX Good Behavior teacher's guide.* Center City: Hazelden.

Embry, D. D., Flannery, D. J., Vazsonyi, A. T., Powell, K. E., & Atha, H. (1996). PeaceBuilders: A theoretically driven, school-based model for early violence prevention. *American Journal of Preventive Medicine, 12,* 91–100.

Espelage, D. L., Low, S., Polanin, J. R., & Brown, E. C. (2013). The impact of a middle school program to reduce aggression, victimization, and sexual violence. *Journal of Adolescent Health, 53*(2), 180–186. doi:10.1016/j.jadohealth.2013.02.021

Fagan, J., & Wilkinson, D. (1998). Social contexts and functions of adolescent violence. In D. Elliott, B. Hamburg, & K. Williams (Eds.), *Violence in American schools* (pp. 55–93). New York: Cambridge University Press.

Farrell, A. D., & Camou, S. (2006). School-based interventions for youth violence prevention. In J. Lutzker (Ed.), *Preventing violence: Research and evidence-based intervention strategies* (pp. 125–145). Washington, DC: American Psychological Association.

Farrell, A. D., & Vulin-Reynolds, M. (2007). Violent behavior and the science of prevention. In D. J. Flannery, A. T. Vazsonyi, & I. D. Waldman (Eds.), *The Cambridge handbook of violent behavior and aggression* (pp. 767–786). New York: Cambridge University Press.

Farrell, A. D., Meyer, A. L., Kung, E. M., & Sullivan, T. N. (2001). Development and evaluation of school-based violence prevention programs. *Journal of Clinical Child Psychology, 30*(2), 207–220. doi:10.1207/S15374424JCCP3002_8

Farrell, A. D., Henry, D. B., & Bettencourt, A. (2013). Methodological challenges examining subgroup differences: Examples from universal school-based youth violence prevention trials. *Prevention Science, 14*(2), 1–13. doi:10.1007/s11121-011-0200-2

Felner, R. D., Favazza, A., Shim, M., Brand, S., Gu, K., & Noonan, N. (2001). Whole school improvement and restructuring as prevention and promotion: Lessons from STEP and the Project on High Performance Learning Communities. *Journal of School Psychology, 39*(2), 177–202. doi:10.1016/S0022-4405(01)00057-7

Fixsen, D. L., Naoom, S. F., Blase, K. A., Friedman, R. M., & Wallace, F. (2005). *Implementation research: A synthesis of the literature. Louis de la Parte Florida Mental Health Institute, National Implementation Research Network (FMHI Publication #231).* Tampa: University of South Florida. http://nirn.fmhi.usf.edu/resources/publications/Monograph/pdf/monograph_full.pdf

Fixsen, D. L., Blase, K. A., Naoom, S. F., & Wallace, F. (2009). Core implementation components. *Research on Social Work Practice, 19*(5), 531–540. doi:10.1177/ 1049731509335549

Flaspohler, P., Stillman, L., Duffy, J. L., Wandersman, A., & Maras, M. (2008). Unpacking capacity: The intersection of research to practice and community centered models. *American Journal of Community Psychology, 41*(3–4), 182–196. doi:10.1007/s10464-008-9162-3

Forman, S. G., Shapiro, E. S., Codding, R. S., Gonzales, J. E., Reddy, L. A., Rosenfield, S. A., Sanetti, L. M., & Stoiber, K. C. (2013). Implementation science and school psychology. *School Psychology Quarterly, 28*(2), 77–100. doi:10.1037/spq0000019

Gottfredson, D. C. (1984). *Environmental change strategies to prevent school disruption.* Report prepared for the Conference on Student Discipline Strategies of the Office of Educational Research and Improvement. Washington, DC: U.S. Department of Education.

Gottfredson, D. C. (2001). *Schools and delinquency.* New York: Cambridge University Press.

Gottfredson, G. D., & Gottfredson, D. C. (2001). What schools do to prevent problem behavior and promote safe environments. *Journal of Educational & Psychological Consultation, 12*(4), 313–344. doi:10.1207/S1532768XJEPC1204_02

Gottfredson, D. C., & Gottfredson, G. D. (2002). Quality of school-based prevention programs: Results from a national survey. *Journal of Research in Crime and Delinquency, 39*(1), 3–35. doi:10.1177/002242780203900101

Gottfredson, G. D., & Gottfredson, D. C. (2007). School violence. In D. J. Flannery, A. T. Vazsonyi, & I. D. Waldman (Eds.), *Cambridge handbook of violent behavior and aggression* (pp. 344–358). New York: Cambridge University Press.

Greenberg, M. T., Weissberg, R. P., O'Brien, M. U., Zins, J. E., Fredericks, L., Resnik, H., & Elias, M. J. (2003). Enhancing school-based prevention and youth development through coordinated social, emotional, and academic learning. *American Psychologist, 58*(6–7), 466–474. doi:10.1037/0003-066X.58.6-7.466

Guerra, N. G., & Bradshaw, C. P. (2008) *Core competencies to prevent problem behaviors and promote positive youth development.* Hoboken: John Wiley & Sons.

Halgunseth, L. C., Carmack, C., Childs, S. S., Caldwell, L., Craig, A., & Smith, E. P. (2012). Using the interactive systems framework in understanding the relation between general program capacity and implementation in afterschool settings. *American Journal of Community Psychology, 50*(3–4), 311–320. doi:10.1007/s10464-012-9500-3

Han, S. S., & Weiss, B. (2005). Sustainability of teacher implementation of school-based mental health programs. *Journal of Abnormal Child Psychology, 33*(6), 665–679. doi:10.1007/ s10802-005-7646-2

Harn, B., Parisi, D., & Stoolmiller, M. (2013). Balancing fidelity with flexibility and fit: What do we really know about fidelity of implementation in schools? *Exceptional Children, 79*(2), 181–193.

Hawkins, J. D., Oesterle, S., Brown, E. C., Monahan, K. C., Abbott, R. D., Arthur, M. W., & Catalano, R. F. (2012). Sustained decreases in risk exposure and youth problem behaviors after installation of the Communities That Care prevention system in a randomized trial. *Archives of Pediatrics & Adolescent Medicine, 166*(2), 141–148. doi:10.1001/archpediatrics.2011.183

Hulleman, C. S., Rimm-Kaufman, S. E., & Abry, T. (2013). Innovative methodologies to explore implementation: Whole-part-whole—construct validity, measurement, and analytical issues for intervention fidelity assessment in education research. In T. Halle, A. Metz, & I. Martinez-Beck (Eds.), *Applying implementation science in early childhood programs and systems* (pp. 65–93). Baltimore: Brookes.

Johnson, K., Hays, C., Center, H., & Daley, C. (2004). Building capacity and sustainable prevention innovations: A sustainability planning model. *Evaluation and Program Planning, 27*(2), 135–149.

Johnston, L. D., O'Malley, P. M., Bachman, J. G., & Schulenberg, J. E. (2013). *Monitoring the future national results on drug use: 2012 overview, key findings on adolescent drug use.* Ann Arbor: Institute for Social Research, University of Michigan.

Kam, C., Greenberg, M. T., & Walls, C. T. (2003). Examining the role of implementation quality in school-based prevention using the PATHS curriculum. *Prevention Science, 4*(1), 55–63. doi:10.1023/A:1021786811186

Kelly, B., & Perkins, D. F. (Eds.). (2012). *Handbook of implementation science for psychology in education.* Cambridge: Cambridge University Press.

McLeod, B. D., Southam-Gerow, M., & Weisz, J. R. (2009). Conceptual and methodological issues in treatment integrity measurement. *School Psychology Review, 38*(4), 541–546.

McLeod, B. D., Southam-Gerow, M. A., Tully, C. B., Rodríguez, A., & Smith, M. M. (2013). Making a case for treatment integrity as a psychosocial treatment quality indicator for youth mental health care. *Clinical Psychology: Science & Practice, 20*(1), 14–32. doi:10.1111/cpsp.12020

Meyer, A. L., Farrell, A. D., Northup, W. B., Kung, E. M., & Plybon, L. (2000). Adaptation of RIPP for cultural and community differences. In A. L. Meyer (Ed.), *Promoting nonviolence in early adolescence* (pp. 97–115). New York: Springer.

Multisite Violence Prevention Project (MVPP). (2009). The ecological effects of universal and selective violence prevention programs for middle school students: A randomized trial. *Journal of Consulting & Clinical Psychology, 77*(3), 526–542. doi:10.1037/a0014395

Nation, M., Crusto, C., Wandersman, A., Kumpfer, K. L., Seybolt, D., Morrissey-Kane, E., & Davino, K. (2003). What works in prevention: Principles of effective prevention programs. *American Psychologist, 58*(6–7), 449–456. doi:10.1037/0003-066X.58.6-7.449

Olweus, D. (2004). The Olweus Bullying Prevention Programme: Design and implementation issues and a new national initiative in Norway. In P. K. Smith, D. Pepler, & K. Rigby (Eds.), *Bullying in schools: How successful can interventions be?* (pp. 13–36). Cambridge: Cambridge University Press.

Pianta, R. C., & Rimm-Kaufman, S. (2006). The social ecology of the transition to school: Classrooms, families, and children. In K. McCarthy & D. Phillips (Eds.), *Handbook of early child development* (pp. 490–507). Oxford: Blackwell.

Reinke, W. M., Sprick, R., & Knight, J. (2009). Coaching classroom management. In J. Knight (Ed.), *Coaching: Approaches and perspectives* (pp. 91–112). Thousand Oaks: Corwin Press.

Reyes, M. R., Brackett, M. A., Rivers, S. E., Elbertson, N. A., & Salovey, P. (2012). The interaction effects of program training, dosage, and implementation quality on targeted student outcomes for the RULER approach to social and emotional learning. *School Psychology Review, 41,* 82–99.

Roberts-Gray, C., Gingiss, P. M., & Boerm, M. (2007). Evaluating school capacity to implement new programs. *Evaluation and Program Planning, 30*(3), 247–257.

Rogers, E. M. (2003). *Diffusion of innovations* (5th ed.). New York: Free Press.

Sanetti, L. M. H., & Fallon, L. M. (2011). Treatment integrity assessment: How estimates of adherence, quality, and exposure influence interpretation of implementation. *Journal of Educational and Psychological Consultation, 21*(3), 209–232. doi:10.1080/10474412.2011.595163

Sanetti, L. M. H., & Kratochwill, T. R. (2009). Treatment integrity assessment in the schools: An evaluation of the treatment integrity planning protocol. *School Psychology Quarterly, 24*(1), 24–35. doi:10.1037/a0015431

Sholomskas, D. E., Syracuse-Siewert, G., Rounsaville, B. J., Ball, S. A., Nuro, K. F., & Carroll, K. M. (2005). We don't train in vain: A dissemination trial of three strategies of training clinicians in cognitive-behavioral therapy. *Journal of Consulting and Clinical Psychology, 73*(1), 106–115. doi:10.1037/0022-006X.73.1.106

Sullivan, T. N., Sutherland, K. S., Farrell, A. D., Taylor, K. A., Doyle, S. T., & Ulmer, L. J. (2013). Evaluation of combined individual-level skill-building and school environment interventions: The role of gender and disability status. Manuscript in preparation.

Sutherland, S., & Katz, S. (2005). Concept mapping methodology: A catalyst for organizational learning. *Evaluation and Program Planning, 28*(3), 257–269.

Sutherland, K. S., McLeod, B. D., Conroy, M. A., & Cox, J. R. (in press). Measuring treatment integrity in the implementation of evidence-based programs in early childhood settings: Conceptual issues and recommendations. *Journal of Early Intervention.*

Trochim, W. (1989). An introduction to concept mapping for planning and evaluation. *Evaluation and Program Planning, 12*(1), 1–16. doi:10.1016/0149-7189(89)90016-5

U.S. Surgeon General. (2001). *Youth violence: A report of the surgeon general*. Washington, DC: U.S. Department of Health and Human Services.

van Lier, P. A., Muthén, B. O., van der Sar, R. M., & Crijnen, A. A. (2004). Preventing disruptive behavior in elementary schoolchildren: Impact of a universal classroom-based intervention. *Journal of Consulting and Clinical Psychology, 72*(3), 467–478. doi:10.1037/0022-006X.72.3.467

Vo, A., Sutherland, K. S., & Conroy, M. A. (2012). Best in Class: A classroom-based model for ameliorating problem behavior in early childhood settings. *Psychology in the Schools, 49*(5), 402–414. doi:10.1002/pits.21609

Wandersman, A. (2003). Community science: Bridging the gap between science and practice with community-centered models. *American Journal of Community Psychology, 31*(3–4), 227–242. doi:10.1023/A:1023954503247

Wilson, S. J., Lipsey, M. W., & Derzon, J. H. (2003). The effects of school-based intervention programs on aggressive behavior: A meta-analysis. *Journal of Consulting and Clinical Psychology, 71*(1), 136–149. doi:10.1037/0022-006X.71.1.136

Winter, S. G., & Szulanski, G. (2001). Replication as strategy. *Organization Science, 12*(6), 730–743. doi:10.1287/orsc.12.6.730.10084

Wolery, M. (2011). Intervention research: The importance of fidelity measurement. *Topics in Early Childhood Special Education, 31*(3), 155–157. doi:10.3102/0034654307313793

Chapter 11
Conducting Prevention Research and Evaluation in Schools

Kimberly Kendziora, Allison Dymnicki, Ann-Marie Faria, Amy Windham and David Osher

The desire for school participation in research is high and growing. Schools have always been a popular setting for prevention and intervention research, since (to paraphrase the bank robber Willie Sutton) that is where the children are. Many researchers are attracted to schools because interventions that are successful in educational settings have the potential to become policy and improve outcomes for thousands or even millions of students.

The pace of education reform has increased quickly in the past decade, to the point where many educators find it challenging to accommodate any more policy changes. The US Department of Education has used high-dollar grant competitions (such as Race to the Top and Investing in Innovation) as well as the promise of flexibility from No Child Left Behind Act (2001) accountability requirements to leverage major policy changes in states and districts (No Child Left Behind 2014).

K. Kendziora (✉) · A. Dymnicki · A.-M. Faria · A. Windham · D. Osher
American Institutes for Research, Washington, DC 20007, USA
e-mail: kkendziora@air.org

A. Dymnicki
e-mail: adymnicki@air.org

A.-M. Faria
e-mail: afaria@air.org

A. Windham
e-mail: amy.windham@truvenhealth.com

D. Osher
e-mail: dosher@air.org

© Springer Science+Business Media New York 2015
K. Bosworth (ed.), *Prevention Science in School Settings,*
Advances in Prevention Science, DOI 10.1007/978-1-4939-3155-2_11

Some of these shifts include adopting college and career-ready standards (such as the Common Core State Standards and associated new achievement assessments) and instituting new teacher and principal evaluation systems. Almost every funding vehicle is accompanied by an evaluation requirement; so the number of surveys that schools are asked to administer each year has grown tremendously. All of this has led to innovation fatigue, and this fatigue has presented increasing challenges for school-research partnerships.

It is important, then, that research with schools not just be presented as aligned with educators' mission and practice, but that it is *actually* aligned with mission and practice. In recent years, the US Department of Education has emphasized research-practice partnerships and has encouraged researchers to take seriously the unanswered questions and evidentiary needs felt by frontline educator, community, and family stakeholders. If care is taken in the conceptualization of research questions so that they are relevant to the people involved in carrying out the research, it will be easier to establish authentic partnerships.

In this chapter, we aim to share some "derived wisdom" regarding some real-world challenges and solutions. We begin by describing the critical initial process of building partnerships with schools. We move on to details of recruitment and data collection, and also describe some considerations in maintaining the integrity of experimental designs in schools.

This chapter is organized around a four-phase process for conducting research with schools: (1) planning, (2) recruitment, (3) data collection, and (4) communication. At each phase, it is important for researchers to be open to educators' ideas and ensure that the research serves the educators' mission as well as the researcher's goals.

11.1 Planning with Districts and Schools

Perhaps the first part of planning is being able to match the schools or districts with the research goals and criteria. For example, testing a curriculum that is only available in English may not be appropriate in a school that has a large population of students who are English language learners. The ability to identify appropriate research partners is greatly enhanced when a researcher has a network of personal relationships. If a researcher is settled in a geographic location, it may be helpful to attend local, county, district, or state-level meetings, school board meetings, as well as to volunteer for small projects with educators. Researchers should follow district issues in the press and be familiar with school board policies in relevant areas. Organizations that implement or advocate for the work the researcher wishes to study should be engaged, and may be helpful in identifying allies who can ease entry into the education system. A recommendation from a trusted person can often open doors that might otherwise be closed.

Initial marketing or publicity about the proposed research should lead with how the study will address the concerns of the constituents in the education sphere. This may mean how it may advance the school's or district's mission, or how it may help develop useful knowledge for unions, family advocates, or other groups whose partnership is desired. Most districts have well-specified strategic plans to advance outcomes such as college and career readiness, graduation, achievement, attendance, and employability skills; these are generally well publicized and available on web sites. Not only should any initial informational materials lead with how the research opportunity may help educators achieve their own aims, but these materials should also be brief. E-mails should not require any scrolling to read in their entirety. Letters should be limited to a single page with short sentences and bullet points to highlight key ideas. An honest assessment of benefits and costs of participation may be helpful, but details can wait for the more personal contacts we describe during the recruitment stage.

Once the desired host site is identified, the critical process of engagement begins. When true engagement is established, school partners will try hard to protect the integrity of the study design. For example, they will adhere to randomization procedures, facilitate collection of consent, and support data collection procedures. Response rates will be higher and results will be more valid.

Building strong partnerships among schools, the research team, and the broader community requires establishing collaboration based on mutually shared interests. Using terms like "buy-in" and "cooperation" can undermine a spirit of true collaboration because they imply that the researcher's goal is to get the school partners to do what the researcher wants them to do, as opposed to developing a true partnership. When partners can articulate mutually shared interests, they can own the work equally and share the responsibility for carrying it out.

Perhaps the most pernicious enemy to school-research partnerships is an attitude on the part of some researchers that educators do not value good evidence. We have found over the years that educators have a very strong interest in doing their best for students, and many are committed to reflective practice and lifelong learning. It is usually straightforward to establish that schools do not want to waste time on programs that do not work, and the need for good, relevant research and evaluation can be readily established.

Engagement must be a priority for all research team members and it must extend across all levels of a school-research partnership. Schools and research teams both have hierarchical structures, and a well-functioning partnership has relationships built across every level. The principal investigator must relate to the superintendent and/or principal. The study coordinator must relate to point of contact in the school responsible for facilitating the intervention and/or data collection. The study's analytic team must connect with the research/accountability staff in the district or school. Every member of the research team must relate to the school secretary, who is a critical gatekeeper. This is one of the most valuable relationships researchers need to develop.

The first stage in partnership building occurs during the recruitment process, which we describe in the following section. Partnerships are based on human connection, and can extend beyond single research projects to encompass ongoing and mutually fulfilling collaborations.

11.2 Recruitment

Despite its centrality to any school-based prevention or intervention research project, recruitment of school districts, individual schools, teachers, students, and families has received surprisingly little attention in the literature (McCormick et al. 1999). Although this issue is addressed in several disciplines such as social work, psychotherapy, and health research (Holden et al. 1993; Jackson et al. 1996; Berman et al. 1998), there is little research addressing participant recruitment as a stand-alone issue (see McCormick et al. 1999 for an exception). In larger research projects that recruit multiple school districts, a multistage recruitment may involve the research team engaging with (a) district leaders, (b) leaders (ideally the principal) of each participating school, (c) staff at each school, and (d) students or families who are participating in research and evaluation activities. Different approaches may be used at each of these levels. At each level, researchers may want to examine their own social networks for linkages. We describe recruitment at these levels in the following sections.

11.2.1 Recruitment at the District Level

The first contact with potential participants is critical and affects whether they respond or ignore it; therefore, recruitment materials need to be strategically planned. Personalized recruitment is often more successful than generic correspondence (Schlernitzauer et al. 1998). When possible, include people's names in the correspondence and use handwritten signatures or notes to help build a human connection. Also, using multiple communication approaches (such as mail; e-mail; an informational web site with tabs for "educators," "parents," "students," "community," and "researchers"; notices in professional association newsletters or web sites; or phone calls) allows for potential participants who prefer one communication mode over another to access the information about the study. The goal is to get to a first meeting with district or school leaders where you can explain the project, with an emphasis on engagement and establishing mutual interest.

Prinz et al. (2001) noted that study teams engaged in district or school recruitment should have good listening skills, relate easily to others, adopt a nonjudgmental approach, pay close attention to detail, and be persistent in the face of obstacles. During recruitment, researchers will meet with a wide variety of stakeholders and will need to build trust with a diverse set of potential participants. Therefore, researchers will be most successful when they express nonjudgmental acceptance of people whose perspectives and lifestyles differ from their own (Prinz et al. 2001). It is also important that all recruitment staff communicate the same messages at each point of contact so that district staff, principals, and teachers are not confused. This can be achieved by training recruiters before they are out in the field.

Communication about the project may be particularly important when the study is a randomized controlled trial (RCT) (Chap. 12). For some stakeholders, the words "random assignment" or "experiment" can conjure up images of white coats and lab rats. It may be better to use the term "lottery" since that is associated with winning a prize. When talking with school staff or families, it may minimize their anxiety if the random assignment process is presented as a simple lottery that will decide who gets the program or when they receive it.

Timing of the request matters. A good time to approach school districts that operate on standard calendars is often during January or February before achievement testing occurs (usually from March through May). In the initial meeting, the most important thing the researcher can do is to learn about the needs and priorities of the district or school and how the proposed project will fit into the district's short- and long-term strategic plans. Then, in the context of that understanding, the researcher can provide evidence that (a) the problem being addressed is important to schools (Botvin, Griffin, & Nichols, 2006), (b) the program has been successful with a similar student population (if appropriate), and (c) the research team has established credibility, including funding for the project (Capaldi et al. 1997; Harrington et al. 1997).

If the meeting is successful and the district wishes to proceed, there are generally two strands of activity: one to support the programming that is being studied and the other to support the research. For the programming, it is valuable to identify and develop several liaisons at the district level who will champion the project and who can help create structures to promote collaboration (Cauce et al. 1998; Poduska et al. 2012). One of the authors of this chapter recently worked on a recruitment effort in the Midwest for an RCT on the impact of an early warning system for preventing dropout. For this study, the state-level dropout prevention coordinators were willing to send letters and e-mails in support of the study to eligible school principals. Having the endorsement from a local, well-respected individual can help encourage schools to participate in the study. Conversely, researchers should generally avoid politically charged entities or initiatives during recruitment. Simply mentioning controversial education legislation or policies during recruitment can turn off potential participants.

In our experience, successful liaisons include the superintendent, assistant superintendent, and members of the student support, school, family, and community engagement, or mental health offices. To identify the most appropriate liaisons, it is important to understand the organizational structure of the district. If the superintendent offers to serve in this capacity, we recommend having additional intermediaries because of the many demands on the superintendent's time. It is helpful to have more than one liaison so that the project will not be dramatically affected if a particular staff leaves the district or is unable to continue in the liaison role.

On the research side, the study team will need to engage with staff from the district's office who handles research, assessment, and/or accountability. In most districts, a formal research application, including approvals for the involvement of human research participants and data sharing agreements for any student records, will be required.

It is helpful to engage district leaders in establishing appropriate incentives for teachers, students, and families. Research suggests that cash incentives may be particularly helpful in recruiting families (Capaldi et al. 1997). Depending on the local regulations and the union contract, financial incentives may be either forbidden or required for data collection with teachers. There should always be a discussion of what the researcher could offer that would be valuable, such as school-specific or subgroup-specific reports (e.g., responses by grade), resources (e.g., free program materials), and access to professional development. If school personnel are to be involved in programming, it will be important to negotiate compensation for their time. Once district approvals are secured, including approval from the appropriate district research review or institutional review board (IRB), then school leaders may be contacted.

11.2.2 Recruitment at the School Level

Recruitment can be one of the most expensive and time-consuming phases of a study. Successful recruitment often includes the opportunity to meet face-to-face with school personnel to build rapport and answer any questions the school staff may have about the research—this may require time and travel. In addition, researchers must respect a school's right to say "no" to research, and may need to approach as many as twice the number of schools they need for their study sample. For example, in a study where the research team will need a sample of 75 schools, the researchers should expect to visit at least 150 schools during recruitment. The amount of time and energy required to build school partnerships is frequently underestimated and may take anywhere from a few months to a year or more (Testa and Coleman 2006). Attempts to speed up the process can lead to resistance and may damage the partnership in the long term (Witt 1986).

A large body of literature has identified the school principal as the critical champion in prevention and intervention research (Barth 1990; Bryk et al. 2010; Demir 2008); therefore, in many ways, school recruitment *is* principal recruitment (see Chap. 3). Although recruitment at the school level parallels that at the district level in many ways, there should be a clear emphasis on the benefits of the project to the school and the effect of the program on the everyday routine at the school. A description of the roles and responsibilities of the school staff, the ways in which the research team will minimize burden, and how perceived barriers will be addressed should be clearly outlined for the principal (Harrington et al. 1997; Ji, DuBois, Flay, & Brechling, 2008; Jaycox et al. 2006).

As at the district level, school-level liaisons can be identified to coordinate ongoing research activities in the school (Ellickson 1994; Jaycox et al. 2006). School liaisons can provide expertise about the most feasible ways to deliver the program content (e.g., in a health class and in an afterschool program) and collect data (e.g., in the computer lab and during homeroom).

Story from the Field: Can I Get Your Number?

The study coordinator received a call from a principal telling her that one of the data collectors hired for a study swore at the school librarian. Apparently, there had been a parking lot altercation, in which the data collector was walking slowly and the librarian honked at him. She reported the incident to the principal, who contacted the study director. This was an obvious breach of professionalism, but even if it had been a lesser offense, the standard response would have applied: "We sincerely apologize. Please extend our apologies to your staff member. The staff member will never go into a school for us again. Thank you very much for calling me to let me know. Is there anything else I can do to repair this situation?"

There are two key points in this exchange that reflect the nature of the school-research partnership. The principal (a) knew who the study director was and called her directly and (b) trusted that the coordinator would address the situation. This is evidence of a functional partnership.

If this partnership *had not* been firmly established, this could have had a very different outcome. The principal could have gone up her chain of command to the school district administrators who then would have called the principal investigator, who would have come back down the research chain to the study coordinator. That *might* have worked, but would certainly have been inefficient. Alternatively, the principal could have simply complained about the data collector to her fellow principals, which could create mistrust for the research. Researchers may have found that principals would not take phone calls from the research team, researchers could not get past the school secretary, and the research team may wonder, "Why are they being uncooperative?"

Lessons learned include:

- Be clear on points of contact across every level of the school-research partnership, including contact information.
- Recognize that frontline data collectors represent the entire research project to schools. They need to be carefully selected, connected to the broader vision for the project, and trained that their first responsibility is to maintain the partnership. If they cannot maintain the partnership, they need to be pulled from schools.
- Have educators and parents on the research team so that they can help other researchers understand the culture of schools and what is (and is not) appropriate behavior in that context. We have hired retired teachers to conduct classroom observations and asked them to train interviewers on understanding the school context.

11.2.3   Recruitment at the Teacher Level

Depending on the project, teachers may be implementers, data providers, or both. To engage with teachers, it may be helpful for researchers to hold information sessions (in person or via videoconference) to provide principals and school staff members an opportunity to learn and ask questions about the study and to describe their roles as part of the research partnership (Horowitz et al. 2003; Massetti et al. 2008; Peterson et al. 2000). As Jaycox et al. (2006) wrote, "Whereas some administrators will have consulted the teachers before making decisions to participate, others will not have done so, with the result that some teachers may feel a study is being imposed on them" (p. 327). Given this possibility, it may be particularly important, if not required, for a project team to inform teachers directly about a project. The research team may distribute study materials (e.g., study objectives, what will be expected of the school staff, what supports or incentives staff will receive, ethics guidelines including consent, questionnaires, and other relevant documents) for staff to review. A research team member should be readily available to promptly answer teachers' questions or address concerns. Some researchers have attributed high response rates to having a face-to-face meeting about the study with school staff members and then having that researcher (sometimes called a school liaison in this role) available for follow-up questions (Testa and Coleman 2006).

Some strategies to facilitate school recruitment include taking snacks to faculty meetings or leaving fruit and cheese platters or donuts in the faculty lounge (it helps to know what kind of food staff may prefer). Some researchers have given all participating schools plaques that stated that the school was a partner with the research organization on the (name) project.

11.2.4   Recruitment at the Student Level

Many school-based studies in prevention research require some level of student participation, whether it is attending a program, completing surveys, or allowing the transfer of school records. When these data are anonymous (i.e., there is no way to trace a data point back to an individual student), family consent is not normally required (but may be helpful, particularly if sensitive questions are asked). If identifiers are required to track participants over time, or to link survey data with school records, family consent is almost always required.

Students under age 18[1] generally require family permission to participate in research. A strong partnership with the school is very helpful for student recruitment since families are more likely to pay attention to study information/consent forms

---

[1] There is no federally determined age of majority that is common across states. In Alabama, Delaware, and Nebraska, the age of majority is 19; in Mississippi, it is 21; in six other states, high school graduation may either accelerate (Ohio, Utah) or delay age of majority (Arkansas, Nevada, Tennessee, and Wisconsin).

that arrive on school or district letterhead. When possible, it is helpful to include study consent forms in the packet of material that is distributed to families on the first day of school. Otherwise, sending forms home with students ("backpacking") and potentially following up by mail will be necessary. In some research we have done in New York City and Chicago, we have had some success offering movie passes to students returning family consent forms (regardless of whether or not consent is granted). Arizona's Promoting Healthy Relationships Project offered $1 for consent return. In addition, students received $10 for survey and program completion (Jaycox et al. 2006). Others have had success with class incentives, such as a pizza party or ice cream social for the class if 90 % of the consent forms are returned by a certain date. Researchers may offer incentives to teachers whose classes have reached a certain percent of returned forms by a certain date.

11.2.5 Recruiting Families in School-Based Research

Depending on the project, engaging with families or family representatives to explain the project may be necessary for a research project to be successful. Prior research has supported two strategies for successful family engagement in research: (a) establishing a personal relationship with the family, potentially including a home visit, and (b) generous compensation for the participants' time (Capaldi and Patterson 1987; Liontos 1992; Thompson 1984). These both require considerable time and resources on the part of the researcher and might not be feasible, even if they could help. Families in the Oregon Youth Study, a longitudinal study of boys who were at risk, were paid up to $300 for the first year of participation which required two and a half hours to complete assessments (Capaldi et al. 1997), with only one family dropping out during the initial phase of the study. This is in contrast to a 54 % recruitment and pretest completion rate using telephone recruiting and lower pay in a similar longitudinal study (Spoth and Redmond 1993).

11.2.6 The Use of Incentives in School Research

One way to show respect for participants' time is to offer an incentive or honorarium for participation. Some researchers have examined how the type of incentive (e.g., gift card and cash) and the amount of the incentive ($1, 5, and 10) affect response rates (Capaldi and Patterson 1987; Singer 2001; Singer and Ye 2013). Although the research evidence about the most effective type of incentive is mixed, monetary incentives are usually found to be more effective than nonmonetary incentives for increasing response rates (Singer et al. 1999) and cash incentives are frequently identified as the most effective (Cantor et al. 2008; Dykema et al. 2012). Most of this research has been done with household survey research; cash incentives might not be allowed or appropriate in school-based contexts.

We have worked with schools to develop a range of appropriate incentives, including sending certificates to any school with a return rate above 90%, raffling off one or two iPads to any participant who completed a survey,[2] and awarding the three schools in the district with the highest response rates $200, $100, and $50 gift certificates to an office supply store. Other researchers have found that a complimentary breakfast was very much appreciated while the teachers completed their teacher survey forms (Jaycox et al. 2006).

Tokens of appreciation for district and school staff members who play key roles in research and evaluation activities are also important to consider (Capaldi et al. 1997). We have sent thank-you gifts such as cookies, flowers, coffee mugs, tote bags, and high-quality pens to acknowledge the effort (often outside of work hours) that district and school staff members contributed toward completion of research activities. Such gifts are best accompanied by a handwritten thank-you note to the principal acknowledging the effort and collaboration of school staff.

Teachers also appreciate supplies for their classrooms or general supplies. We have worked with some schools that were so strapped for supplies that by the end of the school year they had run out of copy paper. We would bring packs of paper on school visits. Besides being needed and appreciated, it communicated that we understood their needs and the challenges of working in under-resourced schools. Even in places where district or union rules prohibit direct honoraria or gifts to teachers, providing supplies or gift cards from educational supply companies may be permissible.

One must beware that incentives are not so large that they become coercive. A researcher who wants to administer a 60-min survey must be aware that this is a significant request and represents a substantial loss of instructional time, but offering a school thousands of dollars to make the data collection happen may not be the most ethical approach. In addition, sometimes principals or teachers may express their enthusiasm for the study in inappropriate ways. One physical education teacher told students that if they did not return their study forms, they would have to run laps around the gym.

11.3 Data Collection

Partnership with district and school staff is particularly critical during the data collection phase of research. District and school liaisons can be important thought partners in planning the best approach to data collection, how to communicate to others in the district or school before, during, and after data collection activities, ways to address important ethical or privacy issues, and the appropriate balance between helpful survey reminders and badgering people. School partners can guide researchers about the best time of year, day, class period, length of survey window (we generally use 4–5 weeks but this varies by district), and how many reminders should be sent. Specific strategies we have found helpful include:

---

[2] One district asked us to raffle off an iPad only if the overall survey response rate reached 60%; this goal was not attained in the first year, but was attained in years 2 and 3.

- Sending postcards or e-mails to teachers a week before a survey opens to alert them to the incoming request and remind them how participating in the survey will help students and advance their school's mission
- Including information about upcoming data collection activities in school, district, or union newsletters
- Thanking participants for their participation after the data collection closes
- Providing respondents with information about the results of the data collection or study

Although online surveys are often preferable to paper and pencil surveys because of saving time and money in data entry, these are not always an option in schools with limited technology capacity. When data must be collected in person and the research team is located remotely, more creative ways of collecting data have been developed, including using retired teachers recruited from a local temp agency as data collectors (Poduska et al. 2012). In-person data collection may be subject to vagaries such as fire drills, gas leaks, and other disruptions. Researchers should always have backup plans in place.

11.3.1   Requests for Student Records

Where possible, researchers should consider using publicly available educational data. The National Center for Educational Statistics, the US Department of Education's Office of Civil Rights and Office of Special Education Programs, the federal web site www.data.gov/education, each state's department of education, and many district web sites provide school- or grade-level historical data on outcomes such as achievement, attendance, suspensions, dropout, and graduation. These sources should be thoroughly researched and capitalized on before pursuing student-level data from districts.

Researchers often request identifiable student-level records from school districts for their research. Sometimes, district data may provide important matching, mediator, moderator, or outcome variables for studies. Recent advocacy of rapid, low-cost randomized trials in education and human services has stressed the value of extant data in advancing both knowledge and social policy (Center for Evidence-Based Policy 2014). When considering the inclusion of such data in a study, researchers must be aware that student records are covered by the Family Educational Rights and Privacy Act (FERPA).

FERPA specifically gives families the right to consent to disclosure of student educational records. There is an exception in the regulations (34 CFR § 99.31 (6)) for "organizations conducting studies for, or on behalf of, educational agencies or institutions." Note that the language in the regulations inherently implies partnership. Researchers may access educational records without prior written consent only if the study meets the following conditions:

- It aims to develop, validate, or administer predictive tests; administer student aid programs; or improve instruction.
- It establishes a written agreement between the education agency and the researcher that specifies the purpose, scope, and duration of the study and the personally identifiable information (PII) to be disclosed.
- Access to PII is restricted to the study team.
- PII is used only for the stated purposes.
- PII is destroyed when no longer needed and the research agreement states this time period.
- No education agency is required to agree with or endorse the conclusions or results of the study.

Once permission to obtain such data is granted, some practical considerations should guide researchers' interactions with the district research office. First, researchers should remember that responding to external research requests is generally the lowest priority task for district research staff. These staff members have many federal, state, and other reporting requirements and most district research offices are overworked and understaffed (Capaldi et al. 1997).

If the district has a data request template, be sure to use it. If no template exists, then develop a written document that includes a list of the data elements needed, the years for which data are requested, whether the data need to be linked longitudinally (i.e., to follow the same student across years), and the format of the files (e.g., Excel or SPSS). We have found it valuable to request a data dictionary or codebook up front, given that there are many district-specific acronyms and different ways of coding variables; if not requested initially, it may take several weeks for the district staff to produce. In addition, if there is not a separate data security plan, researchers may find it helpful to include information about how confidentiality will be protected (e.g., encryption protocols, use of masked identifiers, data security training for staff).

Following the written request, it may be helpful to have a phone call with research staff to talk through the request (e.g., identifying other variables to measure the same outcome if the requested variable is not available). The type of data available varies greatly by district and we recommend asking district research partners how they would assess certain outcomes, given their knowledge of the available data. Ask the district about inconsistencies in the way certain data are measured by different schools (e.g., suspension rates) and if they have any concerns about the validity or reliability of certain data sources. If several requests are being made across different studies in the same school district, then requests should be consolidated where possible to minimize demands on district staff.

From our experience, data requests often take 3–6 months and subsequent requests to receive updated data often take 2–4 months (unless there are personnel changes, in which case expect 3–6 months). An additional 1–2 months may be required to address follow-up questions. Most districts are better able to field data requests in the winter or summer, as they tend to be busy with achievement tests in the spring and enrollment in the fall.

Story from the Field: Mashed Potatoes

A new interviewer was nervous and rushed the start of an interview with a young student. The student was visibly disinterested and distracted and resisted answering every question posed to him. The protocol required the interviewer to instruct the student how to mark his answer sheet that used cartoon icons for the question numbers. The interviewer would periodically check to be sure the student was on the right item, for example, by asking "I am on the balloon. Are you on the balloon?"

Several minutes into the interview, the interviewer asked the student which item he was on. The student responded "mashed potatoes." The answer sheet had planes, trains, automobiles, stars, moons, and cows, but no mashed potatoes. The interviewer stopped, put down his pencil, stared blankly at the student, and said flatly, "Did you say mashed potatoes?" The student smiled (finally) and started to giggle. The interviewer pointed to the picture and said, "That's supposed to be a cloud." The student and the interviewer shared a good laugh over mashed potatoes. It relieved the tension and finally broke the ice. From that point forward, the interviewer relaxed, the student participated, and the interview and resulting data were salvaged.

Although this is a simple example with a student, parallel examples could exist at any level of the school-research partnership. Lessons learned from this episode include the following:

- Field test data collection instruments to ensure that they are understandable to and appropriate for the intended audience
- If you attempt to plow forward with your research with a disengaged or resistant partner, you will irritate your partner and get useless results
- Establish rapport by finding a common interest or using humor
- If your school partner seems "resistant," pause and evaluate why you have not been able to successfully engage him or her
- Try and understand the source of your partner's reluctance to move forward on this project

11.3.2   Experiments in Schools

Over the last decade, there has been an explosion of experiments conducted in schools. The establishment of the Institute of Education Sciences in 2002 promoted increased rigor in education research, and many federal programs have mandated that only evidence-based programs may be funded. RCTs provide the highest level of evidence for program impact because only in this design are both observed and unobserved characteristics that may influence outcomes distributed across groups (Myers and Dynarski 2003). RCTs have been used to evaluate the impact of a variety of educational practices and policies, including school vouchers (Peterson et al. 1998), Head Start (U.S. Department of Health and Human Services 2010), and Reading First (Gamse et al. 2008). In the field of education, the US Department of Education's What Works Clearinghouse (http://ies.ed.gov/ncee/wwc) maintains the evidentiary standards for program effectiveness. RCTs are the only research designs that will allow claims of effectiveness to be made "without reservations" (U.S. Department of Education 2014).

Although the research community embraces the use of RCTs in educational settings, there is concern among some educators that randomization may be unethical because it withholds or delays services for some students. Researchers know that many educational or preventive interventions do not work, and until they are tested, it is impossible to know whether a program will actually help students, or even if it may have unintended negative consequences.

It is important in the context of a research-school partnership to acknowledge any hesitation on the part of educators and explore why an educator may be uncomfortable with random assignment. *Have they already participated in research that made the school look unfavorable? Have they been a participant in some other type of experiment outside of the education field? Are they worried that it is unethical to withhold treatment?* Understanding the school partners' perspectives will help allow the researcher to assuage their fears and discuss how random assignment is an ethical and necessary approach for evaluation. One way to make RCTs more acceptable for educators may be to offer delayed treatment. Instead of being randomized to treatment or control, the student, classroom, or school is randomized to receive the treatment now or later; the lottery determines *when* students receive the program. This approach may increase costs, however, since all students receive services and in some cases may preclude longer term follow-up if controls are treated. However, ultimately treating all eligible students or training all teachers is a powerful incentive for districts, schools, and parents (it may even offset recruitment costs).

Two special issues apply to conducting RCTs in schools that we describe in greater detail: contamination and maintaining treatment conditions. Contamination, or crossover, occurs when participants who are assigned to the control group receive services provided to those in the treatment, or when participants who are assigned to the treatment group end up not receiving those same services. Cases that switch treatment status are sometimes referred to as:

- Always-takers: those who receive the intervention regardless of whether they are assigned to treatment or control
- Never-takers: those who will never receive the intervention regardless of whether they are assigned to treatment or control
- Compliers: those who receive treatment if assigned to treatment and do not receive treatment if assigned to control
- Defiers: those who receive treatment if assigned to control and receive no treatment if assigned to treatment (Imbens and Angrist 1994).

Most school-based RCTs experience some level of contamination, and, conventionally, program impact is estimated using the intent to treat approach (ITT) in which impact is based on treatment status as assigned (whether a school is assigned to treatment or control) and not the actual receipt of the services (whether the school ends up being an always-taker, never-taker, complier, or a defier). The ITT approach has long been mandated by the Food and Drug Administration (FDA) as the primary design and analysis strategy for medical clinical trials and is widely used in other government-funded RCTs (Ten Have et al. 2008). An alternative approach is treatment-on-the-treated (TOT) in which impact is estimated based on treatment *as delivered* (not as assigned). TOT estimates account for contamination and crossover and are usually presented as secondary treatment effects along with ITT results (Ten Have et al. 2008)

Crossover can invalidate study results and there are many strategies to combat contamination, although crossover cannot usually be eliminated completely. Strategies begin early in study design. When choosing at which level to randomly assign, researchers can choose designs that are more or less prone to contamination. For example, if a researcher wanted to investigate the impact of a ninth-grade substance abuse prevention program, the researcher could choose to randomly assign schools to implement the program schoolwide, which would minimize contamination but would require many schools; randomly assign health teachers to implement the program or not, which may increase the chances of contamination since most schools have grade-level or department-level professional learning communities that exist in part to share promising innovations; or deliver the program after school.

Maintaining treatment conditions during an RCT is vital for study integrity. Every member of the research team must accept that maintaining treatment conditions is part of their role and responsibility. That said, trade-offs are inevitable. For example, exceptions to random assignment may need to be made to accommodate practices regarding having siblings in the same classroom or repeating students being assigned to the same teacher. Strong partnerships with schools can help in this effort because the more that school partners (at every level) value the importance of the design, the more they will own and protect it.

Keeping schools engaged throughout the duration of the study is also important. If schools drop out, it threatens the experiment's statistical power[3] to detect an impact of the intervention because it reduces the sample size. Even a small amount of attrition can jeopardize validity, but researchers can take the following steps to maintaining a positive and engaged relationship with schools during the life of the trial:

- Engage in regular, positive interactions with school partners (Stouthamer-Loeber et al. 1992).
- Maintain continuity in contact between the study personnel and the participating schools that includes the study staff, information, and procedures.

---

[3] Statistical power is the ability to detect an effect if the effect actually exists.

- Be flexible with scheduling for data collection to minimize burden. Sometimes, flexibility is not possible, but building it into scheduling and project timelines whenever possible will help schools feel that their participation is on their own terms.
- Always be mindful of the district's assessment calendar, the ebb and flow of the school year, and other school or community activities when planning study activities. This shows respect and responsiveness regarding the school partner's context.

11.4   Communication

Another way to keep education partners engaged in research is by sharing results with them in a way that best meets both the researchers' and the educators' needs. All partnerships are different; so one of the topics to be addressed early on in the engagement process is learning how the education partner wants to be involved. Some educators may want the researcher in and out and they have no particular interest in the findings. Giving such partners too much information may alienate them and harm the partnership (and thereby, the project). For others, building trust means regular communication about how the project (program implementation or data collection) is going. Sometimes, when educators use instructional time to administer a survey or when staff participate in interviews, they often expect researchers to share a summary of that information with them in a timely fashion. Unless the design prevents sharing information with schools, we have found that timely sharing of results from surveys (i.e., providing survey reports within 30 days of the survey's closing) is very much appreciated and helps teachers and other informants feel like the survey was worthwhile.

Educators may ask researchers to make presentations to the school board or to other stakeholders about the project, and it may be the case that educators also invite the researchers to provide some professional development to teachers on the topic under study. Researchers must understand that such presentations are not like professional conference presentations, and the audience's needs and background must be taken into consideration. Educators seldom have much training in statistics, and so presentations that emphasize logic, facts, and especially practical application are most appreciated.

Some principals see one of the payoffs for the extra time they spend on research activities is to be able to keep their superiors (superintendent or school board) informed. While some principals prefer researchers to present results, other principals wish to present their school's data themselves. In some cases, after a presenting to the school board, the project receives additional funding or promise of continuing beyond the study period.

At the end of the project, it may be helpful, where possible, to offer the educators an opportunity to review and comment on a draft of the final report. This respects educators' partnership in the project, and their perspective on the findings and potential application (even if they do not accept the invitation to comment). When the report is complete, the researchers should understand that a variety of communication strategies may be necessary to meet some stakeholders' needs. Many stakeholders will not read a full research report. A user-friendly one- or two-page brief may be helpful, or the researcher may offer to write a short article for a superintendent's newsletter or district's web site. A press release that may be shared with local media outlets may be helpful. Most school districts have a communications director whose input should be solicited in determining the best plan for disseminating findings locally.

11.5   Summary

The resource demands on schools are higher than ever, including demands related to research. The key to working through the challenges of introducing a new project to schools is building a school-research partnership that is built upon trust and mutual interest. We summarize below the five cornerstones of developing and maintaining such partnerships.

1. **Respect**
   Schools have their own culture and rhythm. Researchers may want to approach them as if they were visiting a foreign country. If researchers want to be accepted, they need to understand and respect school customs, and need to remember that they are a guest—and not always one who has been invited. Sensitivity regarding timing shows respect, and researchers should know that there are certain times of year they cannot impose: in particular, the weeks surrounding and including standardized testing. Just as a fundamental principle in bioethics is "first, do no harm," a corollary for those who work in schools may be "first, do not get kicked out." Always know that research is done at the sufferance of schools and can be ended at any time.

2. **Patience**
   Research is rarely a school's first priority. Even when schools are enthusiastic partners, day-to-day educational operations can trump research requirements. Schools embrace their role in addressing the social, emotional, and behavioral needs of their students. However, their absolute priority is and always will be educating students. Second to education, they will welcome the intervention team because they bring something of value to their community. Near the bottom of their list of priorities is evaluation. Even when they have agreed on the value of demonstrating effectiveness, collecting data in schools is a major interruption into their primary mission and their daily routine.

3. **Authenticity**
   Interpersonal styles vary, and researchers will naturally connect with some partners more easily than others. What hopefully all will share is the fundamental good intention to improve student outcomes. When real or perceived differences arise, this shared intention can be the platform for planning and action.
   Having a diverse research team matters. Not everyone on the research team will connect with every school team member. However, a diverse research team (e.g., demographic and professional backgrounds and interests) will be able to make

connections across varied personalities and backgrounds. Each school team member needs to be able to relate to someone on the research team.

4. **Persistence**

Engagement is a never-ending process across the life of a study. Some school partners will be more challenging to engage than others, and some relationships take more time and effort. Some school partners will tire of you when they realize the extent of what their commitment requires ("were you not just here?"). Attrition and turnover will occur. To facilitate continuity of the project, researchers can plan for ongoing engagement and communication of the research plan, such as through meetings, e-mailed project updates, and end-of-year celebrations.

5. **Gratitude**

Funding levels typically do not support lavish incentives. Moreover, although financial incentives may be effective short-term rewards/incentives, they are not necessarily effective in sustaining longer term partnerships. Educators do not enter the profession for the money, but most are happy to have their work and effort acknowledged and honored. As described earlier, small tokens of appreciation that communicate (authentic) gratitude for school partners and the time they have taken to support the research can support the development of long-term partnerships. At the conclusion of a project, handwritten thank-you notes to the people directly supporting the work are a must. Acknowledgments sent to direct superiors are also helpful—for example, letters to principals acknowledging the contribution of their school staff, with the superintendent copied on correspondence, or certificates of appreciation signed by the principal or superintendent. Acknowledging the roles that partners played in the research will also help them to remember and speak favorably of the researchers. This will support your ongoing work and ability to engage new partners, and will make conducting research in schools generally more acceptable and productive, contributing to the broader education-research enterprise.

References

Barth, R. S. (1990). *Improving schools from within: Teachers, parents, and principals can make the difference*. San Francisco: Jossey-Bass. doi:10.1002/1520–6807(199301)30:1<99:aid-pits2310300117>3.0.co;2-j.

Berman, B., Grosser, S., & Gritz, E. (1998). Recruitment to a school-based adult smoking-cessation program. *Journal of Cancer Education, 13*, 220–225. http://link.springer.com/journal/13187.

Botvin, G. J., Griffin, K. W., & Nichols, T. R. (2006). Preventing youth violence and delinquency through a universal school-based prevention approach. Prevention Science, 7, 403–408

Bryk, A., Sebring, P., & Allensworth, E. (2010). *Organizing schools for improvement: Lessons from Chicago*. Chicago: University of Chicago Press. doi:10.7208/chicago/9780226078014001.0001.

Cantor, D., O'Hare, B. C., & O'Connor, K. S. (2008). The use of monetary incentives to reduce nonresponse in random digit dial telephone surveys. In J. M. Lepkowski, C. Tucker, J. M. Brick, E. de Leeuw, L. Japec, P. Lavrakas, M. W. Link, & R. L. Sangster (Eds.), *Advances in telephone survey methodology* (pp. 471–498). NY: Wiley. doi:10.1002/9780470173404ch22.

Capaldi., D. M.,& Patterson, G .R. (1987). An approach to the problem of recruitment and retention rates for longitudinal research. Behavioral Assessment. 9, 169–177.

Cauce, A. M., Ryan, K. D., & Grove, K. (1998). Children and adolescents of color, where are you? Participation, selection, recruitment, and retention in developmental research. In V. C. McLoyd & L. Steinberg (Eds.), *Studying minority adolescents: Conceptual, methodological, and theoretical issues* (pp. 147–166). Mahwah: Erlbaum. doi:10.4324/9781410601506.

Center for Evidence-Based Policy. (2014). *Demonstrating how low-cost randomized controlled trials can drive effective social spending.* Washington, DC: Author. http://coalition4evidence. org.

Demir, K. (2008). Transformational leadership and collective efficacy: The moderating roles of collaborative culture and teachers' self-efficacy. *Eurasian Journal of Educational Research, 33,* 93–112. http://www.ejer.com.tr/.

Dykema, J., Stevenson, J., Klein, L., Kim, Y., & Day, B. (2012). Effects of mailed versus e-mailed invitations and incentives on response rates and costs in a web survey of faculty and university administrators. *Social Science Computer Review, 31,* 359–370. doi:10.1177/0894439312465254.

Ellickson, P. L. (1994). Getting and keeping schools and kids for evaluation studies. *Journal of Community Psychology, 22,* 102–116. http://onlinelibrary.wiley.com/journal/10.1002/ (ISSN)1520–6629.

Gamse, B. C., Bloom, H. S., Kemple, J. J., & Jacob, R. T. (2008). Reading first impact study: Interim report (NCEE 2008–4016). Washington, DC: National Center for Education Evaluation and Regional Assistance, Institute of Education Sciences, U.S. Department of Education. ies. ed.gov/ncee/pubs/20084016.

Harrington, K. F., Binkley, D., Reynolds, K. D., Duvall, R. C., Copeland, J. R., Franklin, F., & Raczynski, J. (1997). Recruitment issues in school-based research: Lessons learned from the High 5 Alabama Project. *Journal of School Health, 67,* 415–421. doi:10.1111/j.1746–1561.1997. tb01287.x.

Holden, G., Rosenberg, G., Barker, K., Tuhrim, S., & Brenner, B. (1993). The recruitment of research participants. *Social Work in Health Care, 19*(2), 1–44. doi:10.1300/J010v19n02_01.

Horowitz, J. A., Vessey, J. A., Carlson, K. L., Bradley, J. F., Montoya, C., & McCullough, B. (2003). Conducting school-based focus groups: Lessons learned from the CATS project. *Journal of Pediatric Nursing, 18,* 321–331. doi:10.1016/s0882-5963(03)00104-0.

Imbens, G. W. & Angrist, J. D. (1994). Identification and estimation of local average treatment effects. Econometrica, 62, 467–475.

Institute for Education Sciences. (2014, March). *What Works Clearinghouse procedures and standards handbook, version 3.0.* Washington, DC: U.S. Department of Education. http://ies. ed.gov/ncee/wwc/documentsum.aspx?sid=19.

Institute for Education Sciences. (2014, March). *What Works Clearinghouse procedures and standards handbook, version 3.0.* Washington, DC: U.S. Department of Education. Retrieved from http://ies.ed.gov/nccc/wwc/documentsum.aspx?sid=19

Jackson, R., Chambless, L., Yang, K., Byrne, T., Watson, R., Folsom, A., & Kalsbeek, W. (1996). Differences between respondents and non-respondents in a multi-center community-based study vary by gender and ethnicity. *Journal of Clinical Epidemiology, 49,* 1441–1446. doi:10.1016/0895-4356(95)00047-x.

Jaycox, L. H., McCaffrey, D. F., Ocampo, B. W., Shelley, G. A., Blake, S. M., Peterson, D. J., & Kub, J. E. (2006). Challenges in the evaluation and implementation of school-based prevention and intervention programs on sensitive topics. *American Journal of Evaluation, 27,* 320–336. doi:10.1177/1098214006291010.

Ji, P., DuBois, D. L., Flay, B. R., & Brechling, V. (2008). "Congratulations, you have been randomized into the control group!(?)": Issues to consider when recruiting schools for matched-pair randomized control trials of prevention programs. *Journal of School Health, 78,* 131–139. doi: 10.1111/j.1746-1561.2007.00275.x.

Liontos, L. (1992). *At-risk families and schools becoming partners.* Eugene, OR: University of Oregon, ERIC Clearinghouse of Educational Management.

Massetti, G. M., Lahey, B. B., Pelham, W. E., Loney, J., Ehrhardt, A., Lee, S. S., & Kipp, H. (2008). Academic achievement over 8 years among children who met modified criteria for attention-deficit/hyperactivity disorder at 4–6 years of age. *Journal of Abnormal Child Psychology, 36,* 399–410. doi: http://dx.doi.org/10.1007/s10802-007-9186-4

McCormick, L., Crawford, M., Anderson, R., Gittelson, J., Kingsley, B., & Upson, D. (1999). Recruiting adolescents into qualitative tobacco research studies: Experiences and lessons learned. *Journal of School Health, 69*(3), 95–99. doi:10.1111/j.1746–1561.1999.tb07215.x.

Myers, D., & Dynarski, M. (2003). Random assignment in program evaluation and intervention research: Questions and answers. Washington, DC: U.S. Department of Education, Institute of Education Sciences, National Center for Education Evaluation and Regional Assistance. www.mathematica-mpr.com/PDFs/randomassign.pdf.

No Child Left Behind. (2014). Elementary and Secondary Education Act. http://www2ed.gov/nclb/landing.

Peterson, P. E., Myers, D., & Howell, W. G. (1998). *An evaluation of the New York City School-Choice Scholarships Program: The first year.* Washington, DC: Mathematica Policy Research. http://www.hks.harvard.edu/pepg/PDF/Papers/nylex.pdf.

Peterson, A. V., Mann, S. L., Kealey, K. A., & Marek, P. M. (2000). Experimental design and methods for school-based randomized trials: Experience from the Hutchinson Smoking Prevention Project (HSPP). *Controlled Clinical Trials, 21,* 144–165. doi:10.1016/s0197-2456(99)00050-1.

Poduska, J., Gomez, M. J., Capo, Z., & Holmes, V. (2012). Developing a collaboration with the Houston independent school district: Testing the generalizability of a partnership model. *Administration and Policy in Mental Health and Mental Health Services Research, 39,* 258–267. doi:10.1007/s10488-011-0383-7.

Prinz, R. J., Smith, E. P., Dumas, J. E., Laughlin, J. E., White, D. W., & Barrón, R. (2001). Recruitment and retention of participants in prevention trials involving family-based interventions. *American Journal of Preventive Medicine, 20,* 31–37. doi:10.1016/s0749-3797(00)00271-3.

Schlernitzauer, M., Bierhals, A. J., Geary, M. D., Prigerson, H. G., Stack, J. A., Miller, M. D., & Reynolds, C. F. (1998). Recruitment methods for intervention research in bereavement-related depression: Five years' experience. *American Journal of Geriatric Psychiatry, 6,* 67–74. doi:10.1097/00019442-199802000-00009.

Singer, E. (2001). The use of incentives to reduce nonresponse in household surveys. In R. M. Groves, D. A. Dillman, J. L. Eltinge, & R. J. A. Little (Eds.), *Survey nonresponse* (pp. 163–177). NY: Wiley. http://www.wiley.com/WileyCDA/WileyTitle/productCd-0471396273.html.

Singer, E., & Ye, C. (2013). The use and effects of incentives in surveys. *The Annals of the American Academy of Political and Social Science, 645,* 112–141. doi:10.1177/0002716212458082.

Singer, E., Van Hoewyk, J., Gebler, N., Raghunathan, T., & McGonagle, K. (1999). The effect of incentives on response rates in interviewer-mediated surveys. *Journal of Official Statistics, 15,* 217–230. http://www.websm.org/uploadi/editor/Singer_1999_The_effect_of_incentives.pdf.

Spoth, R., & Redmond, C. (1993). Study of participation barriers in family-focused prevention: Research issues and preliminary results. *International Quarterly of Community Health Education, 13,* 365–388. doi: 10.2190/69LM-59KD-K9CE-8Y8B

Stouthamer-Loeber, M., van Kammen, W., & Loeber, R. (1992). The nuts and bolts of implementing large-scale longitudinal studies. *Violence and Victims, 7,* 1–16. http://www.springerpub.com/product/08866708#.U_O_5vldWSo.

Ten Have, T. R., Normand, S. T., Marcus, S. M., Brown, C. H., Lavori, P., & Duan, D. (2008). Intent-to-treat vs. non-intent-to-treat analyses under treatment non-adherence in mental health randomized trials. *Psychiatry Annals, 38,* 772–783. doi:10.3928/00485713-20081201-10.

Testa, A. C., & Coleman, L. M. (2006). Accessing research participants in schools: A case study of a UK adolescent sexual health survey. *Health Education Research, 21,* 518–526. doi:10.1093/her/cyh078.

Thompson, T. (1984). A comparison of methods of increasing parental consent rates in social research. *Public Opinion Quarterly, 48*(4), 779–787. doi:10.1086/268883.

U.S. Department of Health and Human Services, Administration for Children and Families. (2010, January). Head start impact study. Final report. Washington, DC: Author. www.acf.hhs.gov/sites/default/files/opre/hs_impact_study_final.pdf.

Witt, J. C. (1986). Teachers' resistance to the use of school-based interventions. *Journal of School Psychology, 24,* 37–44.

Chapter 12
School As a Unit of Assignment and Analysis in Group-Randomized Controlled Trials

Katrina J. Debnam, Catherine P. Bradshaw, Elise T. Pas and Sarah Lindstrom Johnson

Given the amount of time youth spend in schools, schools are common settings for preventive interventions addressing a range of behavioral, mental health, health, and educational outcomes (Cohen et al. 2009). Yet, the school setting presents some unique logistic and statistical challenges for designing intervention trials, due in large part to the "clustering" of participants within classrooms, schools, and even districts (Murray 1998). For example, students have shared experiences that can result in similar outcomes (e.g., behavior, academics, and perceptions). As a result, when testing the effectiveness of school-based interventions, one must consider this clustering when assigning participants to treatment, measuring outcomes, and analyzing data (Luke 2004; Merlo et al. 2005; Raudenbush and Bryk 2002). Moreover, some interventions are most appropriately delivered universally to all students in a school (i.e., rather than select students within school), and thus the randomization (i.e., the gold standard; Flay et al. 2005) should occur at the school level. Such designs are typically referred to as *group-randomized trials* (Murray 1998) and are the focus of the current chapter.

K. J. Debnam (✉)
Johns Hopkins Bloomberg School of Public Health,
415 N. Washington St., Rm 501, Baltimore, MD 21231, USA
e-mail: kdebnam1@jhu.edu

E. T. Pas
Johns Hopkins Bloomberg School of Public Health,
415 N. Washington St., Rm 507, Baltimore, MD 21231, USA
e-mail: epas1@jhu.edu

C. P. Bradshaw
Curry School of Education, University of Virginia, 112-D Bavaro Hall,
417 Emmet Street South, PO Box 400260, Charlottesville, VA 22904-4260, USA
e-mail: catherine.bradshaw@virginia.edu

S. Lindstrom Johnson
Arizona State University, Tempe, USA
e-mail: sarahlj@asu.edu

© Springer Science+Business Media New York 2015   247
K. Bosworth (ed.), *Prevention Science in School Settings*,
Advances in Prevention Science, DOI 10.1007/978-1-4939-3155-2_12

In this chapter, we review factors that are important to consider in conducting group-randomized trials where the school is the unit of assignment and analysis. By unit of assignment, we mean that the school, (i.e., as opposed to students, teachers, or classrooms within the school), is randomized to receive the treatment or serve as a comparison. Additionally, when the school is the unit of analysis, the treatment variable is statistically modeled at the school level, even when data are collected from individuals; the individual-level data serve as the outcomes of interest (Murray 1998). Although our focus is on schools, many of the opportunities and challenges discussed here are also relevant for other group-based designs. For example, similar challenges arise when intervening in and studying classrooms or nonschool settings (e.g., clinics, camps, after-school programs, hospitals, and churches). Individuals in these settings similarly interact with each other and are directly or indirectly affected by other participants. Several of the design and methodological issues considered in this chapter are also relevant to nonrandomized designs, such as regression discontinuity studies (Imbens and Lemieux 2008; Thistlewaite and Campbell 1960), where the school still may be the unit of analysis (e.g., Hallberg et al. 2014). The overall aim of this chapter is to provide guidance to researchers examining preventive interventions where schools are the unit of random assignment and analysis. We take a stage-based approach, beginning with study design, and then discussing recruitment and enrollment, measurement, implementation and analysis, and ending with dissemination of findings.

Where appropriate, we draw upon our own experiences with the National Institute of Mental Health-funded *Project Target* group-randomized effectiveness trial (Bradshaw et al. 2010). Project Target was a collaborative effort of the Maryland State Department of Education, five local school districts, Sheppard Pratt Health System, and the Johns Hopkins Center for the Prevention of Youth Violence to evaluate the effects of a school-wide universal prevention model called Positive Behavioral Interventions and Supports (PBIS) in 37 Maryland elementary schools (Carr et al. 2002). Throughout the chapter, we refer to the Project Target trial as a case study of the design and methodological considerations specific to group-randomized controlled trials. We also use this example to highlight the importance of relationship building with stakeholders to enhance buy-in for the research activities and conduct a successful trial.

12.1 Study Design

The term *group,* or *cluster,* randomized controlled trial (GRT) typically describes a type of study in which groups of subjects, as opposed to individuals, are randomized to treatment and control groups (Murray 1998; Spybrook et al. 2011). GRTs are appropriate when testing an intervention that manipulates the physical or social environment, involves social processes, or cannot be delivered to individuals without risk of contamination. GRTs are common in public health (Varnell et al. 2004) and increasingly in education (Hedges and Rhoads 2011). Similar to individual randomized controlled trials, GRTs are considered the gold standard for evaluating school-level interventions because they allow researchers to draw causal inferences (Donner and Klar 2000; Murray 1998; Murray et al. 2004). This section reviews conceptual as well as practical considerations for conducting GRTs; we then briefly review issues related to study design and power.

Conceptual Considerations There are many conceptual reasons for using a GRT design. Some programs operate at a school level rather than individual level, such as a school policy or a school-wide preventive intervention; these programs would be provided school-wide and not to specific individuals within schools, and thus the experimental examination of them would require a school-level treatment assignment. Other programs are ecological by nature and are intended to impact school-level processes and outcomes; therefore, the study of such outcomes also requires the assignment of schools, rather than students or classrooms, to the treatment conditions. Schools are also an appropriate setting to conduct GRTs, given the complex, multilevel, and interactive nature of students, families, and teachers within this context (Bronfenbrenner 1979; Kelly et al. 2000). For example, in schools, the quality of instruction by a teacher influences the interactions with and between students. Similarly, the behaviors of individual students can influence the quality of the classroom educational experience. Given these interactive qualities of the classroom setting, a GRT helps to reduce risk for contamination when students within classrooms are assigned to treatment.

Practical Considerations In addition to considering the intervention's level of implementation, it is also important to consider the type of school to study (i.e., elementary, middle, and high). Certain interventions are specifically developed to address particular grade levels, in which case, this should be the sample of choice. In other instances, the intervention can be tested at any grade level, but some logistical factors of the different settings may come into consideration. For example, in high schools, youth change classes throughout the day, whereas in elementary schools, students remain largely in intact classrooms with exposure to just one or two teachers throughout the day. Middle schools often have a higher level of class exchange than elementary, but the students typically travel as a group to different classrooms. The movement of students across classrooms, and teachers or administrators across schools can have both implementation and measurement implications and is discussed further in those sections of this chapter. Only recently have statistical software programs, such as M*plus* 7.11, allowed for the adjustment of standard errors to vary across time due to changes in group membership over time (see cross-classification; Muthén and Muthén 1998–2012).

ICCs, Design Effects, and Power The intraclass correlation (ICC) is a statistic used to characterize the amount of clustering, or, more specifically, the proportion of the total variance that is between groups. A positive ICC may occur among students nested within the same school, due to commonalities in selection, exposure, shared environment, mutual interaction, or some combination of those factors. A related statistic is the design effect, which takes into consideration both the ICC as well as the number of participants per cluster. A design effect value of 2.0 or larger generally requires careful consideration of the clustering of observations in the analyses (see Eldridge et al. 2006; Murray 1998).

  Ignoring a positive ICC or a large design effect, and the associated problem of limited degrees of freedom (df), can increase the probability of a type I error rate (i.e., false positive). These problems can be avoided by using analytic methods appropriate to the structure of the design and the data (Donner and Klar 2000; Murray 1998). The number of schools needed for sufficient statistical power will vary greatly by the anticipated effect size, the number of levels in the statistical model, the extent of between-school variability on the outcome measures, the number of individuals per cluster, the number of treatment conditions being studied, the amount of attrition (as in the case of longitudinal studies), as well as the type and reliability of outcome measures being used (e.g., binary versus continuous measures; Murray 1998; Schochet 2013). For example, a recent methodological article noted that trials focused on binary outcomes (e.g., dropout, suspension), which typically utilize 40–60 schools, are likely underpowered to detect an intervention effect on the binary outcomes specifically (Schochet 2013). Furthermore, larger design effects (thus requiring greater statistical power to detect effects) result from larger within-cluster sample size; therefore, some researchers advocate for using a sampling approach to assess a subset of students per cluster, rather than assessing all students within a cluster (for further discussion, see Eldridge et al. 2006).

As with any research design, it is important that an appropriate power analysis be conducted prior to sample selection and randomization (Eldridge et al. 2006); in the case of a GRT, the power analysis will determine the number of schools needed to detect a significant intervention effort on the core outcomes of interest. Several tools have been developed to facilitate the process, such as the Optimal Design (v3) Program (Raudenbush et al. 2011b), Monte Carlo simulations in the M*plus* software (Muthén and Muthén 1998–2012), and Murray's (1998) Excel-based approach to power analysis. Each of these techniques can be used to estimate power while accounting for multiple aspects of the design, including ICCs, cluster size, design effects, and reliability of measures. Researchers may need to draw upon similar prior studies to identify estimates for these parameters and thus the minimum detectable effect sizes. Moreover, multiple scenarios should be examined to determine the estimated power for a range of conditions (e.g., cluster size, effect size).

Overview of the Project Target Case Study

Project Target represented the study of an ecological model called Positive Behavioral Interventions and Supports (PBIS), which aimed to improve the systems, use of data, and delivery of programs to staff and students through a school-wide change in leadership and adult behaviors (Sugai and Horner 2006). In the PBIS model, staff work together to improve the school setting by creating a school-wide framework that clearly articulates positive behavioral expectations, provides incentives to students meeting these expectations, promotes positive student–staff interactions, and encourages data-based decision-making by staff and administrators. The model draws upon behavioral, social learning, organizational, and positive youth development theories and promotes strategies that are used by all students and staff consistently across all school contexts (Lewis and Sugai 1999; Lindsley 1992; Sugai and Horner 2002). Given PBIS is designed to influence school-wide practices and staff and student perceptions and behavior, Project Target was designed to be a GRT of the school-wide PBIS model. Specifically, Project Target sought to determine (a) at the school level, if PBIS schools had fewer discipline referrals than comparison schools; (b) at the classroom level, if teachers in PBIS schools had higher ratings of school climate and principal leadership than teachers in the comparison schools; and (c) at the student level, if students in schools implementing PBIS had higher academic achievement and lower aggressive–disruptive behavior problems than students in comparison schools. With a program of this type, that included intervention components occurring at the school level and the targeted outcomes across multiple levels, it was necessary to assign schools, not students, to treatment versus comparison conditions. An initial power analysis was conducted for continuous outcomes and determined that 37 elementary schools provided adequate power to examine the primary research aims.

12.2   Recruitment and Enrollment into GRTs

Given that the school is the unit of analysis within GRTs, it is usually necessary to recruit a large sample of schools to ensure there is enough statistical power to detect significant differences between conditions (Murray 1998; Spybrook et al. 2011). The recruitment and enrollment of schools into GRTs can include several steps to ensure buy-in and commitment to the study; this buy-in is particularly important given the schools will be randomized to either the intervention or comparison condition. The issue of buy-in and commitment must be considered at multiple levels and is often a top-down process, whereby the local education agency (district) and individual schools must be engaged. In studies involving schools across multiple districts, there are even more stakeholders to consider and thus greater recruitment efforts are needed. Once district buy-in is achieved informally or formally through letters of agreement, both administrator and teacher commitment are needed at the school level to ensure high quality implementation (Domitrovich et al. 2008) and a high response rate in data collection efforts.

A key component to facilitating commitment at the district level is to form collaborative relationships with study partners who can play a vital role in the recruitment and sustained buy-in of schools. These individuals and agencies can help serve as "local champions" (Rogers 2002) for the research as well as for the program (Fixsen et al. 2005; Schoenwald and Hoagwood 2001). As an example, our university-based research team has been working in close collaboration with the Maryland State Department of Education and a nonprofit implementation partner (Sheppard Pratt Health System) for over 15 years; this partnership has helped to engage key personnel from multiple districts to commit to and participate in four GRTs of PBIS, such as Project Target (see Bradshaw et al. 2012a for a review; also see Box 2, pp. 256–257).

After securing district commitment, the next step in recruitment includes garnering school principal support and buy-in. District personnel provide great insight on how best to approach and recruit principals for GRTs. Principals establish the goals and climate for the school and thus are instrumental to any change process taking place within a school (Sarason 1996), including participation in a GRT or any other research study. Principal leadership can serve as either a facilitator or barrier to the implementation of the tested intervention as well as to the completion of study-specific measures. Before school staff and students/parents can be asked to participate, initial consent of the principal is needed for school participation. Therefore, it can be helpful to cohost recruitment or informational meetings for administrators with school district partners, who can speak to their commitment to the project and the importance of the rigorous, randomized design. We have often held these events at the district offices to further symbolize the collaborative nature of the project. Transparency regarding the design details is critical, including a clear outline of the randomization process, responsibilities regarding data collection, and the study timeline. All administrators need to see how the project will benefit their staff and students without additional burden on their already-crowded school day.

A major obstacle during the recruitment of administrators for GRTs is alleviating concerns about randomization into the control condition. Randomization ensures a fair process, whereby all schools have an equal chance to be assigned to treatment or control, but those in the control group may still have negative feelings about their control group status (Ainsworth et al. 2010). Common solutions to this problem include using a randomized waitlist design or providing training to the control schools at the end of the study (Ainsworth et al. 2010). These approaches can keep control schools more engaged, as they await their training.

After establishing buy-in from school administrators, it is necessary to identify strategic opportunities to recruit staff and/or students. Just as district personnel can assist in the recruitment of school-based leaders, administrators can provide an insiders' perspective into the school culture in terms of how to provide a clear message to staff about the project and the benefits to participation. When recruiting teachers and school staff, it is important to recognize that a significant barrier can be staff perceptions of research (for examples see Hunninghake et al. 1987; Lovato et al. 1997), which may include past experiences of limited benefit from research and the perception that research will only add burden to the school. Therefore, recruitment sessions should emphasize any additional burdens while balancing this with *immediate* program benefits. Immediate benefits to teachers and school staff may include additional strategies to use in the classroom, reports from data collected, or access to resources (e.g., trainings, classroom materials) that are otherwise not available. Staff will not be motivated to participate if they cannot clearly see how the study will positively impact their daily work. Another important incentive is monetary compensation for staff members' time spent completing study assessments.

When recruiting students, it is often helpful to create a classroom- or school-level incentive for returning completed parental consent forms, irrespective of the parents' decision to participate. This will encourage students to provide parents with study materials and return them in a timely manner. The various types of written consents required for a study are highly individualized and determined by the university's institutional review board (IRB; see next section). In addition, researchers should be considerate of the communities' needs as well as their perceptions of research. Where possible, researchers may find it helpful to incorporate elements of community-based participatory research into their design (Israel et al. 1998), such as conducting needs assessments and soliciting parents' active participation in elements of the study design. Acquiring support from influential school staff members and parent organizers can also enhance the success of recruitment.

IRB and Consent   In addition to the university-based IRB, many school districts have IRBs or a parallel process requiring approval prior to launching a study. Based on the particular study design, intervention, and how data are collected, written consent may be needed from individual school staff and parents. While youth assent from students may be needed, most research with minors requires some form of parental consent (Mammel and Kaplan 1995). Active consent requires a parental signature agreeing that the child can participate in the proposed study and assessments. Some IRBs may waive the requirement of active parental consent, thereby allowing parents to be informed of the study and assessments and providing parents the opportunity to opt their child out of the data collection (Range et al. 2001). The process of obtaining active written consent from parents can be an challenging and costly task, requiring substantial time, research staff, and resources (e.g., Ellickson and Hawes 1989; Range et al. 2001).

Research has shown that active consent can result in much lower response rates and biased samples, where parents of minority students, parents of students who are from lower socioeconomic status (SES), and parents of children who perform poorly in school are less likely to provide consent (Ellickson and Hawes 1989). This challenge should be considered when designing a study; if data are collected in such a way that student identities are not assessed, then it is possible that active consent may not be required (Jason et al. 2001). Specifically, the American Psychological Association ethics code also suggests that consent may not be needed when anonymous questionnaires are collected while evaluating "normal educational activities" that are likely to be the target of prevention-focused GRTs (American Psychological Association 2002). This is in line with the American Educational Research Association's code of ethics and federal regulations, which state that a waiver for consent is possible when specific criteria are met (American Educational Research Association2011; U.S. Department of Health and Human Services 2009).

When using written consent, our research team has found it helpful to present information about the project to stakeholders at multiple school events and to provide a clear, detailed, 1–2 page fact sheet summarizing study requirements. Throughout the trial, but in particular when obtaining informed consent, cultural and linguistic diversity needs to be considered; forms should be written in a clear and understandable fashion, avoiding research jargon that may confuse staff or parents. In addition, researchers should work with the school to determine whether translated forms are needed for specific subpopulations within the school.

Most IRBs require, at a minimum, written consent to participate in the study from the school principal, which documents their approval of the randomization process and understanding of the intervention. In addition to consenting for their school to be randomized, it may also be necessary to secure an agreement of protections against contamination. Although GRTs reduce risk for contamination across individuals within a school, there is still a potential for cross-school contamination associated with staff or school leadership changing schools or interacting at district events. Having principal and/or teachers agree in writing not to share program materials may further reduce risk for contamination.

Sampling When deciding on the sample of schools for a GRT, one would most ideally define the population of interest upon which the results will generalize (Shadish et al. 2002). Once the population of schools and students is defined, a sample is then selected to represent this population. There are several random sampling methods (i.e., simple, cluster, stratified, and systematic) that can be employed to select the population (Trochim and Donnelly 2007). In its most straightforward form, simple random sampling requires first randomly sampling participating schools from the defined population and then randomly assigning the schools to a treatment condition (Shadish et al. 2002). However, this is rarely employed in practice because of the logistical barriers, such as resource limitations associated with conducting a random sampling, recruiting a large enough number of schools to use a random sampling procedure, and working with schools across a large geographical area (Shadish et al. 2002). If random sampling of schools, is not possible, researchers can instead employ other sampling methods and steps to ensure generalization of findings is possible. For example, if the goal is to generalize to an entire state, cluster sampling can be used to divide schools into geographic regions, in which one can sample clusters of schools and collect data from all students in the sampled school clusters (Konstantopoulos 2011). When random sampling methods cannot be employed, an alternative method is to define clearly the population of interest and then measure the defined characteristics within the sample, as a means for demonstrating similarities and differences between the sample included in a study and the broader population of schools (Shadish et al. 2002). In school GRTs, this includes measuring and reporting baseline characteristics of the school and individuals within it (e.g., school size, performance on student academic and behavioral outcomes, student demographics, and characteristics of the teacher body). This issue is expanded upon in the measurement section below.

Once the sample of schools has been selected, it may also be efficient to use random sampling strategies within schools to select participants. For example, if the goal is to generalize to specific subgroups of students (e.g., males, African Americans) within the schools being studied, stratified random sampling can be employed. This method will allow the oversampling of subgroups of students, based on the proportion of their presence in the sample (Balk et al. 2010). The oversampling of particular subgroups within the school is typically practical to not only ensure the ability to generalize about a specific subgroup but also to maintain power in the face of potential attrition (i.e., students transfer or drop out of school) that can occur across longitudinal studies.

As discussed in the power section, a disadvantage of GRTs is that the number of schools (rather than individuals) is a key component to garnering statistical power to detect differences between treatment and control conditions; though, the number of students within a school is also important to consider when designing the study (Eldridge et al. 2006). However, when sampling a large number of schools, the costs and resources associated with data collection increase substantially, especially if every student within the schools is assessed; therefore, researchers may elect only to collect data on a subset of students within a school. Systematic sampling, or the sampling of every kth student in a school, may be especially relevant in high schools, where the numbers of staff and students in each school can be extremely large.

Sampling must also involve a systematic process which prevents duplication but is inclusive of all student input. For example, the schedule of high schools often complicates data collection, thereby resulting in some researchers selecting a specific homeroom, advisory group, or a single subject, such as language, arts to administer survey materials. We recently used language arts classrooms to administer online surveys to students in a 58 high school GRT. Previous power calculations had indicated that a sample of 25 language arts classrooms per school would provide enough power to estimate intervention effects. Interestingly, in some of the smaller schools in the high school GRT, 25 classrooms represented a population-based approach to sampling wherein all students needed to participate to meet the targeted sample size. A potential drawback of sampling a subset of students is that there may be limited power to detect student-level effect modifiers, such as grade level, gender, ethnicity, or other characteristics unless the sampling approach is designed with this purpose in mind.

Another issue to consider when sampling is that students are generally not randomly assigned to classrooms within schools. In fact, teacher characteristics as well as student factors may influence the administrators' assignment of students to classroom. There are some instances of GRTs where the researchers were able to work in partnership with the school and district leadership to randomly assign students to classrooms, and then classrooms to condition (see for example, Kellam et al. 1998). This level of random assignment of students to schools seems unlikely given that students are typically drawn from geographic catchment areas for specific schools. As a result, it is important to keep in mind characteristics of the students and/or teachers, which may influence students' assignment to groups.

Randomization Some sources of bias can be addressed through randomization. For example, as noted above, there is typically nonrandom assignment of students to schools and classrooms; by randomizing to treatment or control conditions, the differences that can result from nonrandomized classrooms should be evenly dispersed across condition, thus helping to address some of this bias. A number of approaches have been proposed for randomizing schools to condition. Common approaches include complete randomization, where schools are assigned to condition at random. In contrast, pretreatment characteristics can be taken into account when blocking groups of schools or direct pair matching schools based on select pretreatment characteristics, such as demographic factors (e.g., school size, ethnic composition, and free/reduced meals rate) or baseline indicators of the target outcome (e.g., suspension rates and academic performance), ensuring that schools with similar characteristics are assigned to the treatment and control conditions.

In the case of a block design, one or more of the schools within the block is randomly selected, whereas in the case of the matched pairs, one school is randomly assigned to each condition (Imai et al. 2009a). Imai, King, and Nall (2009b) note that "most versions of pair matching with a good choice of pretreatment variables would normally represent a tremendous improvement over a complete randomization design with respect to bias, power, efficiency, and robustness" (p. 66). Although there has been some controversy regarding the efficiency and appropriateness of blocking relative to matched pairs, Imai et al. (2009a) stated that "since matching prior to random treatment assignment can greatly improve the efficiency of causal effect estimation, and matching in pairs can be substantially more efficient than matching in larger blocks, *matched-pair, cluster-randomization* (MPCR) would appear to be an attractive design for field experiments" (p. 30).

For small samples with diverse demographics, it may be challenging to ensure a balanced sample. Some researchers advocate for the use of propensity scores to facilitate the matching process prior to randomization (Imai et al. 2009b), whereas others use traditional randomization approaches. Specifically, propensity score matching can create matched pairs, which have greater balance with regard to a broader set of demographic and pretreatment characteristics. It is also recommended that schools are balanced in terms of the number of schools per condition.

Generalizability Despite efforts to reduce bias through randomization, randomization only addresses issues associated with internal validity, or the validity of causal conclusion; external validity, or generalizability of the findings, is not addressed, as it is based largely on the representativeness of the sampling and the extent to which the sample is representative of the broader population of schools. Stuart and colleagues have proposed a number of methods that attempt to address issues of generalizability of GRT findings to the broader population of schools (see Stuart et al. 2011). Recently, the Project Target schools were matched to the broader population of Maryland elementary schools using propensity scores to determine whether the findings generalized to the larger state population (Stuart et al. 2011). Additional work in this area will provide investigators with more methodological approaches for assessing the extent to which GRT findings generalize to the broader population of schools.

Recruitment and Randomization in the Project Target Case Study
In the Project Target trial, 37 Maryland public elementary schools from five school districts (rural and suburban) were successfully recruited to participate. As highlighted earlier, the partnership served as a foundation for research study buy-in. Recruitment sessions were first held with school district personnel and then with school-level administrators in those districts to secure

commitment. Finally, school-level administrators helped to solicit staff buy-in for participating in the study using a survey completed by their staff. The schools were matched on select baseline demographics (e.g., percentage of students receiving free or reduced meals), of which 21 schools were random-ized to the intervention condition and 16 were assigned to the comparison condition. A slightly higher proportion of schools were randomized to the intervention condition to increase the statistical power to examine research questions regarding variations in implementation quality (see Bradshaw et al. 2008, 2009).

12.3   Measurement

The measurement burden for a GRT can be quite large, complicated by the need to assess potential intervention effects at multiple levels (e.g., school, classroom, and individual) as well as potential confounders at each of these levels (see Boxes 3, pp. 259–260 and 5, p. 263). Additionally, it is important to specify the nature of the in-tervention delivered both in terms of the quantity and quality of what was delivered. This section discusses some measurement concerns specific for GRTs with regard to measuring intervention fidelity, intervention outcomes, and covariates.

Intervention Fidelity   To improve claims of causality as well as improve the likeli-hood of translation of results into practice, it is important to measure *intervention fidelity*. Intervention fidelity is broadly defined as "the extent to which core com-ponents of the intervention are delivered as intended by the protocol" (Gearing et al. 2011). Measurement of intervention delivery can include both measures of the behaviors of those implementing the intervention (i.e., frequency of a specific behavior) as well as measures of the amount of the intervention received (i.e., atten-dance logs; Gearing et al. 2011). In GRTs, the measurement of intervention deliv-ery must be assessed at the group level (i.e., the level of intervention). Thus, for a school-level intervention, each school would have one measure of intervention fidelity. Interventions at the classroom level may need to include teacher fidelity measures in all classrooms implementing the intervention (Hulleman and Cordray 2009; Ialongo et al. 1999). This not only introduces additional measurement require-ments, but introduces variability across classrooms. Between-classroom variabil-ity of intervention fidelity is an important factor to consider when evaluating the impact of an intervention. Studies have shown that classroom- and school-level implementation fidelity is a concern and can be influenced by teacher character-istics (e.g., Beets et al. 2008). Intervention fidelity can be more difficult in situa-tions where multiple individuals are tasked with delivering the intervention, as this increases the number of individuals that need to buy-in to the intervention (see the *Recruitment and Enrollment into GRTs* section above) as well as the support needs (see *Implementation* section below).

Multi-perspective assessments (i.e., administrators, teachers, and students) can improve the validity of fidelity assessment regardless of the level of intervention (Flay et al. 2005). In school-wide interventions, as the treatment is diffused throughout the school, different stakeholders may experience different aspects of treatment delivery. For example, in Project Target, individual teachers were expected to teach the school-wide behavioral expectations and reward student adherence to these expectations (Bradshaw et al. 2010). To accurately assess whether this was happening, it was important that we measured administrators', teachers', and students' perceptions of intervention delivery.

With classroom-based interventions, assessments including multiple perspectives may help account for the social desirability bias that may occur when asking teachers to report their fidelity. This bias can also be eliminated through the use of independent observations of intervention fidelity (Mowbray et al. 2003). The introduction of external observers, however, is costly and may leave concerns about the validity of observations, given that it is difficult to keep observers blind to intervention status and the logistical and financial challenges associated with conducting comprehensive external observations. The most comprehensive way to minimize bias is through triangulating multiple sources of data (e.g., both observational measures and self-report measures; Mowbray et al. 2003).

Outcomes In deciding upon outcome measures for a GRT, it is important to select measures that are appropriate, valid, and reliable for each level of implementation (Flay et al. 2005). Data can be collected at multiple levels (e.g., student, classroom, and school) and longitudinally, which constitutes another level of nested data (i.e., repeated measures within individuals) and thus an additional level in the statistical model. This can complicate the measurement, as assessing various indicators across multiple levels requires that the measures' psychometric properties be sound at each level. For example, it may be difficult to demonstrate solid psychometric properties of measures or indicators that are collected at the cluster level due to the relatively small sample sizes. In Project Target, we collected data from teachers and students regarding individual student behaviors, as well as observational data across various locations in the school. As a result, some indicators were student specific, whereas others were school specific thereby requiring different analytic approaches to assess effects at the student versus school levels. In some instances, we also aggregated student-specific data up to a classroom or school level.

It is typically recommended that multiple sources of data be collected to increase confidence in the results as well as the robustness of findings (Flay et al. 2005). While student self-reporting is an obvious source for interventions designed to influence student behavior, staff can also be asked to provide information about intervention effectiveness as well as student characteristics and behaviors. This is typically easier in elementary schools, as a single teacher has the majority of contact with specific students. In middle and high schools, researchers would need to decide which teacher could accurately complete such a measure. Similar concerns about social desirability bias may occur if the teacher is also delivering the intervention, and independent observers may provide a more impartial view of the students' behavior (Flay et al. 2005). Finally, school-collected data (e.g., suspension and truancy rate) can also be used to evaluate the intervention.

Other Explanatory Variables Other data can also be collected to account for some of the variability in the outcomes, thereby increasing the power to detect intervention effects (Schochet 2008). Again, the clustering of individuals precipitates the need to measure other variables (i.e., covariates) at each level of nesting. For example, student demographics and baseline measures of the outcomes may be used to control for variability in these outcomes, if they are hypothesized to be casually related to the outcome. When examining student-level outcomes, one may also want to account for classroom-level covariates. For example, classroom compositional factors may be important to consider statistically because of shared variability among students at the classroom level. This becomes particularly important in higher grade levels (i.e., middle and high school), where the courses are more skill and prerequisite based, and therefore, students are more likely to share academic achievements. Individual student demographic, behavioral, and academic data can be used to create profiles of the participating classrooms (e.g., percent of students of each gender or ethnic/racial group, percent of students proficient in an academic subject, and percent of students with behavioral infractions) and modeled as classroom-level covariates (Raver et al. 2008). Again, the logistics of this at the elementary level (i.e., where students are assigned to the same teacher all day) are easier than in middle and high schools, where students are not only with different teachers but also with different peers throughout the day. This movement of students further complicates the measurement of exposure to and outcomes of interventions.

Classroom- and teacher-level variables are often included at the first or individual level of the multilevel statistical model when teacher-level outcomes are examined (e.g., perceptions of the school). For example, at the individual teacher level, basic demographic factors (i.e., gender, race, and age) and other factors like number of years teaching/working in the specific school and teaching certifications may be important to measure. These variables can greatly influence implementation and uptake of the intervention as well as intervention effects (Domitrovich et al. 2009).

Finally, at the school and district levels, researchers can collect publically available data to account for in the analyses. This may include the location of the school, school size, student–teacher ratio, number of students receiving special education services, and the concentration of students receiving free or reduced-price lunch. All assessed variables can also assist in the comparison of the sample to the target population to determine how the results can be generalized to other populations (Shadish et al. 2002).

Assessment in the Project Target Case Study

Prior to randomization in Project Target, we were able to collect baseline, fidelity and staff self-report data on a range of indicators. Then in the fall shortly following the summer randomization, we collected student data through observations and teacher ratings of student behavior. The data were then collected each spring in participating schools across all 4 years, for a total of five waves of data of fidelity, teacher ratings of students, and staff self-reports. More specifically, schools completed standard PBIS fidelity assessments as a regular part of the statewide PBIS initiative. Assessments included a staff survey related to PBIS components, a school profile that provided demographic information, and an external evaluation of PBIS fidelity, which consisted of interviews with administrators, staff, and students related to school procedures and rules. The staff in Project Target schools also completed a checklist on school organizational characteristics and a behavior checklist on each student in their classroom. Finally, students were asked to report on their perceptions of the school climate. Annual systematic observations were also conducted in various nonclassroom locations across the schools in both conditions. Administrative and archival data were also obtained to examine discipline problems, attendance, academic achievement, as well as school-level covariates.

12.4 Implementation

To evaluate an intervention, and measure the fidelity with which it is implemented, it is important that the critical components of the intervention are known, trained on, and measured (Century et al. 2010). There may be many facets to the intervention that need to be attended to in a GRT, including how well the implementer delivers the message of the program specifically (e.g., Domitrovich and Greenberg 2000), the extent to which an intervention is implemented as indicated by a manual or treatment materials (Beets et al. 2008; Century et al. 2010; Domitrovich and Greenberg 2000), and the amount of the intervention that is given (e.g., how many "lessons," how often the intervention is used; Dusenbury et al. 2003). With these multiple facets and the multiple implementers within a school setting, the quality and consistency of implementation across intervention deliverers can become a concern (Dusenbury et al. 2003; Ringwalt et al. 2003).

When conducting GRTs, it is important to consider issues regarding training, implementation supports, and fidelity monitoring. An advantage of a GRT, as compared to a within-school treatment assignment, is that there is a certain ease with which one can systematically train teachers or staff members in the intervention with limited concerns about contamination. Training can be embedded into other professional development activities that are already within the structure of the school, such as faculty meetings or other school-wide meetings, to ensure that the entire sample of teachers receives the correct dosage of the intervention training. On the other hand, these types of large group trainings can be more difficult to deliver in terms of engaging a large versus small group of participants; they may require more time and resources than trainings for a smaller group. Buy-in is even more important when trying to deliver an intervention across an entire school. In addition, effectively communicating with schools, teachers, administrators, and/or parents for GRTs takes extra time and modalities (e.g., phone, e-mail, and letters). Poor communication with intervention implementers and recipients can hinder implementation fidelity (see Box 4 below, p. 261).

Research, however, shows that ongoing, rather than occasional support and technical assistance is often needed to ensure adequate implementation (Fixsen et al. 2005). Given the number of schools and individuals within the schools involved in GRTs, this extra implementation support can be costly and difficult to consistently to provide, particularly when the intervention is delivered by teachers within the classroom context. One area that has been of increasing interest within implementation science is coaching to promote the implementation of evidence-based practices and interventions (Pas et al. 2014). However, this introduces an additional aspect of implementation that should also be assessed and perhaps considered as a necessary component of the intervention.

Training and Fidelity in the Project Target Case Study

In Project Target, the PBIS (intervention) training and support system were led and coordinated by the Maryland State Department of Education (rather than Johns Hopkins University) following the state of Maryland's PBIS typical training procedures (Barrett et al. 2008). Specifically, each of the 21 schools assigned to receive PBIS training formed internal PBIS teams comprising 6–10 members (e.g., staff, teachers, and administrators), of which 4–5 team members (including an administrator) attended an initial 2-day summer training. Consistent with the PBIS model, each PBIS team identified a member of the school or district staff (e.g., school psychologist, counselor) who could act as a PBIS coach to support the team meetings and help interpret data associated with the intervention on a monthly basis. There was also a PBIS team leader who ran the meetings and provided other leadership within the school. Neither of these staff members was paid for by the grant, rather their responsibilities for PBIS leadership were often built into their job description or taken on as extra work through the school.

To ensure and maintain consistently high levels of implementation fidelity, several communication methods were employed by the study team. First, the study team provided school teams checklists to track their progress in PBIS implementation. This teaming checklist was not a mandatory component of data collection in the study, but it served as a regular reminder to maintain implementation fidelity. PBIS coaches were also provided a checklist to monitor PBIS implementation of their assigned school. The study team used these forms to communicate regularly with school teams about any barriers to implementation and track progress of individual schools. Finally, PBIS school teams participating in this study (like other PBIS schools in the state) attended annual 2-day summer booster training events. These summer booster training events provided an opportunity for the study team to connect, in person, with PBIS schools and to support their development of an action plan for PBIS implementation in the coming school year.

12.5   Considering Design When Analyzing Data

When conducting GRTs, there are some analytic considerations to take into account. First, one must consider the inherent shared variability between students within schools as well as the fact that schools have been assigned to treatment and control conditions. Students within classrooms and schools naturally share some characteristics (e.g., by virtue of living within the same geographical location) as well as shared experiences (i.e., they are exposed to the same school staff and curriculum, the students interact with one another; Murray 1998; Ozer 2006). As a result, when analyzing data regarding students within schools, it is important to account for this shared variability between students (see section above on ICCs and design effects).

Multilevel modeling accounts for both within- and between-school variability and adjusts the estimated standard errors for individuals and thus is an appropriate choice (Luke 2004; Raudenbush and Bryk 2002). When schools are randomly assigned, all students within the same school will have the same treatment status, and therefore, this assignment status cannot be treated as independent across students. In multilevel models, the treatment status can appropriately be treated as a school- (rather than student-) level variable, eliminating the bias and increased type I error that results from treating assignment status as a student predictor. Classroom clustering and compositional factors are also important to consider analytically (Wei and Haertel 2011).

An advantage of GRTs is that when recruiting and collecting data in multiple schools, oftentimes a large student sample is garnered. With a large sample that is also diverse, there is an additional opportunity to examine subgroup differences, such as demographic characteristics (Farrell et al. 2012), patterns of risk, or symptom trajectories (Bradshaw et al. 2012; Cuijpers et al. 2005). Subgroup analyses can be conducted within the same multilevel framework and can incorporate latent class and growth analyses to identify profiles of students, staff, and/or schools; identify trajectories of change in measures; and examine trends in outcomes over time (Conrod et al. 2013). These types of analyses can expand our understanding of the epidemiology of problem behaviors and varying levels of risk, providing additional insight into the implementation of preventive interventions. These approaches may also help identify for whom the interventions are most effective (Cuijpers et al. 2005). Bradshaw, Waasdorp, and Leaf (2012b) conducted this type of multilevel subgroup analysis within the context of Project Target and observed a significant interaction between grade level of first exposure and school intervention status, suggesting that the effects of PBIS were strongest among children who were exposed to PBIS at a younger age. More recent efforts have used latent variable approaches (e.g., latent class analysis) to identify subgroups of students who are most responsive to the PBIS model (Bradshaw et al. 2015).

Several statistical software programs are now available to analyze such multilevel models. Given the complexity of clustering at multiple levels, not all software include programming to manage fixed and random effects, as this requires the program to fit regression models while accounting for variation at each level. Only a few programs are equipped to analyze longitudinal data for GRT, which account for repeated measurements within students over time. Commonly used software programs for multilevel models observed in GRTs include HLM (Raudenbush et al. 2011a), SAS (SAS Institute, Inc. 2011), STATA (StataCorp 2013), SPSS (IBM Corp 2013), and M*plus* (Muthén and Muthén 1998–2012).

Analytic Approach Used in Project Target Case Study

In examining the impacts of PBIS in the context of the Project Target GRT, we employed a variety of statistical approaches. For example, when examining impacts on student behaviors (e.g., Bradshaw et al. 2012b) and staff perceptions across time (Bradshaw et al. 2010), we used three-level models, whereby we accounted for the repeated measures of students or teachers, who were nested within schools. Many of our initial outcome analyses employed an intent-to-treat approach, whereby we analyzed the data from all participants, according to randomized condition, regardless of their compliance with program implementation (i.e., adherence). Given our high participation and completion rate among both students and staff, we were relatively satisfied with this initial approach (cf. Gross and Fogg 2004); however, we have also considered other factors, such as program adherence in conducting outcome analyses (see Bradshaw et al. 2009). For example, we conducted repeated measures analyses at the school level on suspensions and office discipline referrals, as well as academic performance (see Bradshaw et al. 2010). More recently, our team used a multilevel approach to examine variation in use of positive-behavior support strategies across both intervention and comparison schools, and the extent to which that variation was functionally related to school contextual factors, like school climate (Pas et al. 2014).

12.6 Dissemination

Dissemination of study findings is an important component of any GRT. If grounded in the principles of community-based participatory research (Israel et al. 1998), all partners in the GRT have equal involvement and ownership of the design, intervention implementation, analysis, and dissemination of the study findings. Because GRTs within schools generally include multiple stakeholders (e.g., districts, principals, teachers, and parents), it is critical that data are shared regularly and confidentially. Providing annual study updates, in the form of a short presentation to study partners or more formal annual reports, helps keep everyone informed and committed to the study. School-specific reports can help administrators, school staff, and parents see and learn from the data collected and can encourage sustainability and translation of the research conducted. GRTs that include multiple schools from one school district may provide great influence in creating systems change (Fixsen et al. 2005), wherein successful interventions could be adapted and used within additional schools in the district. Finally, coauthored reports of study findings are another way to disseminate results to the scientific community. Our school partners have served as coauthors on several peer-reviewed papers and multiple conference presentations resulting from these projects (e.g., Bradshaw et al. 2014; Bradshaw et al. 2012a).

The Role of Partnerships in the Project Target Case Study
Project Target was a collaborative effort of the Johns Hopkins Center for the Prevention of Youth Violence, Maryland State Department of Education, and Sheppard Pratt Health System. In 1999, this partnership was formed to provide training, support, and evaluation of the PBIS model and related prevention programs throughout the state to improve conditions for learning in Maryland schools (http://www.PBISMarylandlorg). This partnership created the infrastructure needed to provide the ongoing PBIS training and technical assistance for intervention schools in the trial (Bradshaw et al. 2012a). Instead of schools seeing Project Target as another university-sponsored research study, schools were able to place this study within the context of a statewide scale-up of PBIS. Building on our long-standing commitment to this partnership and the schools involved in the study, research staff created annual comprehensive reports summarizing each school's data and making recommendations for high fidelity implementation of PBIS. The research staff also conducted debriefing sessions with the schools and school districts that participated in the trial. The partnership has also been involved in over a dozen presentations at professional conferences reporting the findings from the trial, as well as three peer-reviewed publications and several reports and presentations for the state department of education.

12.7 Conclusion

This chapter highlighted the considerations at multiple stages in the research, planning, and GRT execution. Of particular importance is the planning that goes into each aspect of a GRT (i.e., sample size, comprehensive measurement of key variables, and ways to balance efficiently resources with statistical power) as well as the relationships one builds to execute successfully a GRT. Although we focused on GRTs in schools to demonstrate the structure and utility of GRTs, several of these issues are important to consider in designing and analyzing data from other group-based interventions or nonrandomized school-based research where students are clustered within classrooms and schools.

Acknowledgments Project Target was funded by grants from the National Institute of Mental Health (R01MH067948-03) and the Centers for Disease Control and Prevention awarded to Dr.

Philip Leaf. We would like to thank Dr. Leaf for his support and contribution to this work. The writing of this chapter was supported in part by grants from the U.S. Department of Education, the William T. Grant Foundation, and the Institute of Education Sciences.

References

AERA Code of Ethics. (2011). AERA code of ethics: American Educational Research Association approved by the AERA Council February 2011. *Educational Researcher, 40*(3), 145–156. doi: 10.3102/0013189x11410403.

Ainsworth, H. R., Torgerson, D. J., & Kang'Ombe, A. R. (2010). Conceptual, design, and statistical complications associated with participant preference. *The Annals of the American Academy of Political and Social Science, 628*(1), 176–188. doi:10.1177/0002716209351524.

American Psychological Association. (2002). Ethical principles of psychologists and code of conduct. http://www.apa.org/ethics/code/index.aspx.

Balk, D. E., Walker, A. C., & Baker, A. (2010). Prevalence and severity of college student bereavement examined in a randomly selected sample. *Death Studies, 34*(5), 459–468. doi:10.1080/07481180903251810.

Barrett, S. B., Bradshaw, C. P., & Lewis-Palmer, T. (2008). Maryland statewide PBIS initiative: Systems, evaluation, and next steps. *Journal of Positive Behavior Interventions, 10*(2), 105–114. doi:10.1177/1098300707312541.

Beets, M. W., Flay, B. R., Vuchinich, S., Acock, A. C., Li, K.-K., & Allred, C. (2008). School climate and teachers' beliefs and attitudes associated with implementation of the positive action program: A diffusion of innovations model. *Prevention Science, 9*(4), 264–275. doi:10.1007/s11121-008-0100-2.

Bradshaw, C. P., Reinke, W. M., Brown, L. D., Bevans, K. B., & Leaf, P. J. (2008). Implementation of school-wide Positive Behavioral Interventions and Supports (PBIS) in elementary schools: Observations from a randomized trial. *Education and Treatment of Children, 31*, 1–26.

Bradshaw, C. P., Koth, C. W., Thornton, L. A., & Leaf, P. J. (2009). Altering school climate through school-wide Positive Behavioral Interventions and Supports: Findings from a group-randomized effectiveness trial. *Prevention Science, 10*(2), 100–115. doi:10.1007/s11121-008-0114-9.

Bradshaw, C. P., Mitchell, M. M., & Leaf, P. J. (2010). Examining the effects of schoolwide Positive Behavioral Interventions and Supports on student outcomes: Results from a randomized controlled effectiveness trial in elementary schools. *Journal of Positive Behavior Interventions, 12*(3), 133–148. doi:10.1177/1098300709334798.

Bradshaw, C. P., Pas, E. T., Bloom, J., Barrett, S., Hershfeldt, P., Alexander, A., & Leaf, P. J. (2012a). A state-wide partnership to promote safe and supportive schools: The PBIS Maryland initiative. *Administration and Policy in Mental Health and Mental Health Services Research, 39*(4), 225–237. doi:10.1007/s10488-011-0384-6.

Bradshaw, C. P., Waasdorp, T. E., & Leaf, P. J. (2012b). Effects of school-wide Positive Behavioral Interventions and Supports on child behavior problems. *Pediatrics, 130*(5), e1136–e1145. doi:10.1542/peds.2012-0243.

Bradshaw, C. P., Waasdorp, T. E., & Leaf, P. J. (2015). Examining variation in the impact of school-wide Positive Behavioral Interventions and Supports: Findings from a randomized controlled effectiveness trial. *Journal of Educational Psychology, 101*(2), 546–557. doi:10.1037/a0037630.

Bradshaw, C. P., Debnam, K. J., Lindstrom Johnson, S., Pas, E., Hershfeldt, P., Alexander, A., Barrett, S., & Leaf, P. J. (2014). Maryland's evolving system of social, emotional, and behavioral interventions in public schools: The Maryland Safe and Supportive Schools Project. *Adolescent Psychiatry, 4*(3), 194–206.

Bronfenbrenner, U. (1979). *The ecology of human development: Experiments by nature and design*. Cambridge: Harvard University Press.

Carr, E. G., Dunlap, G., Horner, R. H., Koegel, R. L., Turnbull, A. P., Sailor, W., Anderson, J., Albin, R. W., Koegel, L. K., & Fox, L. (2002). Positive behavior support: Evolution of an applied science. *Journal of Positive Behavior Interventions, 4*(1), 4–16. doi:10.1177/109830070200400102.

Century, J., Rudnick, M., & Freeman, C. (2010). A framework for measuring fidleity of implementation: A foundation for shared language and accumulation of knowledge. *American Journal of Evaluation, 31*(2), 199–218. doi:10.1177/1098214010366173.

Cohen, J., McCabe, L., Michelli, N. M., & Pickeral, T. (2009). School climate: Research, policy, practice, and teacher education. *Teachers College Record, 111*(1), 180–213.

Conrod, P. J., O'Leary-Barrett, M., Newton, N., Topper, L., Castellanos-Ryan, N., Mackie, C., & Girard, A. (2013). Effectiveness of a selective, personality-targeted prevention program for adolescent alcohol use and misuse: A cluster randomized controlled trial. *JAMA Psychiatry, 70*(3), 334–342. doi:10.1001/jamapsychiatry.2013.651.

Cuijpers, P., van Lier, P. A. C., van Straten, A., & Donker, M. (2005). Examining differential effects of psychological treatment of depressive disorder: An application of trajectory analyses. *Journal of Affective Disorders, 89*(1–3), 137–146. doi:10.1016/j.jad.2005.09.001.

Domitrovich, C. E., & Greenberg, M. T. (2000). The study of implementation: Current findings from effective programs that prevent mental disorders in school-age children. *Journal of Educational and Psychological Consultation, 11*(2), 193–221. doi:10.1207/S1532768XJ-EPC1102_04.

Domitrovich, C. E., Bradshaw, C. P., Poduska, J., Hoagwood, K. E., Buckley, J., Olin, S. S., & Ialongo, N. S. (2008). Maximizing the implantation quality of evidence based preventive interventions in schools: A conceptual framework. *Advances in School Mental Health Promotion: Training and Practice, Research and Policy, 1*, 6–28. doi:10.1080/1754730X.2008.9715730.

Domitrovich, C. E., Gest, S. D., Gill, S., Bierman, K. L., Welsh, J. A., & Jones, D. (2009). Fostering high-quality teaching with an enriched curriculum and professional development support: The Head Start REDI program. *American Educational Research Journal, 46*(2), 567–597. doi:10.3102/0002831208328089.

Donner, A., & Klar, N. (2000). *Design and analysis of cluster randomization trials in health research*. London: Arnold.

Dusenbury, L., Brannigan, R., Falco, M., & Hansen, W. B. (2003). A review of research on fidelity of implementation: Implications for drug abuse prevention in school. *Health Education Research, 18*(2), 237–256. doi:10.1093/her/18.2.237.

Eldridge, S. M., Ashby, D., & Kerry, S. (2006). Sample size for cluster randomized trials: Effect of coefficient of variation of cluster size and analysis method. *International Journal of Epidemiology, 35*(5), 1292–1300. doi:10.1093/ije/dyl129.

Ellickson, P. L., & Hawes, J. A. (1989). An assessment of active versus passive methods for obtaining parental consent. *Evaluation Review, 13*(1), 45–55. doi:10.1177/0193841x8901300104.

Farrell, A. D., Henry, D. B., & Bettencourt, A. (2012). Methodological challenges examining subgroup differences: Examples from universal school-based youth violence prevention trials. *Prevention Science, 14*(2), 121–133. doi:10.1007/s11121-011-0200-2.

Fixsen, D. L., Naoom, S. F., Blase, K. A., Friedman, R. M., & Wallace, F. (2005). *Implementation research: A synthesis of the literature*. (FMHI Publication No. 231). Tampa: University of South Florida, Louis de la Parte Florida Mental Health Institute, National Implementation Research Network.

Flay, B. R., Biglan, A., Boruch, R. F., Gonzalez Castro, F., Gottfredson, D., Kellam, S., & Ji, P. (2005). Standards of evidence: Criteria for efficacy, effectiveness and dissemination. *Prevention Science, 6*(3), 151–175. doi:10.1007/s11121-005-5553-y.

Gearing, R. E., El-Bassel, N., Ghesquiere, A., Baldwin, S., Gillies, J., & Ngeow, E. (2011). Major ingredients of fidelity: A review and scientific guide to improving quality of intervention research implementation. *Clinical Psychology Review, 31*(1), 79–88. doi:10.1016/j.cpr.2010.09.007.

Gross, D., & Fogg, L. (2004). A critical analysis of the intent-to-treat principle in prevention research. *Journal of Primary Prevention, 25*(4), 475–489. doi:10.1023/B:JOPP.0000048113.77939.44.

Hallberg, K., Wing, C., Wong, V., & Cook, T. D. (2014). Experimental design for causal inference: Clinical trials and regression discontinuity designs. In T. D. Little (Ed.), *The oxford handbook of quantitative methods* (Vol. 1, pp. 223–236). New York: Oxford University Press.

Hedges, L. V., & Rhoads, C. H. (2011). Correcting an analysis of variance for clustering. *British Journal of Mathematical and Statistical Psychology, 64*(1), 20–37. doi:10.1111/j.2044-8317.2010.02005.x.

Hulleman, C. S., & Cordray, D. S. (2009). Moving from the lab to the field: The role of fidelity and achieved intervention strength. *Journal of Research on Educational Effectiveness, 2*(1), 88–110. doi:10.1080/19345740802539325.

Hunninghake, D. B., Darby, C. A., & Probstfield, J. L. (1987). Recruitment experience in clinical trials: Literature summary and annotated bibliography. *Controlled Clinical Trials, 8*(4), 6–30. doi:10.1016/0197–2456(87)90004-3.

Ialongo, N. S., Werthamer, L., Kellam, S. G., Brown, C. H., Wang, S., & Lin, Y. (1999). Proximal impact of two first-grade preventive interventions on early risk-behaviors for later substance abuse, depression, and antisocial behavior. *American Journal of Community Psychology, 27*(5), 599–641. doi:10.1023/A:1022137920532.

IBM Corp. Released. (2013). *IBM SPSS Statistics for Windows, Version 22.0*. Armonk: IBM Corp.

Imai, K., King, G., & Nall, C. (2009a). The essential role of pair matching in cluster-randomized experiments, with application to the mexican universal health insurance evaluation. *Statistical Science, 24*(1), 29–53. doi:10.1214/08-STS274.

Imai, K., King, G., & Nall, C. (2009b). Rejoinder: Matched pairs and the future of cluster-randomized experiments. *Statistical Science, 24*(1), 65–72. doi:10.1214/09-STS274REJ.

Imbens, G. W., & Lemieux, T. (2008). Regression discontinuity designs: A guide to practice. *Journal of Econometrics, 142*(2), 615–635. doi:10.1016/j.jeconom.2007.05.001.

Israel, B. A., Schulz, A. J., Parker, E. A., & Becker, A. B. (1998). Review of community-based research: Assessing partnership approaches to improve public health. *Annual Review of Public Health, 19*, 173–202. doi:10.1146/annurev.publhealth.19.1.173.

Jason, L. A., Pokorny, S., & Katz, R. (2001). Passive versus active consent: A case study in school settings. *Journal of Community Psychology, 29*(1), 53–68. doi:10.1002/1520-6629(200101)29:1.

Kellam, S. G., Ling, X., Merisca, R., Brown, C. H., & Ialongo, N. (1998). The effect of the level of aggression in the first grade classroom on the course and malleability of aggressive behavior into middle school. *Development and Psychopathology, 10*(2), 165–185.

Kelly, J. G., Ryan, A. M., Altman, B. E., & Stelzner, S. P. (2000). Understanding and changing social systems: An ecological view. In J. Rappaport & E. Seidman (Eds.), *Handbook of community psychology* (pp. 133–159). New York: Kluwer/Plenum.

Konstantopoulos, S. (2011). Optimal sampling of units in three-level cluster randomized designs: An ANCOVA framework. *Educational snd Psychological Measurement, 71*(5), 798–813. doi:10.1177/0013164410397186.

Lewis, T. J., & Sugai, G. (1999). Effective behavior support: A systems approach to proactive schoolwide management. *Focus on Exceptional Children, 31*(6), 1–24.

Lindsley, O. R. (1992). Why aren't effective teaching tools widely adopted? *Journal of Applied Behavior Analysis, 25*(1), 21–26. doi:10.1901/jaba.1992.25-21.

Lovato, L. C., Hill, K., Hertert, S., Hunninghake, D. B., & Probstfield, J. L. (1997). Recruitment for controlled clinical trials: Literature summary and annotated bibliography. *Controlled Clinical Trials, 18*(4), 328–352. doi:10.1016/S0197-2456(96)00236-X.

Luke, D. A. (2004). *Multilevel modeling*. Thousand Oaks: Sage.

Mammel, K. A., & Kaplan, D. W. (1995). Research consent by adolescent minors and institutional review boards. *Journal of Adolescent Health, 17*(5), 323–330. doi:10.1016/1054-139X(95)00176-S.

Merlo, J., Chaix, B., Yang, M., Lynch, J., & Rastam, L. (2005). A brief conceptual tutorial of multilevel analysis in social epidemiology: Linking the statistical concept of clustering to the idea of contextual phenomenon. *Journal of Epidemiology and Community Health, 59*(6), 443–449. doi:10.1136/jech.2004.023473.

Mowbray, C. T., Holter, M. C., Teague, G. B., & Bybee, D. (2003). Fidelity criteria: Development, validation, and measurement. *American Journal of Evaluation, 24*(3), 315–340. doi:10.1177/109821400302400303.

Murray, D. M. (1998). *Design and analysis of group-randomized trials.* New York: Oxford University Press.

Murray, D. M., Varnell, S. P., & Blitstein, J. L. (2004). Design and analysis of group-randomized trials: A review of recent methodological developments. *Journal Information, 94*(3), 393–399. doi:10.2105/AJPH.94.3.423.

Muthén, L., & Muthén, B. O. (1998–2012). *Mplus user's guide. Version 7.* Los Angeles: Muthén & Muthén.

Ozer, E. J. (2006). Contextual effects in school-based violence prevention programs: A conceptual framework and empirical review. *Journal of Primary Prevention, 27*(3), 315–340. doi:10.1007/s10935-006-0036-x.

Pas, E. T., Bradshaw, C. P., & Cash, A. (2014). Coaching classroom-based preventive interventions. In M. Weist, N. Lever, C. Bradshaw, & J. Owens (Eds.), *Handbook of school mental health,* (2nd ed., pp. 255–268). New York: Springer.

Pas, E., Waasdorp, T., & Bradshaw, C. P. (2014). Examining contextual influences on classroom-based implementation of positive behavior support strategies: Findings from a randomized controlled effectiveness trial. *Prevention Science.* doi:10.1007/s11121-014-0492-0.

Range, L., Embry, T., & MacLeod, T. (2001). Active and passive consent: A comparison of actual research with children. *Ethical Human Sciences and Services, 3*(1), 23–31.

Raudenbush, S. W., & Bryk, A. S. (2002). *Hierarchical linear models: Applications and data analysis methods* (2nd ed.). Thousand Oaks: Sage.

Raudenbush, S. W., Bryk, A. S., Cheong, Y. F., Congdon, R., & du Toit, M. (2011a). *HLM statistical software: Version 7. [Computer software].* Lincolnwood: Scientific Software International, Inc.

Raudenbush, S. W., Spybrook, J., Congdon, R., Liu, X., Martinez, A., Bloom, H., & Hill, C. (2011b). Optimal design plus empirical evidence (Version 3.0) [Computer Software]. www.wtgrantfoundation.org.

Raver, C. C., Jones, S. M., Li-Grining, C. P., Metzger, M., Champion, K. M., & Sardin, L. (2008). Improving preschool classroom processes: Preliminary findings of a randomized controlled trial implemented in Head Start Settings. *Early Childhood Research Quarterly, 63*(3), 10–26. doi:10.1016/j.ecresq.2007.09.001.

Ringwalt, C. L., Ennett, S., Johnson, R., Rohrbach, L. A., Simons-Rudolph, A., Vincus, A., & Thorne, J. (2003). Factors associated with fidelity to substance use prevention curriculum guides in the nation's middle schools. *Health Education and Behavior, 30*(3), 375–391. doi:10.1177/1090198103030003010.

Rogers, E. M. (2002). Diffusion of preventive innovations. *Addictive Behaviors, 27,* 989–993.

Sarason, S. B. (1996). *Revisiting "the culture of the school and the problem of change.".* New York: Teachers College Press.

SAS Institute Inc. (2011). *Base SAS® 9.3 Procedures Guide.* Cary: SAS Institute Inc.

Schochet, P. Z. (2008). Statistical power for random assignment evaluations of education programs. *Journal of Educational and Behavioral Statistics, 33*(1), 62–87. doi:10.3102/1076998607302714.

Schochet, P. Z. (2013). Estimators for clustered education RCTs using the Neyman model for casual inference. *Journal of Educational and Behavioral Statistics, 38*(3), 219–238. doi:10.3102/1076998611432176.

Schoenwald, S. K., & Hoagwood, K. (2001). Effectiveness, transportability, and dissemination of interventions: What matters when? *Psychiatric Services, 52*(9), 1190–1197. doi:10.1176/appi.ps.52.9.1190.

Shadish, W. R., Cook, T. D., & Campbell, D. T. (2002). *Experimental and quasi-experimental designs for generalized causal inference.* Boston: Houghton Mifflin Company.

Spybrook, J., Bloom, H., Congdon, R., Hill, C., Martinez, A., & Raudenbush, S. W. (2011). Optimal design for longitudinal and multilevel research: Documentation for the Optimal Design Software Version 3.0. www.wtgrantfoundation.org.

StataCorp. (2013). *Stata statistical software: Release 13*. College Station: StataCorp LP.

Stuart, E. A., Cole, S. R., Bradshaw, C. P., & Leaf, P. J. (2011). The use of propensity scores to assess the generalizability of results from randomized trials. *The Journal of the Royal Statistical Society, Series A, 174*(2), 369–386. doi:10.1111/j.1467-985X.2010.00673.x.

Sugai, G., & Horner, R. (2002). The evolution of discipline practices: School-wide positive behavior supports. *Child and Family Behavior Therapy, 24*(1–2), 23–50. doi:10.1300/J019v24n01_03.

Sugai, G., & Horner, R. H. (2006). A promising approach for expanding and sustaining the implementation of school-wide positive behavior support. *School Psychology Review, 35*(2), 245–259.

Thistlethwaite, D. L., & Campbell, D. T. (1960). Regression-discontinuity analysis: An alternative to the ex post facto experiment. *Journal of Educational Psychology, 51*(6), 309–317. doi:10.1037/h0044319.

Trochim, W. M., & Donnelly, J. P. (2007). *Research methods knowledge base*. Mason: Atomic Dog.

Varnell, S. P., Murray, D. M., Janega, J. B., & Blitstein, J. L. (2004). Design and analysis of group-randomized trials: A review of recent practices. *Journal Information, 94*(3), 393–399.

Wei, X., & Haertel, E. (2011). The effect of ignoring classroom-level variance in estimating the generalizability of school mean scores. *Educational Measurement: Issues and Practice, 30*(1), 13–22. doi:10.1111/j.1745-3992.2010.00196.x.

U.S. Department of Health and Human Services. (2009). Code of Federal Regulations, Title 45 Public Welfare, Part 46 Protection of Human Subjects (45 CFR 46). http://www.hhs.gov/ohrp/humansubjects/guidance/45cfr46.html.

Part IV
Relationships Between Education and Prevention Science—Parallel Tracks

Chapter 13
School Culture and Classroom Climate

Adam Fletcher

Childhood and youth are critical stages in the life course for improving population-level health and reducing health inequalities because multiple health-risk behaviors, such as smoking, drinking, and drug use (hereafter described collectively as "substance use"); violence; and sexual risk, cluster together among the most disadvantaged youth (Kipping et al. 2012; Marmot 2004). During the twentieth century as youth substance use increased dramatically across the youth population, so too did political and public concerns about adolescent health and risk-taking behavior. This has been particularly true in high-income countries such as the USA and the UK, where harmful patterns of substance use often emerge during early adolescence and contribute to the increasing burden of chronic disease and disability later in the life course (Donaldson 2008; Liao et al. 1999). Youth drinking and drug use are also associated with many acute health risks and other problematic behaviors, such as self-harm, suicide, sexual risk taking, traffic risk behaviors, and violence (Beautrais et al. 1999; Calafat et al. 2009; Fletcher et al. 2010).

The limits of individually focused behavioral interventions, such as classroom-based educational curricula and mass media education campaigns, are now well known. In isolation, school-based health education is rarely an effective means of preventing youth health-risk behavior, and any effects that have been observed tend not to be sustained, especially when the wider school environment does not support the changes (Bonell et al. 2007). Consequently, the US Institute of Medicine now emphasizes the importance of taking an *ecological* perspective to public health improvement (Institute of Medicine 2001; Smedley and Syme 2000), an approach which recognizes the social determinants of health that are beyond the immediate control of individuals. New, multilevel universal preventive interventions are therefore urgently needed. Changing school cultures and climates provides a highly complementary approach to traditional, individual-level health education and other prevention programs in schools in order to promote adolescent health more effec-

A. Fletcher (✉)
DECIPHer, School of Social Sciences, Cardiff University,
1-3 Museum Place, Cardiff, CF10 3BD, UK
e-mail: FletcherA@cardiff.ac.uk

© Springer Science+Business Media New York 2015   273
K. Bosworth (ed.), *Prevention Science in School Settings*,
Advances in Prevention Science, DOI 10.1007/978-1-4939-3155-2_13

tively. This chapter outlines the evidence and policy frameworks supporting such school-level interventions and provides evidence-based case studies of approaches from the USA, Australia, and the UK that have shown effects on substance use and other health-risk behaviors through changing the school culture and classroom climate.

13.1   School Effects on Students' Behavior

The idea of fostering a positive school culture to improve student outcomes is certainly not a new one. In the 1970s, Professor Michael Rutter and colleagues (1979) studied "school effects" in London, demonstrating that the institutional features of secondary schools varied markedly and that differences in students' academic attainment and behavior between schools were associated with these institutional-level cultural and contextual factors. They concluded:

> The total pattern of findings indicates the strong probability that the associations between school process and outcome reflect in part a causal process. In other words, to an appreciable extent children's behavior and attitudes are shaped and influenced by their experiences at school and, in particular, by the qualities of the school as a social institution. (Rutter et al. 1979, p. 179)

This study and much subsequent educational research (e.g., Arnot et al. 1998; Mortimer et al. 1988) suggest that these school qualities are likely to involve inclusiveness and positive student–teacher relations that facilitate a more positive school culture and supportive classroom climate; these features can explain some, if not all, of these significant school effects.

Building on this educational research, West et al. (2004) found evidence of significant school effects on health-risk behaviors in their research with young people in Scotland. After adjusting for students' socio-demographic characteristics, neighborhood environment, and prior health-risk behaviors, significant variations remained between overall rates of substance use in Scottish secondary schools. Those schools with the most engaged students, strong pupil–teacher relationships, and a positive culture had the lowest rates of substance use. Other subsequent multilevel studies examining the effects of the school environment on student health outcomes in the UK and the USA have also found that inclusive and supportive school cultures are associated with lower rates of substance use (Bonell et al. 2013).

Large-scale national surveys have also consistently found that poor school experiences and educational disengagement are strongly correlated with risky health behaviors such as substance use. For example, using cross-sectional survey data from 10 European countries, Canada, and Australia, Nutbeam et al. (1993) found a strong, consistent relationship between "alienation" at secondary school and "abusive behaviors," such as smoking and drinking; they famously warned, "schools can damage your health." Further analysis of these data revealed that students' perceptions of being treated fairly, being safe at school, and receiving teacher support were all related to substance use outcomes (Samdal et al. 1998). Analyses of the Belfast Youth Development Study cohort also found that certain school-related variables were consistently and independently associated with subsequent substance use—for example, positive pupil–teacher relationships at age 13 reduced the risk of daily smoking by 48%, weekly drunkenness by 25%, and weekly cannabis use by 52% at age 16 (Perra et al. 2012). Research carried out in Australia has also found that school disengagement is strongly associated with persistent and problematic drug use (Spooner 2005).

At the same time as this evidence of harmful school effects has emerged, trials of traditional classroom-based health education interventions designed to improve knowledge, develop skills, and modify peer norms have tended to report only relatively small, inconsistent, and short-term effects (Faggiano et al. 2005; Foxcroft et al. 2002; Thomas and Perera 2006). Though necessary to promote students' literacy about health risks and to support the development of peer-resistance skills, health education teaching and learning is not likely to be sufficient on its own for changing youth behavior and substantially reducing substance-use-related harm at a population level. Prevention activities in schools therefore also need to address the whole school environment, especially those institutional features that have been consistently associated with lower rates of substance use, such as an inclusive school culture and positive student–teacher relationships. These features of schools also support the delivery of effective health education. For these reasons, new whole-school, settings-based strategies have emerged to address institutional influences on young people's behavior.

13.2   Settings-Based Approaches to Prevention in Schools

Settings-based approaches to health promotion in schools undoubtedly have their roots in the World Health Organization's (WHO) Health for All Initiative and the Ottawa Charter for Health Promotion (WHO 1986). The Ottawa Charter argued strongly that health is influenced by where people "learn, work, play and love" and heralded the start of more ecologically oriented thinking about how to address individual-level, social, and environmental determinants of health in combination. Subsequent WHO initiatives, such as the Jakarta Declaration, also argued that the social and cultural environment in which young people learn is a vital feature of health promotion:

> Comprehensive approaches to health development are the most effective…. Particular settings offer practical opportunities for the implementation of comprehensive strategies. These include mega-cities, islands, cities, municipalities, local communities, markets, schools, the workplace, and health care facilities. (WHO 1997, p. 3)

Key principles regarded as necessary to achieve the status of a "health promoting setting" are the creation of a healthy physical and social environment; the integration of health-promotion principles into the daily activities of the setting; and development of the capacity to reach out, beyond the setting, into the broader community to support health if necessary (Baric 1993). Health promoters have now applied this approach to a wide range of settings, but most prominently of all, to schools, to support and improve existing prevention strategies. Following a WHO conference in 1989, the Scottish Health Education Group published a report entitled *The Healthy School* (Young and Williams 1989) on behalf of the WHO. Arguing that the whole life and environment of a school can become a health-promoting force, this report advocated strongly for "whole school" approaches to prevention that involved not only traditional health education but also changes in the school environment to foster better relationships both at school and between the school and parents or the wider community.

These approaches that modify the whole school environment have received continued policy support from the WHO, as well as through international networks such as the European Network of Health Promoting Schools and the International School Health Network. If the Ottawa Charter was the beginning of the journey toward settings-based health promotion, then the WHO's framework for Health Promoting Schools was introduced to help operationalize this philosophy. Various government policies around the world have supported such an approach. For example, the UK Department of Health has recognized the importance of the whole-school setting in preventing the onset of health-risk behaviors (Department of Health 1999, 2004). These policy frameworks have also been supported by many educators as such work is increasingly regarded as producing dual benefits in terms of both contributing to health gain and raising levels of student academic achievement.

However, there remains little practical guidance for educators and other school staff seeking to achieve such institutional change. This is not say that we need new standardized, top-down programs that governments, or their public health department, should impose on schools; and therefore, this chapter describes examples, first, of locally adaptable approaches that involve young people in changing their school's organization and culture and, second, of school-wide systems that can be implemented to improve everyday practices and relationships within the school classroom.

13.3   Prevention Through Addressing the School Culture

Systematic reviews have identified several effective interventions that make changes to a school's organization, environment, and institutional culture to deter youth substance use (e.g., Bonell et al. 2013; Fletcher et al. 2008). Among these are innovative new universal approaches that can be adapted to operate in a range of school settings and have been found to reduce a wide range of health-risk behaviors through improving relationships at schools and preventing disengagement, conflict, and unhappiness at school, all of which are features that may lead to substance use and other adverse adolescent health outcomes (Fletcher et al. 2009). Three universal school culture interventions that have been evaluated, namely, the *Gatehouse*

Project, the *Ayan Aba Youth Project*, and the *Healthy School Ethos project*, are described next. All these share three core features that appear to be vital for fostering a more positive institutional culture to promote students' health. First, the process of reviewing and, where necessary, revising a school's systems and practices to ensure the school environment is inclusive and emotionally and physically safe. Second, promoting positive student–teacher relationships to ensure students feel respected, cared for, and have a sense of belonging and commitment to school, and, ultimately, better health outcomes. Third, the importance of setting healthy norms, behaviors, and relationships during early adolescence is clear.

13.3.1   The Gatehouse Project, Australia

The *Gatehouse Project* was implemented and evaluated in high schools that varied according to their level of neighborhood deprivation, in the state of Victoria, Australia, between 1996 and 2001 (Bond et al. 2001). Informed by attachment theory, the project aimed to improve health outcomes via changing high school cultures to promote students' security, self-esteem, and positive communication with staff and other students. The project lasted for 2 school years. At the start of the project, participating schools administered student surveys to assess young people's views on local needs and priorities. Institutional action teams composed of a range of staff and students were then established in each school to review policies and promote a more positive school environment. It was facilitated by an external "critical friend" and directly informed by the data from student surveys. The project also included professional training for teachers and a new student curriculum to promote social and emotional skills.

Evaluated using a cluster randomized controlled trial (RCT) design and compared to schools that continued with their standard practice, the Gatehouse Project produced consistent reductions in composite measures of risky behaviors, including substance use, antisocial behaviors, and risky sexual behavior (Bond et al. 2004; Patton et al. 2006). Some of the most positive findings were for student substance use outcomes: for example, 3 years after the start of the project, fewer young people in the intervention group reported having used cannabis in the past 6 months and there were nonsignificant but consistent 3–5 % protective risk differences for drinking alcohol in the past month, smoking in the past month, and smoking regularly.

The evaluation also suggested that addressing students' early experiences of secondary/high school might be particularly important, further increasing the preventative potential of such an approach: findings from the follow-up study conducted 4 years after the start of the project reported even stronger protective effects for subsequent cohorts of new students at Gatehouse Project schools compared to the comparison group (Patton et al. 2006). The process evaluation also found that the use of multiple different intervention components (in particular, the needs assessment survey, the action team, the external critical friend, and staff training) functioned synergistically to modify the school culture and teacher practices, and these processes were acceptable and adaptable across different school contexts.

13.3.2 The Aban Aya Youth Project, USA

The *Aban Aya Youth Project* (AAYP), another multilevel intervention involving both school environment change and a social skills curriculum component, was conducted in the Chicago public high school system in the late 1990s (Flay et al. 2004). AAYP aimed to reduce health-risk behaviors by "rebuilding the village" in disadvantaged schools, often serving largely African American communities. Goals were to enhance students' sense of community and belonging, and to increase social support, within these schools. Like the Gatehouse Project, AAYP was strongly informed by theories of school and peer attachment which postulate that increasing social ties and cultural pride in schools can reduce rates of aggression, substance use, and other problem behaviors (Flay and Petraitis 1994). The intervention involved a standardized process of school change through convening a local, institutional task force involving staff, students, parents, and local residents to examine and amend school policies relating to young people's health, behavior, and the school ethos; developing new links with community organizations and businesses; and training teachers to develop more interactive and culturally appropriate teaching methods to improve relationships at school.

In the trial, schools were assigned to one of three groups. Schools in the first group participated in the process of whole-school cultural change (school task force and teacher training) plus the new social-skills curriculum. Those in the second group received the curriculum only. In the final group there was no new intervention at all and standard policies and practices continued in those schools. For boys, the whole-school intervention was associated with a 34% reduction in a composite measure of alcohol, tobacco, and cannabis use compared to the comparison group, suggesting that school-level cultural change was a highly effective preventative strategy in these disadvantaged urban school environments (Flay et al. 2004). The intervention also reduced violent acts, bullying, truancy, and school suspension for boys.

13.3.3 The Healthy School Ethos Project, England

Informed by these projects in Australia and the USA, an exploratory trial of a similar approach to youth substance use prevention through promotion of a more inclusive school culture was undertaken in English secondary schools (Bonell et al. 2010a, b). Like its predecessors, this project did not entail the delivery of highly standardized intervention activities enforced on all schools. Rather, schools initiated a structured change process involving a student needs assessment survey, deployment of an expert adviser, establishment of a staff and student action team to review and revise policies and rules using the survey data, and staff training to improve communication at school. This study was exploratory, undertaken across four schools, but it clearly indicated such a flexible, whole-school approach to building a health-promoting climate was feasible and acceptable to the school staff. The results also showed positive short-term effects at 9-month follow-up, as students in intervention schools reported less hurting and teasing of others and were more likely to report feeling safe at school (Bonell et al. 2010a). Substance use outcomes suggested intervention benefits, but results were not significant due to the lack of statistical power in this small-scale study.

An integrated process evaluation suggested that the following are likely to be key ingredients for successfully modifying a school's culture in order to promote a sense of inclusion and reduce substance use and other risky behaviors:

- Involving students in the process of whole-school change
- Deploying an experienced school adviser
- Establishing a new action group involving both students and staff
- Linking resources to progress to incentivize action
- Ensuring a strong focus on actions to benefit the most disengaged students
- Ensuring the project combines actions that are responsive to local needs with common core components (e.g., new staff training, student curricula).

The school that appeared to have the greatest success in changing their policies and practices via this approach reported that their expert adviser's experience as a former head teacher had enabled them to convene for the first time an effective action team involving a range of staff and students. This fact, combined with the freedom to adopt locally determined actions, was welcomed by the school management team and the members of the action group. This project provided the impetus for the school's new action group to review and revise all their peer-mediation policies and practices, using student survey data to inform their actions. The main barriers reported were time, resources, and competing priorities, although schools in this study also reported that they recognized the potential reciprocal benefits of heath improvement on educational attainment, attendance, and student behavior.

Furthermore, qualitative research was undertaken in the UK alongside this project to explore how schools could address substance use at an institutional level. Findings suggested that the following are likely to be important pathways: (a) making changes to improve relationships at school and reduce disengagement and truancy in order to reduce incentives to use substances as a source of "anti-school" identity and bonding; (b) improving safety at school to reduce pressure on students to seek safety by fitting in with substance-using peer groups; and (c) reducing student anxiety and subsequent use of substances as "self-medication" (Fletcher et al. 2009). This qualitative research draws attention to the centrality of promoting positive classroom climates and changing the overall school organization and culture to address teacher–student conflict and student disengagement, student safety, and student stress and anxiety.

13.4   The Centrality of the Classroom Climate

School-based prevention efforts aiming to address important institutional-level determinants must also pay close attention to the routine classroom climate, which includes staff and student attitudes, standards, and tone of communication in the classroom on an everyday basis. A negative classroom climate—especially if it is a relatively normal condition—can feel hostile, chaotic, and out of control, which can lead to conflict and academic disengagement. In contrast, a positive classroom climate feels safe, respectful, welcoming, and supportive of student learning. New school culture approaches, such as those described earlier, are vital for changing the overall organization and ethos of a school—particularly in terms of ensuring that young people's voices are heard and changes are made responsively to address local organizational needs—but many young people's experience of schooling may not be improved greatly if approaches focus merely on macro-level institutional policies and largely ignore the routine practices and behaviors in the classroom that shape students' everyday lived experiences (Rowe et al. 2007).

Although the aforementioned examples do include some components to improve routine communication and classroom climate via staff training and new curricula to promote students' social and emotional competencies, other evidence-based methods are specifically designed for developing and reinforcing positive behaviors to support a positive classroom climate as the norm. By creating safe, engaging learning environments for all students, these methods in turn support school cultural change to promote a more positive, inclusive ethos. In other words, "school culture" and "classroom climate" interventions should be seen as mutually supportive, and equal attention should be given to both in order to prevent substance use and other adolescent health-risk behaviors. Clear classroom rules can also give highly disadvantaged students from challenging family backgrounds clear boundaries and opportunities to practice self-regulation and make good choices. Two examples are described here: the Incredible Years teacher classroom management project; and Positive Behavioral Interventions and Supports (PBIS).

The Incredible Years The Incredible Years training is aimed primarily at teachers who are having difficulties in managing some students' aggressive, hyperactive, and noncompliant behaviors in the classroom (Webster-Stratton et al. 2008). If these behaviors are ignored, or if teachers only give them negative attention, they will continue to increase and likely spread to other students, potentially increasing school disengagement, conflict with staff, and even substance use across the whole school (Fletcher et al. 2009). Randomized evaluations of the Incredible Years teacher training resources undertaken by the intervention developer, Carolyn Webster-Stratton, and her colleagues at the University of Washington report significant increases in teachers' use of praise and encouragement, and reductions in their use of criticism and harsh discipline, following implementation of the program. The following student benefits were also observed: increased cooperation with teachers, more positive interactions with peers and engagement with school activities, and reduced aggression in the classroom (Webster-Stratton et al. 2008). This suggests that it is both feasible and effective for health promoters to work with school staff and train them to adopt new practices and norms.

Positive Behavioral Interventions and Supports (PBIS) PBIS has been introduced school-wide in a range of American and international school contexts and grade levels. The aim is to improve both student academic and behavior outcomes by ensuring all students receive the most effective and accurately implemented instructional and behavioral practices. PBIS is an evidence-based systems approach to support school administrators and staff in establishing not only a more positive school culture but also more positive routine behavioral supports.

The premise of PBIS is that "the discipline process should help students accept responsibility, place high value on academic engagement and achievement, teach alternative ways to behave, and focus on restoring a positive environment and social relationships in the school" (Sprague and Horner 2012, p. 450). Rather than discipline revolving around rule infractions, PBIS establishes a small set of positively worded behavioral expectations, upon which a behavior matrix specific to each context in the school day is constructed. Students receive explicit instruction about how to follow these expectations, with reinforcement for compliance and a clear discipline protocol establishing consistent consequences for misbehavior. Regular data collection enables monitoring of discipline challenges, which may be addressed through environmental modification as well as refinements in the behavior matrix. Following a public health model, PBIS is designed to implement universal interventions for all students, with targeted interventions for students who show risk behaviors or need additional support to follow the behavioral expectations.

This approach is likely to be highly relevant at schools that need to address general classroom management and disciplinary issues (e.g., attendance and antisocial behavior) as well as to support students whose behaviors require more specialized assistance (e.g., those with emotional and behavioral disorders). Where such support does not happen, and truancy and anti-school behavior escalate, substance use is also likely to increase (Fletcher et al. 2008). A randomized controlled trial has found that implementation of school-wide PBIS was associated with reductions in discipline referrals and suspensions, and with improved academic performance (Bradshaw et al. 2010). In another trial, teachers reported improvements in their classroom climate and reductions in aggressive behaviors (Waasdorp et al. 2012).

Although these methods have been found to have positive effects, it has also been suggested that classroom environments and teacher–student relationships may also need to be addressed through the "reclassification" of pedagogic boundaries between teachers and students (Bernstein 2000; Markham and Aveyard 2003), which would require longer-term changes in teacher training and education policies. When strong boundaries are maintained between teachers and students, as is the case in the UK secondary school education system, the opportunities for students to gain insight into the lives and personalities of teachers and school administrators, and vice versa, are diminished, and there may be less scope for developing high-quality relationships and connections. These relationships are vital, as Marzano (2003) found that schools with good-quality teacher–student relationships have 31% fewer behavioral problems over the course of the school year. Yet, the dominant educational orientation toward performance, standards, and outcomes has arguably created more "distant, depersonalized and dehumanising relationships between leaders, teachers and students" (Harris 2008, p. 369).

13.5 The Future of Prevention in Schools

Childhood and youth have always been—and will remain—critical stages in the life course for substance use prevention, and schools have long been recognized as an important site for this intervention. School-based efforts make sense for several reasons, not only because the years young people spend at school are the formative period in their "health career" during which patterns of substance use often develop. Where schools provide universal education, the vast majority of young people have access to it. In turn, students spend a significant amount of time at school—it has been estimated that young people in the industrialized world spend more than 15,000 hours at school (Rutter et al. 1979). Evidence that substance use prevention is beneficial in terms of improving students' achievement and behavior in school has encouraged schools and education policy makers to engage with these activities.

However, health education and health services in schools are insufficient on their own. The importance of the whole school environment—particularly the school culture and classroom environments—in shaping health behaviors, has now been extensively documented. Of the constellation of institutions that influence youth behavior, schools are certainly among the most critical—perhaps because they are the first formal, public institution that young people engage with, or perhaps because of the degree of exposure youth have to them. The success of the interventions described here provides further evidence that there is a strong causal association between, on the one hand, modifying the school environment to increase student participation, improve relationships, promote a positive school ethos, and address disengagement and, on the other hand, reduced student substance use and other health-risk behaviors. These new universal prevention strategies should now be rolled out more widely, with a strong focus on improving students' experiences of school during early adolescence. A stronger focus is also needed on educational policies that promote school connectedness, a documented protective factor for adolescent health (McNeely et al. 2002).

The case studies described in this chapter highlight the key steps to promoting a healthy high school/secondary school culture. First, start by assessing local needs, as all schools are different and priorities will vary. Second, involve young people by using an action group consisting of both students and staff to review and revise policies and practices based on the needs assessment data. Third, ensure that action groups have adequate resources to take responsive actions, monitor these actions, and evaluate change. Because teacher–student relationships are one of the most important determinants of health risk, organizational changes should be supplemented by systems for training and supporting teachers in the use of positive interventions and behavioral supports in the classroom on a routine basis. Together, these school environment interventions can promote inclusivity and school connectedness more effectively and, in turn, help deliver the step change in prevention science and education practices necessary to promote lifelong health.

References

Arnot, M., Gray, J., James, M., Rudduck, J., & Duveen, G. (1998). *Recent research on gender and educational performance*. London: OFSTED.

Baric, L. (1993). The settings approach—Implications for policy and strategy. *Journal of the Institute of Health Education, 31*(1), 17–24. doi:10.1080/03073289.1993.10805782.

Beautrais, A. L., Joyce, P. R., & Mulder, R. T. (1999). Cannabis abuse and serious suicide attempts. *Addiction, 94*(8), 1155–1164. doi:10.1046/j.1360–0443.1999.94811555.x.

Bernstein, B. (2000). *Pedagogy, symbolic control and identity: Theory, research, critique*. Lanham: Rowman & Littlefield.

Bond, L., Glover, S., Godfrey, S., Godfrey, C., Butler, H., & Patton, G. C. (2001). Building capacity for system-level change in schools: Lessons from the Gatehouse Project. *Health Education & Behavior, 28*(3), 368–383. doi:10.1177/109019810102800310.

Bond, L., Patton, G., Glover, S., Carlin, J. B., Butler, H., Thomas, L., & Bowes, G. (2004). The Gatehouse Project: Can a multilevel school intervention affect emotional well-being and health risk behaviors? *Journal of Epidemiology & Community Health, 58*(12), 997–1003. doi:10.1136/jech.2003.009449.

Bonell, C., Fletcher, A., & McCambridge, J. (2007). Improving school ethos may reduce substance misuse and teenage pregnancy. *BMJ, 334*, 614–616. doi:10.1136/bmj.39139.414005.AD.

Bonell, C., Sorhaindo, A., Allen, E., Strange, V., Wiggins, M., Fletcher, A., Oakley, A., Bond, L., Flay, B., Patton, G., & Rhodes, T. (2010a). Pilot multi-method trial of a school-ethos intervention to reduce substance use: Building hypotheses about upstream pathways to prevention. *Journal of Adolescent Health, 47*(6), 555–563. doi:10.1016/j.jadohealth.2010.04.011.

Bonell, C., Sorhaindo, A., Strange, V., Wiggins, M., Allen, E., Fletcher, A., Oakley, A., Bond, L., Flay, B., Patton, G., & Rhodes, T. (2010b). A pilot whole-school intervention to improve school ethos and reduce substance use. *Health Education, 110*(4), 252–272. doi:10.1108/09654281011052628.

Bonell, C., Jamal, F., Harden, A., Wells, H., Parry, W., Fletcher, A., Campbell, R., & Whitehead, M. (2013). Systematic review of the effects of schools and school environment interventions on health: Evidence mapping and synthesis. *Public Health Research, 1*(1). doi:10.3310/phr01010.

Bradshaw, C., Mitchell, M., & Leaf, P. (2010). Examining the effects of school-wide positive behavioral interventions and supports on student outcomes: Results from a randomized controlled effectiveness trial in elementary schools. *Journal of Positive Behavior Interventions, 12*(3), 133–148. doi:10.1177/1098300709334798.

Calafat, A., Blay, N., Juan, M., Adrover, D., Bellis, M. A., Hughes, K., Stocco, P., Siamou, I., Mendes, F., & Bohrn, K. (2009). Traffic risk behaviors at nightlife: Drinking, taking drugs, driving, and use of public transport by young people. *Traffic Injury Prevention, 10*(2), 162–169. doi:10.1080/15389580802597054.

Department of Health (UK). (1999). *Saving lives: Our healthier nation*. London: Stationery Office.

Department of Health (UK). (2004). *Choosing health: Making healthier choices easier*. [Public Health White Paper]. London: Author.

Donaldson, L. (2008). *Tackling the health of the teenage nation: 2007 Annual report of the chief medical officer on the state of public health*. London: Department of Health. http://info.wirral.nhs.uk/document_uploads/Annually-Produced-Reports/2007CMOreport.pdf.

Faggiano, F., Vigna-Taglianti, F. D., Versino, E., Zambon, A., Borraccino, A., & Lemma, P. (2005). School-based prevention for illegal drugs' use. *Cochrane Database of Systematic Reviews, 2*, art. no. CD003020. doi:10.1002/14651858.CD003020.pub2.

Flay, B. R., & Petraitis, J. (1994). The theory of triadic influence: A new theory of health behavior with implications for preventive interventions. In G. Albrecht (Ed.), *Advances in medical sociology: A reconsideration of health behavior change models* (pp. 19–44). Greenwich: JAI Press.

Flay, B. R., Graumlich, S., Segawa, E., Burns, J. L., Holliday, M. Y., & Aban Aya Investigators (2004). Effects of 2 prevention programs on high-risk behaviors among African American youth: A randomized trial. *Archives of Pediatrics & Adolescent Medicine, 158*(4), 377–384. doi:10.1001/archpedi.158.4.377.

Fletcher, A., Bonell, C., & Hargreaves, J. (2008). School effects on young people's drug use: A systematic review of intervention and observational studies. *Journal of Adolescent Health, 42*(3), 209–220. doi:10.1016/j.jadohealth.2007.09.020.

Fletcher, A., Bonell, C., Sorhaindo, A., & Strange, V. (2009). How might schools influence young people's drug use? Development of theory from qualitative case-study research. *Journal of Adolescent Health, 45*(2), 126–132. doi:10.1016/j.jadohealth.2008.12.021.

Fletcher, A., Calafat, A., Pirona, A., & Olszewski, D. (2010). Young people, recreational drug use and harm reduction. In European Monitoring Centre for Drugs and Drug Addiction (Ed.), *Harm reduction: Evidence, impacts and challenges* (pp. 357–378). Luxembourg: Publications Office of the European Union.

Foxcroft, D. R., Ireland, D., Lowe, G., & Breen, R. (2002). Primary prevention for alcohol misuse in young people. *Cochrane Database of Systematic Reviews, 3*, art. no. CD003024. doi:10.1002/14651858.CD003024.

Harris, B. (2008). Befriending the two-headed monster: Personal, social and emotional development in schools in challenging times. *British Journal of Guidance and Counselling, 36*(4), 367–383. doi:10.1080/03069880802364494.

Institute of Medicine. (2001). *Health and behavior: The interplay of biological, behavioral and societal influences*. Washington, DC: National Academy Press.

Kipping, R. R., Campbell, R. M., MacArthur, G. J., Gunnell, D. J., & Hickman, M. (2012). Multiple risk behaviour in adolescence. *Journal of Public Health, 34*(s1), i1–i2. doi:10.1093/pubmed/fdr122.

Liao, Y., McGee, D., Kaufman, J., Cao, G., & Cooper, R. (1999). Socioeconomic status and morbidity in the last years of life. *American Journal of Public Health, 89*(4), 569–572. doi:10.2105/AJPH.89.4.569.

Markham, W., & Aveyard, P. (2003). A new theory of health promoting schools based on human functioning, school organization and pedagogic practice. *Social Science & Medicine, 56*(6), 1209–1220. doi:10.1016/S0277-9536(02)00120-X.

Marmot, M. (2004). Creating healthier societies. *Bulletin of the World Health Organization, 82*(5), 320. http://www.who.int/bulletin/volumes/82/5/320.pdf.

Marzano, R. (2003). *What works in schools: Translating research into action*. Vancouver: ASCD.

McNeely, C. A., Nonnemaker, J. M., & Blum, R. W. (2002). Promoting school connectedness: Evidence from the National Longitudinal Study of adolescent health. *Journal of School Health, 72*(4), 138–146. doi:10.1111/j.1746-1561.2002.tb06533.x.

Mortimer, P., Sammons, P., Stoll, L., Lewis, D., & Ecob, R. (1988). *School matters: The junior years*. London: Open Books.

Nutbeam, D., Smith, C., Moore, L., & Bauman, A. (1993). Warning! Schools can damage your health: Alienation from school and its impact on health behaviour. *Journal of Paediatrics & Child Health, 29*(s1), S25–S30. doi:10.1111/j.1440-1754.1993.tb02256.x.

Patton, G. C., Bond, L., Carlin, J. B., Thomas, L., Butler, H., Glover, S., Catalano, R., & Bowes, G. (2006). Promoting social inclusion in schools: A group-randomized trial of effects on student health risk behavior and well-being. *American Journal of Public Health, 96*(9), 1582–1587. doi: 10.2105/AJPH.2004.047399.

Perra, O., Fletcher, A., Bonell, C., Higgins, K., & McCrystal, P. (2012). School-related predictors of smoking, drinking and drug use: Evidence from the Belfast Youth Development Study. *Journal of Adolescence, 35*(2), 315–324. doi:10.1016/j.adolescence.2011.08.009.

Rowe, F., Stewart, D., & Patterson, C. (2007). Promoting school connectedness through whole school approaches. *Health Education, 107*(6), 524–542. doi:10.1108/09654280710827920.

Rutter, M., Maughan, B., Mortimer, P., & Ouston, J. (1979). *Fifteen thousand hours: Secondary schools and their effects on children.* Somerset: Open Books.

Samdal, O., Nutbeam, D., Wold, B., & Kannas, L. (1998). Achieving health and educational goals through school—A study of the importance of the school climate and the student's satisfaction with school. *Health Education Research: Theory and Practice, 13*(3), 383–397. doi:10.1093/her/13.3.383.

Smedley, B. D., & Syme, S. L. (2000). *Promoting health: Intervention strategies from social and behavioral research.* Washington, DC: National Academy Press.

Spooner, C. (2005). Structural determinants of drug use—A plea for broadening our thinking. *Drug and Alcohol Review, 24*(2), 89–92. doi:10.1080/09595230500102566.

Sprague, J. R., & Horner, R. H. (2012). School-wide positive behavioral interventions and supports: Proven practices and future directions. In S. R. Jimerson, A. B. Nickerson, M. J. Mayer, & M. J. Furlong (Eds.), *Handbook of school violence and school safety: International research and practice* (2nd ed., pp. 447–467). New York: Routledge.

Thomas, R., & Perera, R. (2006). School-based programs for preventing smoking. *Cochrane Database of Systematic Reviews, 3,* art. no. CD001293. doi:10.1002/14651858.CD001293.pub2.

Waasdorp, T. E., Bradshaw, C. P., & Leaf, P. J. (2012). The impact of schoolwide positive behavioral interventions and supports on bullying and peer rejection: A randomized controlled effectiveness trial. *Archives of Pediatrics & Adolescent Medicine, 166*(2), 149–156. doi:10.1001/archpediatrics.2011.755.

Webster-Stratton, C., Reid, M. J., & Stoolmiller, M. (2008). Preventing conduct problems and improving school readiness: Evaluation of the incredible years teacher and child training programs in high-risk schools. *Journal of Child Psychology & Psychiatry, 49*(5), 471–488. doi:10.1111/j.1469-7610.2007.01861.x.

West, P., Sweeting, H., & Leyland, A. (2004). School effects on pupils' health behaviours: Evidence in support of the health promoting school. *Research Papers in Education, 19*(3), 261–291. doi:10.1080/02671522.2004.10058645.

World Health Organization (WHO). (1986). *The Ottawa charter for health promotion.* Copenhagen: WHO. http://www.who.int/healthpromotion/conferences/previous/ottawa/en/.

World Health Organization (WHO). (1997). *Jakarta declaration on leading health promotion into the 21st century.* Geneva: WHO. http://www.who.int/healthpromotion/conferences/previous/jakarta/declaration/en/.

Young, I., & Williams, T. (1989). *The healthy school.* Edinburgh: Scottish Health Education Group.

Chapter 14
Social and Emotional Learning (SEL): A Framework for Academic, Social, and Emotional Success

Jessica Newman and Linda Dusenbury

14.1 Skills for Success in School, Work, and Life

Young people will face many challenges in the decades to come, including global problems such as climate change as well as competition for oil, water, and other natural resources. Knowledge of math and science will be important, but knowledge alone will not be sufficient to prepare young people to meet these challenges. Solutions to these and other problems will demand teamwork and problem solving. In addition, the accelerating rate of information growth and the constant development of new technologies will require young people to have the requisite skills to learn independently, so that they can master new information throughout their lives.

In the future, students will also need different intra- and interpersonal skills to succeed both academically and socially in a variety of learning environments. For example, intrapersonal skills in the area of self-management will allow them to focus on tasks. Interpersonal skills such as social awareness and communication skills are necessary in order to plan collaboratively with others and work effectively in teams with people who come from different backgrounds and have diverse skill sets. The most successful individuals in the future will likely be those who are able to constantly seek and independently learn new information. In fact, two recent reports—one produced jointly by the Conference Board, Partnership for 21st Century Skills, Corporate Voices for Working Families, and the Society for Human Resource Management (2006), and the other by the American Management Association (2012)—both reveal that employers consider it critical that their employees have skills in the areas of critical thinking, problem solving, collaboration,

J. Newman (✉)
American Institutes for Research (AIR), 20 N. Wacker Drive, Suite 1231, Chicago,
IL 60606, USA
e-mail: jnewman@air.org

L. Dusenbury
Collaborative for Academic, Social, and Emotional Learning, 720 Barber Rd.,
Southern Pines, NC 28387, USA
e-mail: lindadusenbury@gmail.com

© Springer Science+Business Media New York 2015   287
K. Bosworth (ed.), *Prevention Science in School Settings*,
Advances in Prevention Science, DOI 10.1007/978-1-4939-3155-2_14

and communication. Likewise, more than 600 teachers in a national survey indicated that they endorse social and emotional learning (SEL) for all students as something that merits more attention in school, improves academic performance, increases positive social behaviors, and prepares students for learning in the real world (Bridgeland et al. 2013).

14.2 History of SEL as a Framework for Academic, Social, and Emotional Success

In the past few decades, public education has faced increasing prevalence of issues that challenge students' healthy growth and development (Greenberg et al. 2001), including rising poverty, academic failure, school dropout, bullying, substance abuse, and violence. During the same time, schools have faced increasing demands to meet student needs and promote academic performance, leading to the implementation of a large number of prevention and intervention efforts addressing a variety of concerns. For example, the past 20 years has witnessed a series of academic innovations designed to improve student performance in core content areas such as reading and mathematics, along with a growing number of empirically supported programs that prevent risky behaviors such as drug use, violence, and bullying; promote character development, service learning, and positive behavior support, or both (see Catalano et al. 2002; Cicchetti et al. 2000; Durlak 1997; Greenberg et al. 2001; Weissberg and Greenberg 1998).

As schools attempt to implement an increasing number and variety of school-wide prevention and health-promotion initiatives, many efforts may lack the necessary coordination or support from key stakeholders, leading to poor quality and often only short-term implementation. Not surprisingly, educators reportedly suffer from "initiative fatigue" and often view programs as piecemeal add-ons that are easily abandoned when priorities shift.

It is however possible to coordinate and organize these important prevention efforts, in order to combat multiple barriers to student learning in a manner that is feasible and sustainable. Although the concepts, competencies, and skills behind what we now know as SEL had been receiving increased attention for years, the field lacked a unifying vocabulary or framework to tie everything together. The Fetzer Institute convened the leading minds in education research and practice for a meeting in 1994, where they coined the term *SEL*. SEL, as a new term and concept, would serve as a unifying framework for addressing a broad range of competencies and skills (Elias et al. 1997; Greenberg et al. 2003). These experts believed that addressing SEL as a developmental process would enable youth to develop important competencies that would likely not only reduce or prevent problem behaviors but also enhance young people's existing strengths and skills.

As a result of this Fetzer Institute, the Collaborative for Academic, Social, and Emotional Learning (CASEL) was officially formed "to make evidence-based SEL an integral part of education from preschool through high school" (CASEL n.d.).

CASEL has defined SEL as "the processes through which children and adults acquire and effectively apply the knowledge, attitudes, and skills necessary to understand and manage emotions, set and achieve positive goals, feel and show empathy for others, establish and maintain positive relationships, and make responsible decisions." SEL consists of "five interrelated sets of cognitive, affective, and behavioral competencies: self-awareness, self-management, social awareness, relationship skills, and responsible decision-making" (CASEL 2012, p. 9). Although many other definitions encompassing a variety of personal and social skills have been proposed, we define SEL according to the five competency sets as originally presented by Elias et al. in 1997 and further refined in related works by Payton et al. (2000) and CASEL (2003, 2012). At the time of this writing, this is the most widely used research- and evidence-based set of competencies in the field of SEL. These competencies have been used in a wide variety of ways: They served as the defining criteria in the only comprehensive review of SEL programs (CASEL 2012) and as a basis for state learning standards for SEL in Illinois (2005), Kansas (2012), and Pennsylvania (2012). They have also been codified in proposed bipartisan federal legislation supporting SEL for students, specifically, the Academic, Social, and Emotional Learning Acts of 2009 (H.R. 4223), 2011 (H.R. 2437), and 2013 (H.R. 1875). Table 14.1 displays the five competency domains, with examples of skills standards at pre-K, elementary-, middle-, and high-school levels. These developmental examples are intended to be illustrative rather than definitive.

Over the past three decades, the concept of SEL has served as an umbrella framework for a variety of approaches to positive youth development (Schonert-Reichl and Hymel 2007). Recent education movements, including 21st Century Learning, Career Readiness, and Association for Supervision and Curriculum Development (ASCD)'s Whole Child, are designed in part to prepare students to succeed in the global future. Not surprisingly, these movements converge on a similar set of goals for students that center on the development of social and emotional competencies. As mentioned earlier, a number of reports have also identified competencies and skill sets related to SEL that will be important for success in the future (see, e.g., American Management Association 2012; US Department of Labor 1991; and Wilstrom-Ahlstrom et al. 2011). For example, a recently released National Research Council report recommends an educational approach the authors call "deeper learning" and highlights the importance of twenty-first century skills in three critical domains: cognitive, interpersonal, and intrapersonal. Cognitive competencies include critical thinking, problem solving, and reasoning; interpersonal skills include communication and collaboration with others; and intrapersonal competencies include metacognition, conscientiousness, and self-direction (Pellegrino and Hilton 2012). The partnership for twenty-first century skills (2011) has developed a framework that includes *learning and innovation skills* such as creativity and innovation, critical thinking and problem solving, communication, and collaboration; and *life and career skills* that include flexibility and adaptability, initiative and self-direction, social and cross-cultural skills, productivity and accountability, and leadership and responsibility.

Table 14.1 Sample social and emotional learning (SEL) competencies and skills at key developmental periods

Skill domain	Definition[a]	Example competency and skill standards[b]			
		Preschool	Elementary school	Middle school	High school
Self-awareness	Accurately recognizing one's emotions and thoughts, and their influence on behaviors, assessing one's strengths and limitations, and possessing a well-grounded sense of confidence and optimism	Recognize and label basic emotions, describe oneself using several basic characteristics, show initiative, self-direction, and independence in actions	Describe a range of emotions and the situations that cause them, identify personal skills and interests that one wants to develop, identify personal strengths and weaknesses, ask clarifying questions	Analyze factors that create stress or motivate successful performance, describe benefits of various personal qualities	Analyze how thoughts and emotions affect behavior, generate ways to develop more positive attitudes, implement a plan to build on a strength, meet a need, or address a challenge
Self-management	Regulating one's emotions, thoughts, and behaviors effectively in different situations	Express feelings that are appropriate to the situation, understand and follow rules, identify and develop techniques to manage emotions	Identify goals for academic success and classroom behavior, describe the steps in setting and working toward goal achievement	Apply strategies to manage stress and to motivate successful performance, set a short-term goal and make a plan for achieving it	Analyze cause/effect relationships, evaluate how expressing more positive attitudes influences others
Social awareness	Demonstrating the ability to take the perspective of and empathize with others from diverse backgrounds and cultures; to understand social and ethical norms for behavior; and to recognize family, school, and community resources and supports	Recognize the feelings of others, show sympathy and caring for others	Describe ways that people are similar and different, predict how one's own behavior affects the emotions of others	Explain how individual, social, and cultural differences may increase vulnerability to stereotyping and identify ways to address this	Demonstrate ways to express understanding of those who hold different opinions

Table 14.1 (continued)

Skill domain	Definition[a]	Example competency and skill standards[b]			
Relationship skills	Establishing and maintaining healthy relationships with diverse individuals and groups, communicating clearly, listening actively, cooperating with others, resisting inappropriate social pressure, negotiating conflict constructively, and seeking and offering help when needed	Demonstrate attachment to familiar adults, develop positive relationships with peers, engage in cooperative group play	Describe approaches for making and keeping friends, identify approaches to resolving conflicts constructively	Demonstrate cooperation and teamwork to promote group effectiveness	Evaluate the application of communication and social skills in daily interactions with peers, teachers, and families
Responsible decision-making	Making constructive and respectful choices about personal behavior, social interactions, and school based on consideration of ethical standards, safety concerns, social norms, the realistic evaluation of consequences of various actions, and the well-being of oneself and others	Discuss why rules exist, follow rules and make good choices about behavior, begin finding alternative solutions to problems	Identify a range of decisions that students make at school; identify and apply the steps of systematic decision-making	Analyze the short- and long-term outcomes of safe, risky, and harmful behaviors, evaluate one's participation in efforts to address an identified need in one's local community	Analyze one's responsibilities as an involved citizen of a democratic society, work cooperatively with others to plan, implement, and evaluate a project that addresses an identified need in the broader community

[a] Definitions from CASEL (2012, p. 9)
[b] Examples from Anchorage School District 2004/2013; Illinois State Board of Education 2005; Kansas State Department of Education 2012)

In the past decade, state learning standards have also begun moving in the direction of articulating standards for SEL that will prepare students for present and future success. This goal is reflected in the Common Core State Standards developed by the National Governors Association Center for Best Practices and the Council of Chief State School Officers (2010), organizations which represent all the states. The Common Core Standards articulate what students should know and be able to do in the areas of mathematics and English language arts at each grade. However, they go beyond knowledge acquisition to describe the underlying learning skills (many of which are social and emotional competencies) students will need to master these subject areas, including skills in problem solving, speaking, and listening. These were previously called "habits of mind" and are now referred to as the "capacities of a literate individual" for English language arts and "standards of mathematical practice" for mathematics. Capacities of a literate individual include demonstrating independence, building strong content knowledge, responding to varying demands, comprehending and critiquing, and valuing evidence. Standards of mathematical practice include making sense of problems and persevering in solving them, reasoning abstractly, constructing viable arguments, using appropriate tools strategically, and reasoning (National Governors Association Center for Best Practices & Council of Chief State School Officers 2010).

A number of programs have been developed over the years to promote social and emotional competencies. In the sections that follow, we discuss programs currently available to schools and to afterschool and expanded learning programs, the research that supports the efficacy of these programs, and common elements of SEL programs.

14.3 SEL Programs

SEL programming has typically been delivered within the school setting during the day; however, research suggests that providing high-quality SEL instruction in afterschool or expanded learning programs could also be an effective way to strengthen students' social, emotional, and academic skills (Durlak and Weissberg 2007; Durlak et al. 2010; Miller 2003). In fact, given the limited time during the school day and the current emphasis in public education on core academic content areas and high-stakes testing, programs designed for delivery outside the instructional day or in settings other than school may have excellent potential for enriching the lives of youth.

As we use the term, "SEL programs" encompasses any educational activities and pedagogy designed to promote the development of social and emotional skills and behaviors. The SEL framework has been applied in programming intended to address a wide variety of goals, including to support positive youth development broadly defined; to promote health and character development; and to prevent substance abuse, violence, and other risk behaviors. SEL "programs" have also taken a variety of forms, for example, some out-of-the-box lesson-based curricula focus explicitly on developing social and emotional skills, whereas others seek to integrate social and emotional skill development within a core academic subject area, such as language arts or social studies. Other approaches involve training and professional development initiatives designed to influence teacher and staff pedagogy and emphasize responsive practices.

14.3.1   Impact of SEL Programs

Over the past few decades, the field of SEL has advanced in terms of both the quality of programming and the growing evidence base to support the effectiveness of SEL instruction. Two recent developments are (a) a meta-analysis of 213 research studies of SEL programs (Durlak et al. 2011) and (b) a comprehensive review of 23 evidence-based SEL programs currently available for use in preschool and elementary schools (CASEL 2012). These and other studies indicate that social and emotional competencies and skills are teachable, that regular classroom teachers can effectively develop those competencies and skills in their students (Cohen 2006; Durlak et al. 2011; Kress and Elias 2006) and in themselves; and that, when implemented with fidelity, SEL programs can improve social behavior and academic performance and reduce conduct problems and emotional distress (Durlak et al. 2011). Many educators now believe that SEL is "the missing piece" in education and a critical factor in student success both in and out of the classroom (Bridgeland et al. 2013).

The *2013 CASEL Guide: Effective Social and Emotional Learning Programs: Preschool and Elementary Edition* is a comprehensive review developed by a large team of researchers, of which we were a part. A companion edition covering programs for middle-school and high-school ages is in development as of 2013. The release of this guide was an important development, because it set a new standard for the minimum level of evidence required for SEL programs to be considered effective. Specifically, at least one evaluation using a pretest/posttest, control group design must have demonstrated that the program had a desired effect on at least one of four key outcomes: academic performance, positive social behavior, emotional distress, or conduct problems (CASEL 2012). A total of 23 programs were found to meet these criteria, with many having more than one qualifying evaluation or influencing more than one outcome of interest.

Although the *2013 CASEL Guide* is the only review to focus specifically on SEL programs, several other systematic reviews of evidence-based prevention programs exist, including the US Department of Education, Institute of Education Sciences's *What Works ClearinghouseTM)*, the US Department of Health and Human Services' Substance Abuse and Mental Health Services Administration (SAMHSA) *National Registry of Evidence Based Programs and Practices (NREPP)*, the Center for the Study and Prevention of Violence *Blueprints for Healthy Youth Development*, the California Healthy Kids *Research-Validated Programs*, and the US Department of Justice's *Office of Juvenile Justice and Delinquency Prevention (OJJDP) Model Programs Guide*. Each of these guides has slightly different review criteria. For example, some assess quality of evaluation studies in terms of characteristics of the sample, study design, analysis procedures, and reported outcomes (e.g., *What Works Clearinghouse (WWC), NREPP*). Others (e.g., California Healthy Kids *Research-Validated Programs*) focus on specific outcomes of interest in addition to requiring adequate study design. Still others examine programmatic features that occurred during the evaluation (e.g., *NREPP, OJJDP Model Programs Guide*) such as fidelity of implementation or quality of training and implementation support. Many of the effective SEL programs have also met the criteria for inclusion in these other sources, and descriptions of them can be found there. Because the *2013 CASEL Guide* is the only source to focus exclusively on SEL, however, we base our following discussion of effective programs on the set of programs listed therein.

Based on evaluation studies conducted to date and reported in the *CASEL Guide*, preschool-level SEL programs have had the greatest effect in reducing conduct problems, with lesser effects in the areas of academic performance, positive social behavior, and emotional distress; elementary-level programs are equally likely to reduce conduct problems and increase positive social behaviors (e.g., Domitrovich et al. 2007; Hennessey 2007; Schonert-Reichl and Lawlor 2010; Webster-Stratton et al. 2001; Webster-Stratton et al. 2008). However of the ten programs with multiple evaluations, all of them were shown to affect more than one of the four desired outcomes. One longitudinal study of the High Scope Preschool Program followed students for 37 years, finding a range of important long-term educational and economic outcomes, including greater high-school graduation rates, delayed childbearing, and higher-socioeconomic status (Muennig et al. 2009).

An extensive research literature at the middle- and high-school levels suggests that programs promoting social and emotional development (often called "life skills" in the research literature) can reduce a range of adolescent risk behaviors, including substance use and violence. Substance-abuse-oriented programs focus on emphasizing refusal skills, building self-esteem, and promoting a sense of personal responsibility. Many also develop a range of communication skills such as assertiveness, communicating wants and needs effectively and directly, and negotiating with peers (see, e.g., Botvin et al. 1990; Dusenbury et al. 1989; Eisen et al. 2003; Pentz et al. 1989). Other SEL programs take a social cognition approach to reducing youth violence (Farrell et al. 2001; Farrell et al. 2003). These emphasize conflict-resolution strategies, problem-solving processes, and understanding emotions.

14.3.2 Characteristics of Effective SEL Programs

SEL programs appear to be most effective when they have four primary characteristics, which Durlak et al. (2011) refer to as *SAFE features* (a) a *S*equenced training approach; (b) *A*ctive forms of learning to practice new skills; (c) a *F*ocus on skill development; and (d) *E*xplicit definitions of the social and emotional skills the program is seeking to promote. In addition, all programs with proven effectiveness contain certain design elements in common, such as providing opportunities for behavioral practice, and integrating SEL concepts into the classroom and throughout the school day (CASEL 2012). Note that these features largely overlap with SAFE. Next, we discuss each of these principles, many of which are applicable to other types of prevention programming as well.

Effective Programs Are Comprehensive Effective programs can be used with a variety of populations and are comprehensive in terms of age, culture, language, and skill development. Effective programs also support social and emotional development across multiple grade levels (CASEL 2012)—ideally providing developmentally appropriate coverage of all age groups or grades, preschool through high school (Greenberg et al. 2003; Nation et al. 2003). Such programs are sequenced in a way that scaffolds skill development year over year so that programming builds on what students learned in years past while also enhancing these skills and developing new ones. For example, a lesson on patience in week 15 might expand skills taught during the week 6 lesson on self-calming strategies such as deep breathing or counting to ten. A sixth-grade lesson on peer pressure might build on lessons that taught self-respect and assertive communication during fifth grade.

Because the landscape of our education system is diverse, it is important that programs are appropriate for, and sensitive to, diverse populations. Research has shown that programs are more effective when they not only address linguistic competence but also the cultural contexts in which students live (Gay 2000, 2002).

Effective programs are also comprehensive in that they develop a range of competencies and skills that serve a variety of purposes, including both academic achievement and social adjustment, with specific competencies playing roles individually and collectively (Durlak et al. 2011; Elias 2006; Greenberg et al. 2003; Nation et al. 2003; Payton et al. 2000; Zins et al. 2004). SEL programs are structured to systematically develop a broad range of skills because research and developmental theory emphasize the integration of emotion, cognition, communication, and behavior (Crick and Dodge 1994; Lemerise and Arsenio 2000). Developing skills separately without attending to how those skills interact may reduce program effectiveness and produce only short-term gains (Osher et al. 2013).

Effective Programs Use a Variety of Methodologies to Develop Social and Emotional Competencies and Skills All 23 effective programs demonstrated positive effects on student behavior, and every program promoted all five of the social and emotional skill domains; namely, self-awareness, self-management, social awareness, relationship skills, and responsible decision-making (CASEL 2012). However, the methodology through which these competencies and skills were developed varied. Four emerging approaches were identified, with some programs utilizing a combination of these: (a) explicit skill development that occurs through freestanding practice, (b) explicit skill development that integrates with core academic content, (c) skill development that occurs implicitly through teacher practices and pedagogy, and (d) skill development that occurs implicitly through project- or service-based learning (CASEL 2012).

The most common type of SEL program is a free-standing, "out-of-the-box" curriculum with scripted lessons explicitly designed to promote specific skills; 5 of 7 effective preschool-level programs and 15 of 19 elementary programs used this approach (some programs have components for both preschool and elementary levels so are counted twice). These programs address social and emotional skills that can be broadly applied to a variety of situations, such as making friends, working cooperatively with others, coping with stress, making decisions about engaging in potentially risky behaviors, and resolving interpersonal conflicts. They may also cover specific health promotion or problem prevention domains (e.g., engaged citizenry, violence prevention, drug prevention).

Many programs, including some of the aforementioned programs that emphasize explicit skills instruction, provide additional strategies for integrating newly developed skills within core academic content areas or for enhancing teacher practices. Of the 23 effective programs, all but four provided *optional* academic integration strategies. The remaining four programs were intentionally structured to incorporate social and emotional skill development into academic content, and thus were even more integrative (CASEL 2012). The academic content areas most frequently targeted for integration with SEL are English language arts and history, though integration with science, physical education, arts, and mathematics instruction is incipient. It is reasonable to expect that integration of academic content with SEL would be a greater focus at the secondary school level, so that as effective programs are identified at this level, integration will be a more prominent feature.

Another emerging movement among SEL programs is a focus on instructional and pedagogical processes that promote positive dynamics in the classroom or afterschool program to actively engage students in learning while simultaneously supporting social and emotional development. This approach not only creates a climate where young people feel safe and connected but also improves student–teacher relations, thus fostering better conditions for learning (Allen et al. 2011). Research on the quality of teacher–student interactions and the instructional practices that take place within the classroom suggests that they are two critical factors for student academic performance and social adjustment (Hamre and Pianta 2007; Mashburn and Pianta 2006). This approach to SEL involves training teachers in a variety of classroom management techniques, such as using positive discipline or creating shared group norms, as well as how to be emotionally responsive to students' needs.

SEL Programs Provide Opportunities to Develop Skills Through Active Practice It is critical that young people have opportunities to practice and apply developing skills, not only with support and scaffolding from a teacher or other adult, but also in real-life situations, which may be even more important for learning (Bond and Carmola-Hauf 2004; Hawkins et al. 2004; Nation et al. 2003; Weare and Nind 2011). Youth interventions are more successful when they use interactive strategies such as coaching or role-playing, and provide feedback on individuals' progress toward specific goals (DuBois et al. 2002; Tobler et al. 2000).

Skill Development Is Reinforced in a Variety of Settings Skill building occurs not only through active practice but also through generalization and reinforcement of the targeted skills to a variety of settings and aspects of daily life beyond the specific skills instruction time—in the classroom, throughout the school, with families, and in the community. Durlak et al. (2011) suggest that "interventions are unlikely to have much practical utility or gain widespread acceptance unless they are effective under real-world conditions," and that "interventions that combined components within and outside of the daily classroom routine would yield stronger effects than those that were only classroom based," which is "grounded in the premise that the broader ecological focus of multicomponent programs that extend beyond the classroom should better support and sustain new skill development" (Tolan et al. 1995, as cited in Durlak et al. 2011, p. 407). All 23 effective programs are designed to reinforce SEL in a variety of ways beyond the structured instruction.

Many Programs Incorporate Practices That Extend Program Concepts and Skill Development into the Regular Classroom Routine There is a critical need to balance the focus on academic performance with the development of key social and emotional skills both in and out of school (McCombs 2004). Morning meetings, peace centers, and daily check-ins are routines that help promote relationship building, develop conflict resolution skills, and build trust in the classroom or other setting. SEL programs also make use of similar school- or building-wide practices that foster more and better relationships among students, teachers, staff, and families. These practices can facilitate SEL integration and extend the impact of SEL programs through consistent reinforcement of the target values, beliefs, and behaviors.

Many programs have structures for collaboration, whether that be by planning activities across different groups or grade levels or by engaging nonteaching personnel in activities they would not otherwise take part in. Research suggests that when school principals and other administrators endorse the use of SEL practices throughout the school building and model those behaviors themselves, implementation is stronger and more effective (Elias et al. 2006; Kam et al. 2003). Every youth–adult interaction is a potential opportunity to model skills and reinforce positive social behaviors, from the front office staff to the bus driver, from classroom teachers to paraprofessional staff.

Family and Community Involvement Can Be Supported in Multiple Ways Communication with parents and caregivers occurs in a variety of ways: Letters for home with updates and information about the daily or weekly lessons, as well as suggestions for home practice; parent/caregiver workshops that increase awareness and may even promote skill development; and homework activities and suggestions for how students can practice skills in "real life." Involving families ensures that social and emotional competencies and skills—which cannot be taught in isolation (Mart et al. 2011)—are consistently reinforced in both the school and home environments (Albright and Weissberg 2010).

Only 4 of the 23 programs contained opportunities to connect with the community via community service and awareness activities such as visits and guest presentations, volunteer work, or community projects. Service learning is increasingly being viewed as a complementary activity that may increase the effectiveness of SEL programming (Billig 2000). Billig (2000) notes that the act of service without the learning lacks impact for youth. It is when service is integrated with socially and emotionally relevant activities (e.g., reflection) that it becomes effective.

Effective Programs Are Implemented with Fidelity and Provide Support for Implementation The most critical component of an effective SEL program is appropriate implementation (Abbott et al. 1998; Aber et al. 2003; Battistich et al. 1996; Durlak et al. 2011; Greenberg et al. 2005). The most effective programs provide support for implementation, including ongoing professional development, technical assistance, and training (Botvin et al. 1990; Ringwalt et al. 2002; Ross et al. 1991; Tappe et al. 1995). As Durlak et al. (2011) pointed out in their meta-analysis, programs produced positive effects only when they had SAFE features and were implemented with fidelity.

Many programs offer initial training for frontline staff that will be implementing the programs, and some programs also offer training specific to principals, paraprofessionals, and other staff who support the program. Ongoing and follow-up training, along with additional supports (hotlines, online forums, e-mail reminders), may also be offered throughout program implementation. Especially those programs that focus on teacher training and improving pedagogy offer a deep and detailed professional development series designed to increase understanding, build familiarity, and strengthen social and emotional skills in the adult implementers.

Ongoing Assessment and Evaluation Promote Continuous Program Improvement It goes without saying that a key means for ensuring that any type of education or prevention program remains effective is to structure implementation in a way that promotes continuous program improvement through ongoing assessment and evaluation. Ongoing evaluation is critical for program monitoring and identifying whether and how to adjust programming to ensure that it is having the desired effect (Cohen 2006; Nation et al. 2003). Many SEL programs recommend a continuous improvement process and offer tools for monitoring implementation and measuring youth outcomes. These may involve formative assessments conducted over the course of the program, pre- and post-implementation youth surveys, or fidelity checklists for teachers or staff to complete during the course of implementation.

14.4 SEL in Practice

As we mentioned before, hundreds of prevention and intervention programs ranging in style, focus area, and implementation are available in the market, and the majority have been evaluated, with many demonstrating success. How then does one determine whether SEL is the way to go? The reasons vary from teacher to teacher, school to school, and even district to district.

14.4.1 Respect and Responsibility Program: A Homegrown SEL Initiative

In the case of Community Consolidated School District 181, in a southwestern suburb of Chicago, Illinois, the decision to focus on developing social and emotional skills was a much-needed positive response to increasing problems with bullying. In 2001, a few years after the mass shooting at Columbine High School, a group of parents started paying attention to the climate of their elementary school. They had begun to notice a change in the mood of the school and the ways students treated one another, particularly that bullying was occurring at earlier ages. In response, a small group of parents joined together, developed a set of lessons they called the "Respect and Responsibility Program," and started to implement it. Calling themselves "Kindness Ambassadors," the parents came into the classrooms each quarter and conducted workshops focusing on social skills like making friends and dealing with bullying. The Kindness Ambassadors focused on keeping these lessons positive, upbeat, and strengths based, because they believed this was the best way of getting through to students. They also sent notes home about the importance of social and emotional skills and how parents could help.

The Kindness Ambassadors chose the route of developing social and emotional skills instead of focusing solely on bullying prevention because they felt that promoting social skills was a positive approach to prevention, unlike the approach of the other drug and violence prevention programs being implemented in the district, with little effect. The parents also valued an approach that offered a variety of tools and strategies that students could learn and practice regularly in order to deal with challenges in a constructive way. The Kindness Ambassadors' workshops were effective in creating a caring learning community, and their efforts soon came to the attention of the district superintendent, who decided to expand the Respect and Responsibility Program into a district-wide initiative.

Toward that end District 181 engaged CASEL in 2002 to provide guidance around implementing and scaling up the program. CASEL's primary recommendation to the district was to implement an evidence-based program that would not only enable the district to increase the number of students who participated in programming but would also offer a variety of supports for implementation, such as standardized materials, training, and evaluation materials. CASEL staff worked with members of the district team to review evidence-based programs (CASEL 2003) and identify one that was a good match for the district's needs. The district selected the Lions Quest program based on a variety of factors (e.g., current implementation of the Respect and Responsibility Program, feasibility of implementation, cost, and fit with the district's students). Although the program has changed over the years, the district is still implementing Lions Quest at the time of this publication.

Around the same time, the Illinois Children's Mental Health Act of 2003 was enacted, leading shortly thereafter to the establishment of state learning standards for SEL—the first such standards in the country. This was a time of rapid expansion for SEL in Illinois, and District 181 was ahead of the curve. The legislation and standards served to support the work they were already doing and to guide its evolution and strengthening over the subsequent decade.

14.4.2   The Humanware Initiative: A Systemic Approach to SEL

Since 2002, SEL has seen many advances, particularly in terms of how we think about implementation. What was once a field of mostly classroom-based, off-the-shelf SEL curricula emphasizing direct skills instruction is now characterized by systemic efforts, standards, and rigor. There is increasing evidence that SEL is most effective and longest lasting when implemented systemically—that is, not tied to a specific program, classroom teacher, or school but rather aligned and integrated at every level from pre-K through secondary school and with support from a variety of stakeholders (Devaney et al. 2006).

Research on systemic SEL is still limited, but a notable development is the CASEL Collaborating Districts Initiative, a demonstration program in eight urban school districts around the country. The initiative began in 2011 with an initial cohort of three districts (Anchorage School District, AK; Austin Independent School District, TX; Cleveland Metropolitan School District (CMSD), OH), and in 2012 a second cohort of five districts was added (Chicago Public Schools, IL; Metropolitan Nashville Public Schools, TN; Oakland Unified School District, CA; Sacramento City Unified School District, CA; Washoe County School District, NV). The main goal is for these districts to strengthen their capacity to promote SEL for all students through providing administrative leadership, improving instruction, and building a culture of connections and continuous improvement to support SEL (CASEL 2013). These districts have gone beyond the standard program-based approach to SEL to establish SEL standards, allot dedicated planning time for SEL, and integrate SEL into academic instruction throughout the school day.

CMSD, which is now a member of the CASEL Collaborating Districts Initiative, had begun making drastic changes to school policy and conditions for learning in favor of promoting SEL as early as 2007. Like District 181 in Illinois, CMSD officials chose SEL in response to what they saw as a climate issue, in this case a school shooting that rattled the district. The superintendent increased security measures and developed a district-wide school safety strategy that included a comprehensive evaluation of the conditions for learning. The evaluation, conducted by the American Institutes for Research (AIR), identified eight factors that contributed to unruly student behavior and negative school climate: chronic poverty, lead poisoning/effect, harsh and inconsistent approaches to discipline, reactive and punitive approaches to discipline, unclear and inconsistently implemented disciplinary codes, poor adult supervision and role modeling, limited school and family connections, and student mental health needs that exceeded the school's capacity to provide services (Osher et al. 2008).

The findings of this evaluation led CMSD to launch its districtwide "Humanware" initiative in 2008 (see CMSD n.d.). Humanware—conceived as the opposite of hardware—focused on increasing student safety through promoting positive social skills. Humanware fosters four conditions for learning in all schools: "a caring environment where students are connected to others in learning; social and emotional instruction, promotion, and support; positive behavioral supports; and engaged instruction, using high-academic standards and inclusive supports for all" (CMSD 2000–2014). Shortly after implementation of the Humanware initiative began, CMSD joined the Collaborating Districts Initiative to address the social and emotional instruction core component of their conditions for learning (CASEL 2013).

One of several strategies supporting CMSD's Humanware Initiative, which spans all grades across the district, is implementation of the Promoting Alternative THinking Strategies (PATHS) program in the elementary grades. Findings from a recent implementation and outcomes evaluation indicate that CMSD students receiving PATHS improved in both social and emotional competence and improved attentiveness in each of the school years from 2010 to 2012. Furthermore, students' level of improvement was associated with how well teachers implemented the program (Faria et al. 2013). Efforts like those in District 181 and in Cleveland show that educators are at the forefront of what works in SEL, and that SEL works even under the less-than-ideal conditions of the "real world."

14.5   Conclusion

Youth will need to know and be able to do many things if they are to thrive in our fast-changing, complex, and interconnected world, and it is clear that social and emotional skills are a critical part of what they will require. There are a variety of ways effective SEL can promote social competence while reducing antisocial behavior (Durlak et al. 2011). Evidence-based SEL programs and systemic SEL programming are proven methods of positively influencing youth attitudes, behaviors, and skills. The experiences in Community Consolidated School District 181 in Illinois and CMSD in Ohio suggest that it is possible for SEL to be implemented on a wide scale, with the potential to help communities organize and coordinate their educational efforts in strategic ways that prepare youth for success in the future.

References

Abbott, R. D., O'Donnell, J., Hawkins, J. D., Hill, K. G., Kosterman, R., & Catalano, R. F. (1998). Changing teaching practices to promote achievement and bonding to school. *American Journal of Orthopsychiatry, 68*(4), 542–552. doi:10.1037/h0080363.
Aber, J. L., Brown, J. L., & Jones, S. M. (2003). Developmental trajectories toward violence in middle childhood: Course, demographic differences, and response to school-based intervention. *Developmental Psychology, 39*(2), 324–348. doi:10.1037/0012-1649.39.2.324.

Academic, Social, and Emotional Learning Act of 2009, H.R. 4223, 111th Cong. (2009–2010). http://www.govtrack.us/congress/bills/111/hr4223.

Academic, Social, and Emotional Learning Act of 2011, H.R. 2437, 112th Cong. (2011–2013). http://www.govtrack.us/congress/bills/113/hr1875.

Academic, Social, and Emotional Learning Act of 2013, H.R. 1875, 113th Cong. (2013). http://www.govtrack.us/congress/bills/113/hr1875.

Albright, M. I., & Weissberg, R. P. (2010). School-family partnerships to promote social and emotional learning. In S. Redding, M. Murphy, & P. Sheley (Eds.), *Handbook on family and community engagement* (pp. 246–265). Lincoln: Academic Development Institute. http://www. schoolcommunitynetwork.org/downloads/FACEHandbook.pdf.

Allen, J. P., Pianta, R. C., Gregory, A., Mikami, A. Y., & Lun, J. (2011). An interaction-based approach to enhancing secondary school instruction and student achievement. *Science, 333*, 1034–1037. doi:10.1126/science.1207998.

American Management Association. (2012). *AMA 2012 critical skills survey*. New York: American Management Association. http://www.amanet.org/uploaded/2012-Critical-Skills-Survey.pdf.

Anchorage School District. (2004/2013). *Social and emotional learning (SEL) standards and benchmarks for the Anchorage School District*. http://www.asdk12.org/media/anchorage/globalmedia/documents/sel/SEL_Standards.pdf.

Battistich, V., Schaps, E., Watson, M., & Solomon, D. (1996). Prevention effects of the child development project: Early findings from an ongoing multisite demonstration trial. *Journal of Adolescent Research, 11*, 12–35. doi:10.1177/0743554896111003.

Billig, S. H. (2000). Research on K–12 school-based service-learning: The evidence builds. *Phi Delta Kappan, 81*, 658–664.

Bond, L. A., & Carmola-Hauf, A. M. (2004). Taking stock and putting stock in primary prevention: Characteristics of effective programs. *Journal of Primary Prevention, 24*(3), 199–221. doi:10.1023/B:JOPP.0000018051.90165.65.

Botvin, G. J., Baker, E., Dusenbury, L., Tortu, S., & Botvin, E. M. (1990). Preventing adolescent drug abuse through a multimodal cognitive-behavioral approach: Results of a 3-year study. *Journal of Consulting and Clinical Psychology, 58*(4), 437–446. doi:10.1037/0022-006X.58.4.437.

Bridgeland, J., Bruce, M., & Hariharan, A. (2013). *The missing piece: A national teacher survey on how social and emotional learning can empower children and transform schools*. Chicago: Collaborative for Academic, Social and Emotional Learning. http://casel.org/themissingpiece.

California Healthy Kids Resource Center. (n.d.). *Research-validated programs*. http://www.californiahealthykids.org/rvalidated.

Catalano, R. F., Berglund, M. L., Ryan, J. A., Lonczak, H. S., & Hawkins, J. D. (2002). Positive youth development in the United States: Research findings on evaluations of positive youth development programs. *Prevention & Treatment, 5*(1), 15a.

Center for the Study and Prevention of Violence. (2012–2014). *Blueprints for healthy youth development*. http://www.blueprintsprograms.com/.

Cicchetti, D. E., Rappaport, J. E., Sandler, I. E., & Weissberg, R. P. (2000). *The promotion of wellness in children and adolescents*. Washington, DC: Child Welfare League of America.

Cleveland Metropolitan School District (CMSD). (2002–2014). *CMSD Humanware frequently asked questions*. http://clevelandmetroschools.org/Page/587.

Cleveland Metropolitan School District (CMSD). (n.d.a). *CMSD Facts*. http://www.cmsdnet.net/en/AboutCMSD/Facts.aspx. Accessed 25 June 2013

Cleveland Metropolitan School District (CMSD). (n.d.b). *Humanware*. http://www.clevelandmetroschools.org/Page/398.

Cohen, J. (2006). Social, emotional, ethical, and academic education: Creating a climate for learning, participation in democracy, and well-being. *Harvard Educational Review, 76*, 201–237.

Collaborative for Academic, Social, and Emotional Learning (CASEL). (2003). *Safe and sound: An educational leader's guide to evidence-based social and emotional learning (SEL) programs*. Chicago: CASEL.

Collaborative for Academic, Social, and Emotional Learning (CASEL). (2012). *2013 CASEL guide: Effective social and emotional learning programs, preschool-elementary edition.* Chicago: CASEL.

Collaborative for Academic, Social, and Emotional Learning (CASEL). (2013). *Implementing systemic district and school social and emotional learning.* Chicago: CASEL.

Collaborative for Academic, Social, and Emotional Learning (CASEL). (n.d.). Organization mission statement. http://www.casel.org/about.

Conference Board, Partnership for twenty-first Century Skills, Corporate Voices for Working Families, and Society for Human Resource Management. (2006). *Are they really ready to work? Employers perspectives on the basic knowledge and applied skills of new entrants to the twenty-first century U.S. workforce.* http://www.p21.org/storage/documents/FINAL_REPORT_PDF09-29-06.pdf.

Crick, N. R., & Dodge, K. A. (1994). A review and reformulation of social information processing mechanisms in children's social adjustment. *Psychological Bulletin, 115,* 74–101. doi:10.1037/0033-2909.115.1.74.

Devaney, E., O'Brien, M. U., Resnik, H., Keister, S., & Weissberg, R. P. (2006). *Sustainable schoolwide social and emotional learning: Implementation guide and toolkit.* Chicago: CASEL.

Domitrovich, C. E., Cortes, R., & Greenberg, M. T. (2007). Improving young children's social and emotional competence: A randomized trial of the preschool PATHS curriculum. *Journal of Primary Prevention, 28*(2), 67–91. doi:10.1007/s10935-007-0081-0.

DuBois, D. L., Holloway, B. E., Valentine, J. C., & Cooper, H. (2002). Effectiveness of mentoring programs for youth: A meta-analytic review. *American Journal of Community Psychology, 30,* 157–197. doi:10.1023/A:1014628810714.

Durlak, J. A. (1997). *Successful prevention programs for children and adolescents.* New York: Plenum.

Durlak, J. A., & Weissberg, R. P. (2007). *The impact of after-school programs that promote personal and social skills.* Chicago: CASEL.

Durlak, J. A., Weissberg, R. P., & Pachan, M. K. (2010). A meta-analysis of after-school programs that seek to promote personal and social skills in children and adolescents. *American Journal of Community Psychology, 45*(3–4), 294–309. doi:10.1007/s10464-010-9300-6.

Durlak, J. A., Weissberg, R. P., Dymnicki, A. B., Taylor, R. D., & Schellinger, K. B. (2011). The impact of enhancing students' social and emotional learning: A meta-analysis of school-based universal interventions. *Child Development, 82,* 405–432. doi:10.1111/j.1467-8624.2010.01564.x.

Dusenbury, L., Botvin, G. J., & James-Ortiz, S. (1989). The primary prevention of adolescent substance abuse through the promotion of personal and social competence. *Prevention in Human Services, 7,* 201–224.

Eisen, M., Zellman, G. L., & Murray, D. M. (2003). Evaluating the Lions-Quest "Skills for Adolescence" drug education program: Second year behavior outcomes. *Addictive Behaviors, 28,* 883–897. doi:10.1016/S0306-4603(01)00292-1.

Elias, M. J. (2006). The connection between academic and social-emotional learning. In M. J. Elias & H. Arnold (Eds.), *The educator's guide to emotional intelligence and academic achievement: Social-emotional learning in the classroom* (pp. 4–14). Thousand Oaks: Corwin Press.

Elias, M. J., Zins, J. E., Weissberg, R. P., Greenberg, M. S., Frey, K. S., Haynes, N. M., & Shriver, T. P. (1997). *Promoting social and emotional learning: Guidelines for educators.* Alexandria: ASCD.

Elias, M., O'Brien, M. U., & Weissberg, R. P. (2006). Transformative leadership for social-emotional learning. *Principal Leadership, 7*(5), 10–13.

Faria, A. M., Kendziora, K., Brown, L., O'Brien, B., & Osher, D. (2013). *PATHS implementation and outcome study in the Cleveland Metropolitan School District: Final report.* Washington, DC: American Institutes for Research.

Farrell, A. D., Meyer, A. L., & White, K. S. (2001). Evaluation of responding in peaceful and positive ways (RIPP): A school-based prevention program for reducing violence among urban adolescents. *Journal of Clinical Child Psychology, 30,* 451–463 doi:10.1207/S15374424JC-CP3004_02.

Farrell, A. D., Meyer, A. L., Sullivan, T. N., & Kung, E. M. (2003). Evaluation of the responding in peaceful and positive ways (RIPP) seventh grade violence prevention curriculum. *Journal of Child & Family Studies, 12,* 101–120. doi:10.1023/A:1021314327308.

Gay, G. (2000). *Culturally responsive teaching: Theory, research, and practice.* New York: Teachers College Press.

Gay, G. (2002). Preparing for culturally responsive teaching. *Journal of Teacher Education, 53,* 106–116. doi:10.1177/0022487102053002003.

Greenberg, M. T., Domitrovich, C., & Bumbarger, B. (2001). Preventing mental disorder in school-aged children: Current state of the field. *Prevention & Treatment, 4,* 1–64. doi:10.1037/1522-3736.4.1.41a.

Greenberg, M. T., Weissberg, R. P., O'Brien, M. U., Zins, J. E., Fredericks, L., Resnik, H., & Elias, M. J. (2003). Enhancing school-based prevention and youth development through coordinated social, emotional, and academic learning. *American Psychologist, 58*(6–7), 466–474. doi:10.1037/0003-066X.58.6–7.466.

Greenberg, M. T., Domitrovich, C. E., Graczyk, P. A., & Zins, J. E. (2005). *The study of implementation in school-based preventive interventions: Theory, research, and practice* (Vol. 3). Rockville: Center for Mental Health Services, SAMHSA.

Hamre, B. K., & Pianta, R. C. (2007). Learning opportunities in preschool and early elementary classrooms. In R. Pianta, M. Cox, & K. Snow (Eds.), *School readiness and the transition to kindergarten in the era of accountability* (pp. 49–84). Baltimore: Brookes.

Hawkins, J. D., Smith, B. H., & Catalano, R. F. (2004). Social development and social and emotional learning. In J. E. Zins, R. P. Weissberg, M. C. Wang, & H. J. Walberg (Eds.), *Building academic success on social and emotional learning: What does the research say?* (pp. 135–150). New York: Teachers College Press.

Hennessey, B. A. (2007). Promoting social competence in school-aged children: The effects of the Open Circle program. *Journal of School Psychology, 45*(3), 349–360. doi:10.1016/j.jsp.2006.11.007.

Illinois State Board of Education. (2005). *Comprehensive system of learning supports.* http://www.isbe.state.il.us/learningsupports.

Kam, C., Greenberg, M. T., & Walls, C. T. (2003). Examining the role of implementation quality in school-based prevention using the PATHS curriculum. *Prevention Science, 4,* 55–63. doi:10.1023/A:1021786811186.

Kansas State Department of Education. (2012). *Kansas social, emotional, and character development model standards.* http://www.ksde.org/Portals/0/CSAS/Content%20Area%20(M-Z)/School%20Counseling/Soc_Emot_Char_Dev/Kansas%20Social,%20Emotional,%20and%20Character%20Development%20Model%20Standards.pdf.

Kress, J. S., & Elias, M. J. (2006). School-based social and emotional learning programs. In W. Damon & R. M. Lerner (Series Eds.) and K. A. Renninger & I. E. Sigel (Vol. Eds.), *Handbook of child psychology: Vol. 4. Child psychology in practice* (6th ed., pp 592–618). New York: Wiley.

Lemerise, E. A., & Arsenio, W. F. (2000). An integrated model of emotion processes and cognition in social information processing. *Child Development, 71,* 107–118. doi:10.1111/1467-8624.00124.

Mart, A., Dusenbury, L., & Weissberg, R. P. (2011). Social, emotional, and academic learning: Complementary goals for school-family partnerships. In S. Redding, M. Murphy, & P. Sheley (Eds.), *Handbook on family and community engagement* (pp. 37–44). Lincoln, IL: Academic Development Institute. http://www.schoolcommunitynetwork.org/downloads/FACEHandbook.pdf.

Mashburn, A. J., & Pianta, R. C. (2006). Social relationships and school readiness. *Early Education and Development, 17,* 151–176. doi:10.1207/s15566935eed1701_7.

McCombs, B. (2004). The learner-centered psychological principles: A framework for balancing academic achievement and social-emotional learning outcomes. In J. E. Zins, R. W. Weissberg, M. C. Wang, & H. J. Walberg (Eds.), *Building academic success on social and emotional learning: What does the research say?* (pp. 23–39). New York: Teachers College Press.

Miller, B. M. (2003). *Critical hours: Afterschool programs and educational success.* Quincy: Nellie Mae Educational Foundation. http://www.nmefoundation.org/getmedia/08b6e87b-69ff4865-b44e-ad42f2596381/Critical-Hours?ext=.pdf.

Muennig, P., Schweinhart, L., Montie, J., & Neidell, M. (2009). Effects of a prekindergarten educational intervention on adult health: 37-year follow-up results of a randomized controlled trial. *American Journal of Public Health, 99,* 1431–1437. doi:10.2105/AJPH.2008.148353.

Nation, M., Crusto, C., Wandersman, A., Kumpfer, K. L., Seybolt, D., Morrissey-Kane, E., & Davino, K. (2003). What works in prevention: Principles of effective prevention practice. *American Psychologist, 58*(6–7), 449–456. doi:10.1037/0003-066X.58.6–7.449.

National Governors Association Center for Best Practices & Council of Chief State School Officers. (2010). *Common core state standards.* Washington, DC: National Governors Association Center for Best Practices & Council of Chief State School Officers.

Osher, D. M., Poirier, J. M., Dwyer, K. P., Hicks, R., Brown, L. J., Lampron, S., & Rodriguez, C. (2008). *Cleveland metropolitan school district humanware audit: Findings and recommendations.* Washington, DC: American Institutes for Research.

Osher, D. M., Poirier, J. M., Jarjoura, G. R., Brown, R., & Kendziora, K. (2013). *Avoid simple solutions and quick fixes.* Paper presented at the Closing the School Discipline Gap: Research to Practice Conference, Washington, DC. http://www.air.org/resource/avoid-simple-solutions-and-quick-fixes-improving-conditions-learning.

Partnership for twenty-first Century Skills. (2011). *Framework for twenty-first century learning.* http://www.p21.org/overview.

Payton, J. W., Wardlaw, M. D., Graczyk, P. A., Bloodworth, M. R., Tompsett, C. J., & Weissberg, R. P. (2000). Social and emotional learning: A framework for promoting mental health and reducing risk behavior in children and youth. *Journal of School Health, 70*(5), 179–185. doi:10.1111/j.1746–1561.2000.tb06468.x.

Pellegrino, J. W. E., & Hilton, M. L. E. (2012). *Education for life and work: Developing transferable knowledge and skills in the twenty-first century.* Washington, DC: National Academies Press.

Pennsylvania Department of Education. (2012). *Standards for student interpersonal skills: Grades PreK–12.* http://static.pdesas.org/content/documents/Student_Interpersonal_Skills_Standards.pdf.

Pentz, M. A., MacKinnon, D. P., Dwyer, J. H., Wang, E. Y. I., Hansen, W. B., Flay, B. R., & Johnson, C. A. (1989). Longitudinal effects of the Midwestern prevention project on regular and experimental smoking in adolescents. *Preventive Medicine, 18,* 304–321. doi:10.1016/0091-7435(89)90077-7.

Ringwalt, C. L., Ennett, S., Vincus, A., Throne, J., Rohrbach, L. A., & Simons- Rudolph, A. (2002). The prevalence of effective substance use prevention curricula in U.S. middle schools. *Prevention Science, 3*(4), 257–267. doi:10.1023/A:1020872424136.

Ross, J. G., Luepker, R. V., Nelson, G. D., Saavedra, P., & Hubbard, B. M. (1991). Teenage health teaching modules: Impact of teacher training on implementation and student outcomes. *Journal of School Health, 61*(1), 31–34. doi:10.1111/j.1746–1561.1991.tb07856.x.

Schonert-Reichl, K. A., & Hymel, S. (2007). Educating the heart as well as the mind: Why social and emotional learning is critical for students' school and life success. *Education Canada, 47,* 20–25.

Schonert-Reichl, K. A., & Lawlor, M. S. (2010). The effects of a mindfulness-based education program on pre- and early adolescents well-being and social and emotional competence. *Mindfulness, 1,* 137–151. doi:10.1007/s12671-010-0011-8.

Tappe, M. K., Galer-Unti, R. A., & Bailey, K. C. (1995). Long-term implementation of teenage health teaching modules by trained teachers: A case study. *Journal of School Health, 65*(10), 411–415. doi:10.1111/j.1746–1561.1995.tb08203.x.

Tobler, N. S., Roona, M. R., Ochshorn, P., Marshall, D. G., Streke, A. V., & Stackpole, K. M. (2000). School-based adolescent drug prevention programs: 1998 meta-analysis. *Journal of Primary Prevention, 20,* 275–336. doi:10.1023/A:1021314704811.

U.S. Department of Education, Institute of Education Sciences. (n.d.) What Works Clearing-house™. http://ies.ed.gov/ncee/wwc/.

U.S. Department of Health and Human Services, Substance Abuse and Mental Health Services Administration. (2014). *National registry of evidence-based programs and practices (NREPP).* http://www.nrepp.samhsa.gov/Index.aspx.

U.S. Department of Justice, Office of Justice Programs. (n.d.) *Office of Juvenile Justice and Delinquency Prevention (OJJDP) Model Programs Guide.* http://www.ojjdp.gov/mpg/.

U.S. Department of Labor, Secretary's Commission on Achieving Necessary Skills (SCANS). (1991). *What work requires of schools: A SCANS report for America 2000.* Washington, DC: U.S. Department of Labor, Secretary's Commission on Achieving Necessary Skills (SCANS).

Weare, K., & Nind, M. (2011). Mental health promotion and problem prevention in schools: What does the evidence say? *Health Promotion International, 26*(s1), s29–s69. doi:10.1093/heapro/dar075.

Webster-Stratton, C., Reid, M. J., & Hammond, M. (2001). Preventing conduct problems, promoting social competence: A parent and teacher training partnership in head start. *Journal of Clinical Child Psychology, 30*(3), 283–302. doi:10.1207/S15374424JCCP3003_2.

Webster-Stratton, C., Reid, M. J., & Stoolmiller, M. (2008). Preventing conduct problems and improving school readiness: Evaluation of the Incredible Years teacher and child training programs in high-risk schools. *Journal of Child Psychology and Psychiatry, 49*(5), 471–488. doi:10.1111/j.1469-7610.2007.01861.x.

Weissberg, R. P., & Greenberg, M. T. (1998). School and community competence-enhancement and prevention programs. In W. Damon (Series Eds.) and I. E. Siegel & L. A. Renninger (Vol. Eds.), *Handbook of child psychology: Vol 4. Child psychology in practice* (5th ed., pp. 877–954). New York: Wiley.

Wilstrom-Ahlstrom, A., Yohalem, N., DuBois, D., & Ji, P. (2011). *From soft skills to hard data: Measuring youth program outcomes.* Ypsilanti: Forum for Youth Investment.

Zins, J. E., Weissberg, R. P., Wang, M. C., & Walberg, H. J. (Eds.). (2004). *Building academic success on social and emotional learning: What does the research say?* New York: Teachers College Press.

Chapter 15
Promoting Safe Schools for All Students

Katie Eklund, Kris Bosworth and Sheri Bauman

15.1 Introduction

The second decade in life is one in which, based on arrest records, a disproportionate amount of violence occurs (Puzzanchera and Adams 2011). Researchers have identified a developmental progression of violent behavior with such behavior peaking in adolescence and early adulthood. Although schools are where the vast majority of people in this age range congregate, schools are generally safe places for students and "the safety of America's schools has improved over the past decade" (Mayer and Furlong 2010, p 24). Between 1998 and 2010, schools saw reductions in bullying behaviors and physical fighting among students (Perlus et al. 2014). The majority of students in the USA will not experience peer violence during their K-12 educational experience (Fein et al. 2002). However, due to significant concerns about violence, theft, bullying, and intimidation, and as there are no clear standards for assessing harm, "determination of what constitutes safety remains fluid and relative" (Mayer and Furlong 2010, p. 24). Schools have increasingly engaged in a number of prevention and intervention efforts to ensure student safety over the past decade, and many of these interventions have been shown to reduce violent, unsafe behavior. For example, in a review of 17 violence prevention

K. Eklund (✉)
School Psychology Program, University of Arizona, 1430 E. Second Street,
Tucson, AZ 85721, USA
e-mail: kelund@u.arizona.edu

K. Bosworth
Department of Educational Policy and Practice, University of Arizona, 1430 E 2nd Street,
Tucson, AZ 85721, USA
e-mail: boswortk@email.arizona.edu

S. Bauman
School Counseling Program, University of Arizona, 1430 E. Second Street,
Tucson, AZ 85721, USA
e-mail: sherib@u.arizona.edu

© Springer Science+Business Media New York 2015
K. Bosworth (ed.), *Prevention Science in School Settings,*
Advances in Prevention Science, DOI 10.1007/978-1-4939-3155-2_15

interventions with rigorous evaluation designs, evidence-based violence prevention programs, when developmentally appropriate and implemented with fidelity, "can significantly reduce violent behaviors" (Fagan and Catalano 2013, p. 151).

School administrators are charged with keeping all children and adults within their jurisdiction safe. The vast majority of schools have standard processes that are designed to maintain a safe learning environment. Federal and individual state laws require schools to develop crisis response plans and to generally address student safety concerns. However, school and classroom rules and procedures are determined at the local level and traditionally are shared with students and their families through a student handbook. Minor deviations from these rules are handled in the classroom. Repeated or major behavioral issues are dealt with in the office, usually by a principal or another school administrator. Suspension and expulsion are the last resort for administrators, and total exclusion from school through expulsion usually requires school board action. Criminal offenses on school property are handled by law enforcement.

This system is effective for the majority of students who follow the rules and rarely engage the discipline system. However, some students exhibit behaviors that indicate the need for additional support to function effectively and safely in a learning environment. Extreme behaviors such as drug sales, theft, or engaging in violent behaviors at school are acts that garner the attention of the news media and the community at large. Although these actions are dramatic, especially when considering the ages of the perpetrators and the protected setting of the school environment, schools remain some of the safest places for students in terms of injury or death (Flannery et al. 2013). Although these extremely violent acts are rare, they are complex and have lasting impacts on students, schools, and the community (Anderson et al. 2001), thus requiring analysis and attention.

Some of these fatal and dramatic incidents have led educators to be more conscious of the systems that are in place to ensure safety within a school environment. This chapter will review key safety issues facing educators, policy makers, and communities by reviewing (a) the research on causes and student issues that lead to school safety concerns; (b) school discipline concerns; (c) approaches to prevention; (d) two unique types of violence that threaten school safety, including bullying and relationship/dating violence; and finally, (e) crisis response and threat assessment procedures.

15.2   Secret Service Study

Following the horrific school shooting at Columbine High School in 1999 in which two student shooters killed 12 students and a teacher before killing themselves, the Secret Service and the US Department of Education undertook a large study to investigate pre-attack student behaviors in an effort to prevent future attacks (Vossekuil et al. 2002). This study closely examined 27 incidents of "targeted school shootings" between 1974 and 2000, in which a student purposefully attacked other students and faculty (Vossekuil et al. 2002, p. ii). The findings indicated that there was no "accurate or useful profile of students who engage in targeted school violence" (Vossekuil et al. p. 11), although the majority of shooters demonstrated behaviors preceding the incident that caused concern or indicated a need for help. Nearly three quarters of the 27 shooters felt attacked or bullied by others. One of the most disturbing findings was that in 81 % of the cases, at least one other student had knowledge of the planned attack but only two students reported this to an adult. This implies a climate in which students were fearful of reporting the threat or in which they felt that the administration would take no action. Thus, the report recommends that the climate of the school needs to play a role in preventing such attacks. Additionally, the report recommends that educators become proficient in assessing threats to school safety and regularly gather data to analyze student behavior and communications. Educators are also responsible for creating environments in which students do not fear bullying and intimidation from other students and where students feel comfortable accessing an adult for help and support.

Discipline Even in the most organized and orderly school setting, just as in society at large, students will break rules and display disruptive or aggressive behaviors. Millions of students, primarily in secondary schools, lose classroom time primarily for minor misconduct. Students of color, students with disabilities, and students who identify as lesbian, gay, bisexual or transgendered (LGBT) are disproportionally represented among students who are suspended or expelled from school (Fabelo et al. 2011; Morgan et al. 2014). The motivation behind the events that led to suspension and expulsion can come from a myriad of factors and the rule-breaking behavior may serve a variety of functions (Cornell and Mayer 2010). However, how these behavioral errors and transgressions are handled within the school setting has ramifications not only for the individual but for the entire school community. For example, Thomas and colleagues noted that even a few aggressive children in a classroom could result in increased aggression in the classroom (Thomas and Bierman 2006). Any time out of the classroom has ramifications for learning, but students who are suspended or expelled are forced away from academics for a substantial period of time, which can send them on a trajectory for dropout and involvement with the juvenile justice system (Fabelo et al. 2011; Steinberg et al. 2013).

Approaches to dealing with misbehavior fall roughly into two philosophical orientations: Authoritative and authoritarian (e.g., Baumrind 1996; Walker 2009). Authoritarian discipline or punitive practices and traditional approaches to discipline in schools are highly structured, provide little support to students, and emphasize control and strict obedience. Although widely accepted, such punitive practices do not significantly decrease problem behaviors because students do not automatically link the negative behavior with a positive, more acceptable alternative or with the school's stated behavioral expectations (Skiba and Knesting 2002). Instead, punishment simply may teach students to practice these behaviors when adults are not present.

Authoritative practices in contrast, provide both high structure and high support. In authoritative schools, rules are clearly defined, consistently enforced, and perceived as fair (high structure). Additionally, student–teacher relationships are viewed as positive and students have access to resources when they need assistance to master academic and social behaviors (high support). Students attending authoritative schools report increased feelings of safety and security compared to peers in authoritarian schools (Gregory et al. 2010).

As previously noted, students of color, particularly African American students, have been found to be overrepresented in office discipline referrals and school suspensions (Christle et al. 2004). Skiba and colleagues (2000) found that African American students were particularly overrepresented in referrals for violations such as disrespect or excessive noise, which are subjective, whereas white students were referred for more specific violations such as tardiness, dress code violations, or theft. Suspension (the temporary removal from school) was designed to protect other students from aggressive and violent students who were in danger or who had injured themselves or others (Skiba et al. 2014). However, suspension commonly is the choice for a variety of less severe offenses (Fenning and Rose 2007). Due to high recidivism rates for suspended students, many argue that suspension is an ineffective strategy either to change the behavior of the student or to keep the school population safer from student threats (Christle et al. 2004; McCord et al. 2000; Raffaele-Mendez et al. 2002).

A number of studies have identified characteristics of the school environment and personnel that contribute to high suspension rates and the noted disparities. For example, in a study of school disciplinary codes of conduct, more alternatives to suspensions were offered in schools serving a higher socioeconomic student population compared to schools in lower-income urban areas (Casella 2003). In a study comparing a group of middle schools with high suspension rates to a group with lower suspension rates, schools with high retention rates (repeating a grade) and lower academic achievement demonstrated higher suspension rates (Christle et al. 2004). Additionally, per pupil expenditures were higher in schools with lower suspension rates. From their field notes, the research group concluded that the schools with lower suspension rates, had more positive, caring environments with less yelling at students. Further, academics were more challenging with high expectations and support for academic success. Both school staff and administration at low-suspension schools focused on proactive, positive disciplinary measures in contrast to punitive and reactive approaches (Christle et al. 2004). Skiba and colleagues (2014) investigated several levels of variables to begin to sort out the contributions of each to the differing rates of school exclusion. They found that "*systemic, school-level variables* appear to contribute to disproportionality in out-of-school suspensions far more than either the type of infraction or individual demographics" (p. 664). The authors suggested that prevention be focused on principal orientation to an authoritative approach to discipline, the achievement orientations of the school, and "possible contributions of implicit bias" among school staff (p. 664).

Alternative approaches include utilizing a team approach to developing rules and expectations for the school environment, as well as ongoing monitoring of discipline records so that corrective action can be taken appropriately (Fenning and Rose 2007). Staff development in classroom management and cultural proficiency are suggested remedies for school level predictors. Clearly, district and school policies should be examined to begin to identify opportunities to shift schools to a more pro-active and authoritative approach. This could include restorative justice principles and practices of a framework in a whole-school approach to discipline (Morrison 2003). Engaging students in establishing behavioral expectations and rules and dis-cussions of feelings of safety can contribute significantly to a safer school (Bracy 2010).

15.3 Contemporary Approaches to School Climate and Safety

In the past decade, the focus of school safety and violence prevention has veered away from a focus on the individual, with a move toward population-based, public health approaches to prevention. These approaches are based on changes in the school community or the school environments in which students and staff inter-act on a daily basis (Johnson 2009; Sugimoto-Matsuda and Braun 2014). Some of these changes include school-wide social norms for behavior and problem solving, district and school polices for behavioral expectations and consequences, assessing school climate, and a multitiered approach to providing and coordinating services (Cohen et al. 2009; Cole et al. 1993).

School climate is defined as "the quality and character of school life ... based on patterns of people's experiences of school life and reflecting norms, goals, and values" (Cohen et al. 2009, p. 180). School climate often involves an evaluation of student perceptions of safety, teacher–student interactions, positive youth devel-opment, and student achievement. Five key elements of safe and healthy schools include: (a) positive and productive relationships, (b) awareness of and respect for diversity, (c) transparent and unbiased norms and expectations, (d) a balance be-tween individual value and shared community purpose, and (e) opportunities for growth and achievement (O'Malley and Eklund 2012). These five elements have been found to promote improved school climate, result in lower rates of student problematic behaviors, and positive staff and student outcomes (e.g., Griggs et al. 2009; Hattie 2009). Specific examples of how schools, staff, and teachers can embed these important elements in the classroom and school environment are de-scribed in Table 15.1.

Accordingly, the importance of a positive school climate as a foundation for school safety has been identified in numerous studies. In the study of 12 inner city schools in London, Sir Michael Rutter and colleagues (1979) found that schools with well-organized classrooms, an emphasis on academics, and good personal re-lationships between students and teachers reported fewer student behavior problems in the classroom and less delinquency. The longer students attended such schools, the more significant the decreases in problem behaviors (Rutter et al. 1979). Gott-fredson and Gottfredson (2001) found that schools with weak school leadership and organization, low emphasis on academics, lack of support for students, and unclear

Table 15.1 *Key characteristics of safe and healthy schools.* (adapted with permission from O'Malley and Eklund (2012))

Positive, productive relationships
Social and emotional skill development of youth is supported using evidence-based programs as well as structured, natural opportunities for skill building
Collegial relationships among school staff are supported and encouraged through systematic school planning
Professional development opportunities are provided for staff to support the development of the social and emotional competencies required to work with youth
Caring home and neighborhood adults are encouraged to volunteer in classrooms and shared school spaces
Awareness and respect for diversity
Students can "see" themselves in school materials. Curricula, classroom activities, and wall images represent the demographics of the school
School staff members reflect upon their own potential biases and assumptions
Caring home and neighborhood adults from diverse groups are encouraged to volunteer at school and actively participate in school decision-making activities
Teachers reflect upon the diverse backgrounds (i.e., culture, language, family history, religion) of their students and modify curricula to meet their needs
School adults communicate high expectations for all students, regardless of background
Transparent and unbiased norms and expectations
School policies are applied to all students, regardless of gender, race, socioeconomic privilege, or perceived sexual orientation
Students and caring home and neighborhood adults are provided opportunities to participate in classroom and school-wide norm- and rule-setting activities
School rules and expectations are reiterated on a regular basis and are visible within classrooms and shared spaces
Professional development opportunities are provided for staff to support the development of positive classroom management practices
Individual value and shared purpose
School staff members share a sense of responsibility over school activities and goals
Staff members are given opportunities to inform decisions related to future directions of school activities, including professional development planning
Students are encouraged to participate in governance councils and advisory committees
Students are encouraged to make shared contributions to the school and neighborhood communities through a variety of experiences, including service-learning projects
Opportunities for growth and achievement
Cooperative planning and professional development time for school staff is supported, encouraged, and expected
Curricula are rigorous and meaningful, emphasizing critical thinking, application of knowledge, and self-reflective learning
Academic and professional standards for students and staff are high, but achievable
Achievements of staff and students are celebrated and widely highlighted

rules and norms correlated with higher rates of violence. In the Add Health study, researchers found that in a sample of over 70,000 high school students, student's self-reported feelings of connectedness to school was related significantly to reductions in violence and disruptive behavior (McNeely et al. 2002). School climates that are safe, caring, participatory, and responsive tend to foster greater attachment and bonding to school, and in turn, reduce the prevalence of both victimization and aggression (Gregory et al. 2010; Osterman 2000; Thapa et al. 2013; Wilson 2004). Additionally, a sense of connectedness is linked to lower risk of student substance abuse, truancy, and other acts of misconduct (Hawkins et al. 1992).

A multitiered approach to creating and maintaining safe and supportive climates can provide guidance to educators and program developers (Morrison 2003; Osher et al. 2010). At the *universal level*, the focus is on interventions that are designed for all students regardless of level of risk. Universal strategies influence school climate, rather than individuals, through raising awareness and skills and changing school policies (Orpinas et al. 2003). In particular, strategies that promote a positive and consistent classroom and school climate, along with effective instruction, deter at-risk students from antisocial behavior and other school failures (Reinke and Herman 2002; Task Force on Community Preventive Services 2007). Universal strategies, when implemented effectively, emphasize prevention and address the underlying causes of behavior, in contrast to the traditional discipline approach of treating problem behaviors as discrete events and punishing the perpetrators (Adelman and Taylor 2000). These interventions provide a type of "immunization" from aggressive or violent behavior by creating an environment that is antithetical to violence and aggression and reinforces pro-social behavior (Morrison 2003). At this universal level, teaching students skills such as self-awareness, self-management, social awareness, and relationship skills has been shown to be effective in improving school climate (Osher et al. 2010).

At the *targeted level* students who have identified risk factors are provided with services such as a mentor, additional adult attention, social skills groups, community service, scheduling changes, or counseling (Sugai et al. 2000). For example, transitioning to a new school setting can be a risk factor for all students. Some schools target incoming ninth graders with orientation, mentors, and special events for them to become familiar with and comfortable in the new school setting. Some students do not respond to the interventions at the universal or targeted levels and need additional support. At this *indicated* level, students may receive more intensive evaluation and support through individualized interventions that could include a provision of services through one-on-one counseling, academic support, and/or special education services (Sugai et al. 2000).

A popular example of a multitiered system of support are positive behavior interventions and supports (PBIS); Sprague and Horner 2007). PBIS frameworks have been implemented in many schools across the country to help reduce disciplinary infractions and increase students' sense of safety at school by promoting positive, pro-social behaviors and improving school-wide behavior. The premise of PBIS is that recognizing and rewarding positive student behavior through continual teaching will reduce unnecessary discipline and promote a climate of greater productivity, learning, and safety (Sprague and Horner 2007).

Physical Safety Measures Although police have been present in schools since the 1950s, a rash of school shootings in the 1990s led to a dramatic increase in the presence of law enforcement personnel in school settings (Coon and Travis 2012; Maguire et al. 2002). Additionally, schools and criminal justice officials have responded to these challenges by intensifying their use of other security measures such as the use of video surveillance to monitor students and metal detectors to screen students for weapons (e.g., Barrios et al. 2000; Gottfredson and Gottfredson 2001; National Center for Education Statistics & the Bureau of Justice Statistics 2009). A total of 68 % of the students ages 12–18 report that there are security guards or police officers in their schools, 70 % report the presence of security cameras, and 11 % report the use of metal detectors (Robers et al. 2012). Clearly, increasing physical safety measures in schools has become a prominent activity in many schools across the country.

Crime Prevention Through Environmental Design The architectural design and physical surroundings of the school building is a critical component of ensuring physical safety of school community members. Crime prevention through environmental design is an approach often used by law enforcement, architects, and city planners to prevent crime by designing a physical environment that positively influences human behavior (National Crime Prevention Council n.d.). Three components important for securing a school include natural surveillance, natural access control, and territoriality (Sprague and Walker 2005). *Natural surveillance* includes the ability to ensure effective communication and to be able to see what is happening within and outside the school. This could include a two-way communication system between the school staff and the front office, increasing supervision in hallways and classrooms, as well as hiring school resource officers (SROs; Sprague and Walker 2005).

Natural access control refers to the procedures employed by schools to determine what individuals enter and exit the school building and how they do so. Specific school requirements include having one centralized entrance and exit to the school as well as the use of surveillance cameras to increase school security. *Territoriality* is a final principle that encourages staff and students to have shared ownership of the school so everyone feels empowered to challenge inappropriate behavior or incidents when they occur (Schneider et al. 2000). This can include decorating or painting certain areas of the building to demonstrate school pride or the creation of school policies that promote a positive school climate and clear behavioral expectations.

School Resource Officers With the intention of increasing school safety, law enforcement officers have been deployed to serve in schools. Commonly known as SROs, these individuals have become common in many public schools around the country. SROs are called to serve a multifaceted role, which includes duties such as "law enforcement officer, counselor, teacher, and liaison between law enforcement, schools, families, and the community" (Girouard 2001, p. 1). Indeed, SROs can be seen as a new form of public servant asked to balance security and law enforcement duties while also considering law related education, policies, and practices. Although there is a positive popular perception of SROs, and these positions have the support of educators, law enforcement and other stakeholder groups, the research on the effectiveness of SROs is sparse. Some research suggests that the presence of police officers in schools has led to some students feeling less safe at school, and there are concerns that schools are criminalizing student behavior by moving problematic students into the juvenile justice system rather than disciplining them at school (Jackson 2002; Theriot 2009). Some studies suggest an increasing number of referrals to court for behaviors that could otherwise be treated as school discipline (Kim and Geronimo 2009) and that racial/ethnic minority youth and students with disabilities are disproportionality represented among students referred for criminal delinquency referrals (Advancement Project 2013; Brown 2006. As Na and Gottfredson (2013) concluded from their study of the School Survey on Crime and Safety, "...more rigorous research [needs to] be carried out to assess more carefully the school climate and school safety outcomes related to this popular and costly practice" (p. 1).

Many efforts to increase physical safety measures (e.g., presence of security guards and installing metal detectors) in school have been at the expense of student perceptions of safety, often increasing fear among students (Bachman et al. 2011; Gastic 2011; Schreck et al. 2003). Whereas some SROs take on a more traditional, reactive-oriented approach to student behavior including enforcement of rules and responding to behavioral incidents on campus, prevention-oriented models of practice support the use of trained SROs who are actively involved and integrated with the school community and leadership team.

To improve school safety, each school needs personnel with expertise in recognizing risk factors and warning signs for potentially dangerous events and identified individuals who can serve as first responders in the event of critical incidents. School safety teams include multiple school professionals (e.g., administrators, school psychologists, school counselors, SROs, teachers, administrative staff) who are tasked with ensuring the physical and psychological safety of all students. School safety teams provide the structure and oversight necessary for a comprehensive approach to school safety.

15.4   Evidence-Based Prevention Programs

With the growth in the understanding of prevention science (Chap. 6 in this volume), a number of approaches and programs have been identified through meta-analyses and systematic reviews that reduce violence and aggressive acts and create safer environments for students and adults (Derzon et al. 2006; Fagan and Catalano

2013; Limbos et al. 2007; Wilson and Lipsey 2007). For example, primary prevention such as classes on anger management has been found to be effective in reducing aggression and disruptive behavior (Wilson and Lipsey 2007). Through interviews with a multidisciplinary group of 15 experts in violence prevention, Dusenbury and colleagues (1997) identified nine key components of effective programs. These included programs that are comprehensive, developmentally appropriate, promote personal and social competencies, use interactive techniques, are ethnically and culturally sensitive, support a positive school climate, and foster norms against violence, aggression and bullying. To have the same results as were found in evaluation studies, all programs need to be implemented with fidelity by trained facilitators. Further, effective prevention programs follow a public health model that mobilizes "the knowledge and efforts of multiple fields of science and practice" (Welsh et al. 2014, p. 501).

The Centers for Disease Control and Prevention Task Force on Community Preventive Services reviewed universal school-based programs with published evaluations prior to December 2004 and identified 53 studies that met criteria of rigor. These spanned grades from kindergarten to high school. Developmental differences were clear. In the elementary and middle school interventions, the focus was on disruptive and antisocial behavior with an emphasis on using cognitive skills training. Interventions aimed at middle and high school students shifted focus to target specific forms of violence such as bullying and dating/relationship violence, with an emphasis on changes in cognition, consequential thinking, or affective processes (Hahn et al. 2007).

Park-Higgerson and colleagues (2008) conducted a meta-analysis of 26 school-based violence or aggression prevention programs using randomized control trials. They found that programs that focused on a curriculum-based strategy in schools had better outcomes than programs that focused on selected individuals or included multiple approaches such as involving the community or parents. Comprehensive lists of evidence-based programs and strategies can be found at Blueprints for Healthy Youth Development (http://colorado.edu/csvp/blueprints/) National Registry of Evidence-based Programs and Practices (NREPP; http://nrepp.samhsa. gov/), and What Works Clearinghouse (http://ies.ed.gov/ncee/wcc). The following are selected examples of evidence-based programs that have been shown to reduce student violence, aggressive behavior, or delinquency, and can be found on one or more of these lists.

Child Development Project The elements of the *Child Development Project* comprise a universal intervention for elementary school children that focus on strengthening student's connectedness to school. A core activity is class meetings, in which students discuss issues, make plans for projects and assignments, and foreshadow potential difficult situations. Cross age activities, family activities, and school-wide community building activities engage parents in the school activities and increase student's pro-social skills. Evaluations of this program found that students had a greater sense of school as a caring community, better conflict resolution skills, and less misconduct and delinquency than students in control schools (Battistich et al. 2000).

Coping Power *Coping Power* is a school-based targeted preventive program designed for at-risk late elementary and middle school students in the transition to middle school. Coping Power is counselor driven and includes 34 group sessions over a 15–18 month period along with individual sessions, home visits, and parent education. The content focuses on building social competence, conflict resolution, goal setting, peer relations, and self-regulation skills in students. In a randomized control trial with over 180 aggressive boys, Lochman and Wells (2004) found statistically significant differences in school behavior, as well as decreases in parent-reported alcohol use and delinquency between the treatment and comparison groups.

Good Behavior Game The *Good Behavior Game* (GBG) is a universal behavior management strategy for early elementary classrooms that can be used in academic instruction. Using a game format with teams and rewards, students are socialized to pro-social and nonaggressive behavior through a group contingency model that reinforces positive group and individual behavior. Participation in classrooms in which the GBG was used was significantly related to reduction of aggressive, disruptive behavior, and an increase in on-task behavior by the end of first grade. In a 14-year follow up, researchers found that for males who were aggressive and disruptive in first grade, being part of a GBG classroom had positive long-terms effects on students' mental health and substance abuse behaviors (Grossman et al. 1997; Kellam et al. 2008).

Second Step *Second Step* is a universal social skills curriculum designed for use in kindergarten through middle school classrooms. The goals of the curriculum include reducing aggressive and impulsive behaviors through teaching problem solving, empathy, and goal-setting skills. Recent evaluations demonstrate that when the program was well implemented, children in the Second Step classrooms showed greater declines in antisocial behavior than students in control classrooms (Frey et al. 2005).

Using evidence-based curricula, strategies, and programs can reduce the incidence of violence and aggression in schools and lead to improvements in student connectedness and feelings of safety. To have the predicted impact on positive student outcomes, these programs should be implemented with fidelity by trained facilitators.

15.5   Special Topics in School Violence

15.5.1   Bullying

Bullying is a specific type of aggressive behavior that is defined as intentional, repeated behavior against a target who is less powerful than the perpetrator. It can be physical (e.g., hitting and kicking), verbal (e.g., malicious teasing, name-calling, and threats), or social/relational (e.g., exclusion and rumor-spreading). Bullying in schools has long been a problem, but it is only in the past few decades that the harmful consequences of bullying have been recognized. Bullying is often confused with more general aggression, which means behavior that intentionally harms someone else. Because bullying has received so much publicity, educators, parents and the public in general often incorrectly consider all aggressive acts to be bullying.

Early research on school bullying was largely informed by the work of Dan Olweus of Norway, whose research was initiated after several young children committed suicide as a result of chronic victimization by bullies. The USA ranked 20 out of 40 countries for prevalence of bullying behaviors (Craig et al. 2009). A review of cases of school shootings revealed that in 80% of cases, the perpetrators had been subjected to ongoing teasing and bullying (Leary et al. 2003). With increased awareness of the problem came expectations that schools take a more active role in bullying prevention.

The importance of addressing bullying and victimization is magnified by recent research on the biological foundation of these behaviors. Vaillancourt et al. (2013) reviewed the literature and concluded that victimization has biological as well as psychological effects, and those effects influence future mental and physical health. Victimization was linked to memory impairment for months following incidents, which indicates academic performance is likely to be affected as well. They summarize their findings by saying "the accumulating evidence clearly demonstrates that peer victimization erodes functioning at all levels, perhaps the most important at the level of altering individual physiology" (p. 246).

The most cited study on bullying analyzed data from the 1998 World Health Organization's Health Behaviour in School-Aged Children survey of nationally representative 15,686 students in grades 6–10, and found that 29% of the sample was involved in bullying as perpetrators, targets, or both. Boys were found to be more involved in incidents of bullying than girls, and middle school students more than high school (Nansel et al. 2001). This underscored the need for schools to increase their efforts to address this problem.

Evidence-Based Programs to Combat Bullying Many programs have been developed to reduce bullying in schools. Several studies evaluated the empirical studies on such programs, and found that their impact has been modest at best, with reductions in bullying at about 20–23% and in victimization at 17–20% (Evans et al. 2014; Merrell et al. 2008; Ttofi and Farrington 2011). It is generally agreed that comprehensive, systematic, whole-school programs are most likely to be effective. Whole-school programs aim to increase awareness of bullying, create and publicize clear anti-bullying policies, and include anti-bullying curriculum (Payne and Gottfredson 2004). However, it has been difficult for US schools to devote the time and resources to implementing such programs in sustainable ways. Efforts to improve school climate have found that in schools with high structure and high support, bullying occurred at lower levels (Cornell 2013). This suggests that programs focused on improving school climate may have a positive impact on bullying as well. Related to school climate, studies have examined the role of teachers in bullying prevention and intervention. There is a body of literature that suggests teachers are less efficacious at reducing bullying than they perceive themselves to be (Payne and Gottfredson 2004). See Yoon and Bauman (2014) for a discussion of the role of teachers in creating a classroom and school climate that discourages bullying behavior.

A review of the literature reveals that two anti-bullying programs have been extensively reviewed: The Olweus Bullying Prevention Program (OBPP) and the KiVa Anti-Bullying program. Although the Olweus program has reported significant reductions in bullying in Norway (Olweus 1994, 2003), data from the USA have not found comparable effects (e.g., Limber et al. 2004). As noted by Smith (2014), "OBPP has proved highly effective in Norway, but so far its success in other countries is more variable" (p. 174). The KiVa program in Finland has been carefully researched in Finland (Salmivalli et al. 2011) and the Netherlands (Wienke et al. 2014) with positive results; the English version has not yet been evaluated in the USA.

Ttofi and Farrington (2009, 2011) conducted an exhaustive review and meta-analysis of 53 anti-bullying programs, including only studies that met their criteria for rigorous evaluation. Their findings revealed that in general, anti-bullying programs delivered in schools reduce bullying and victimization by about 20 % in experimental schools when compared to control schools. Effect sizes in most studies were small. Results demonstrate that the most effective program components were parent training, increased supervision on playgrounds, consistently applied firm discipline, school conferences, videos, information for parents, classroom rules, and effective classroom management. Program components involving the use of peers, such as peer mediation, peer mentoring, and bystander intervention, were associated with increases in victimization. Furthermore, the more components included, and the greater the duration and intensity of the programs for students and teachers, the larger the reduction in bullying and victimization. Programs worked best in Norway, and with children who were at least 11 years old. The outcomes in studies conducted in the USA were not as successful as those in Europe.

A subsequent systematic review examined research conducted from 2009 to 2013, a follow-up to the Ttofi and Farrington study, although these researchers limited the studies to those conducted in elementary or middle schools around the world (Evans et al. 2014). Their review included 32 articles evaluating 24 different anti-bullying programs, 15 of which were conducted in the USA. Findings showed that results were mixed, with 50 % of the studies reporting significant reductions in bullying behavior and 67 % reporting significant reductions in victimization. These researchers attempted to validate Ttofi and Farrington's (2009) finding that specific program components were associated with more favorable outcomes, but were unable to identify those components in the studies included in their review. They indicated that some of the newer and more novel programs used components that were not identified in the previous review because they are recent innovations. Similar to Ttofi and Farrington, this review found that positive outcomes were more likely to come from studies conducted outside the USA and with homogeneous samples.

An earlier review of anti-bullying programs can be found in a chapter by Samples (2004). While she did not specify inclusion criteria, Samples stated that studies included in her review used appropriate methodology. Her review examines a variety of studies evaluating the *OBPP, Bullyproof, Bully Proofing Your School, Lions-Quest, Promoting Alternative Thinking Strategies (PATHS), Quit It!, Second Step*, the *Seville Antibullying Project*, and others. Samples highlights programs with promising findings, and concludes there is evidence for "cautious optimism" (p. 220) when considering the results. The author notes that variations in methodological rigor reduced the impact of findings in some of the studies; a necessary first step is changes in school policies whereby bullying is clearly unacceptable.

Cyberbullying Whether cyberbullying (the use of electronic communications technology to deliberately harm another person) is a form of traditional bullying, akin to physical, verbal, and relational bullying, or a qualitatively different phenomenon, is debatable (e.g., Bauman et al. 2013; Tokunaga 2010). What is not debatable is that cyberbullying is a significant problem, although prevalence appears to be lower than rates for traditional bullying. Negative consequences of cyberbullying have been reported, including increased depressive symptomology and suicidal ideation (Bonanno and Hymel 2013; Wang et al. 2011). Experts often focus on the unique features of cyberbullying: perception of anonymity, absence of nonverbal cues, size of audience, constant accessibility, and the permanence of online content in their quest to understand the impact of this phenomenon (Bauman et al. in press). It is also unclear whether schools have the authority to take action against cyberbullying that occurs between students outside of school time using personal (not school-owned) devices. In addition to this policy dilemma, there is evidence that teachers do not feel prepared to deal with cyberbullying (Cassidy et al. 2012).

In summary, bullying and victimization in schools are obstacles to the creation and maintenance of safe and supportive school cultures. Research has found that programs that have been evaluated to date are only modestly successful. It is imperative that future research continues to rigorously evaluate anti-bullying programs, with a goal of identifying specific program elements that account for positive results. These components can then be emphasized in new and developing programs, and components that do not contribute to positive outcomes can be revised or removed so that programs are efficient while being effective. If a conscious and systematic effort to address the long-term problem of bullying is not present, it will be difficult for schools to create a physically and psychologically safe climate that allows students to flourish. It is also worth noting that some initial impressive findings were not sustained over time; a challenge for schools is to maintain energy and enthusiasm so that effective programs are not diluted over time.

15.5.2 Teen Dating Violence

Violence in teen dating relationships has been well documented. Dating violence is characterized by any type of physical, sexual, or psychological violence (Cornelius and Resseguie, 2007). On the Centers for Disease Control and Prevention Youth

Risk Behavior Survey (YRBSS 2011), nearly 10% of high school students reported being hit, slapped, or physically hurt on purpose by their dating partner in the past 12 months. Other studies report females are more often the victims of dating violence as 18–20% adolescent girls reporting being physically and/or sexually hurt by a dating partner (Foshee et al. 2011; Silverman et al. 2001). Serious injuries can also be sustained as 8% of males and 9% of females had been to an emergency department because of an injury in a dating relationship (Foshee et al. 2011).

There is strong evidence that being involved in a violent relationship as a teen is a strong predictor of intimate partner violence in adulthood (Close 2005; Wolfe 2006). Psychological correlates for both the perpetrator and the victim can include lowered self-esteem, increased self-blame, anger, hurt, and anxiety (Cornelius and Resseguie 2007; Jackson et al. 2000). Additional health risks include self-reported increases in binge drinking, marijuana use, suicide attempts, physical fighting, and sexually transmitted diseases (Antle et al. 2011; Foshee et al. 2011; Silverman et al. 2001). If a victim of abuse goes untreated, this may carry over a pattern of abuse into parenting (Leiderman and Almo 2001). In a review of 20 studies with solid methodologies published between 2000 and 2010, Vagi and colleagues (2013) identified 53 risk factors and 6 protective factors. The risk factors fell into broad categories including (a) mental health problems, (b) attitudes such as accepting violence in dating relationships, (c) behaviors including use of aggressive media, substance use, or having antisocial peers, and (d) hostile peer or partner relationships. Protective factors included demonstrating empathy, good grades, average to high verbal IQ, positive maternal relationships, and feeling connected to school (Vagi et al. 2013).

To date, schools have been a primary venue for addressing prevention of teen dating violence, and school staff are called upon to identify strategies and prevention efforts to combat the prevalence of teen dating violence. *Safe Dates* is a widely evaluated dating violence prevention curriculum (Foshee et al. 1998; Foshee et al. 2004). The topics covered in the ten lessons include defining caring relationships, defining abuse, how to help a friend, gender stereotypes, and communications skills. Decreases in relationship violence were found up to 4 years after completing the program (Foshee et al. 2004). *Love U2 Relationship Smarts* is an additional targeted prevention program (Adler-Baeder et al. 2007). This 12–18 session program targets communication skills, conflict resolution skills, and relationship patterns. Evaluation results indicate an increase in knowledge about the curriculum content and a reduction in verbal aggression. These and other promising school-based programs provide educators options for providing students with dating violence prevention.

15.6   School Crisis Response

Crisis events in schools can take many forms, from a natural disaster such as flooding from a recent storm to a cheerleading coach dying from a heart attack in the middle of practice. The most extreme crisis events could include an act of violence with deadly force on school grounds. Each of these crises threatens the safety of students, educators, and potentially other community members. However, effective school safety is a day-in, day-out commitment that is infused into every aspect of school life, not just when a crisis event takes place. The National Association of School Psychologists (NASP) encourages school mental health professionals and other educators to become more unified, vocal advocates for policies that support what schools *can* do effectively, which in turn supports our schools' primary mission of learning (NASP 2013). It is important that adequate learning supports and policies are present to provide a continuum of services that respond to the needs of *all* students as well as structures that can effectively deal with a full range of crises when they occur. An active school safety and/or crisis team can focus on continual efforts to promote a safe, positive school culture while minimizing the impact of school crises when they occur.

Before considering any crisis prevention, response, or recovery strategies, it is important to understand the characteristics that make up a crisis event. Those events that may require a school crisis response are described as being extremely negative, uncontrollable, and unpredictable because they have the potential to generate a significant amount of emotional or physical pain (Brock 2002, 2006a, b). Within schools, a student or staff member's perception of the crisis event is especially important as the more negatively an individual views the event and its impact on the community, the more significant the personal crisis becomes (Bryant et al. 2007; Shaw 2003). Second, the crisis events generate feelings of helplessness or powerlessness, as individuals often report feelings of losing control (APA 2000). And finally, when crisis events occur unexpectedly or without warning, there is little time for individuals to adapt or adjust to the problem generated by the crisis. This can make the event highly traumatic for some individuals. In fact, research has demonstrated that very sudden and unpredictable events (e.g., school shooting, car accident) typically generate more traumatic stress than those that are gradual and more predictable (e.g., death following a long-term illness; Brock et al. 2009).

It is customary for schools to have crisis teams trained and ready to respond in the event of a crisis situation. In fact, the No Child Left Behind Act of 2001 requires local school systems that receive federal funding (under Title IV, Part A, Safe and Drug-Free Schools and Communities) to have school crisis plans in place. In addition, 92 % of states require districts or schools to have a crisis plan (Kann et al. 2007) or other laws requiring components such as prevention programming or annual crisis response training in place.

However, the need for school crisis intervention services are often determined by the extent to which school crisis team members are impacted by the crisis event. Further, "a crisis event should prompt *consideration* of the need to provide a school crisis response, an event itself is insufficient to justify *provision* of the response" (Brock et al. 2009, p. 8). One of the key functions of the school crisis team is to understand what circumstances signal the need to activate appropriate crisis intervention services as well consider what level of response is needed. For example, the death of a parent within a school community may require a minimal response (e.g., only the child of that parent and close friends may have known the individual or feel impacted by the event) whereas another parent well known to the school community could precipitate a more significant building or district-level crisis response, bringing in outside resources and supports to better meet the needs of affected students and teachers.

The U S Department of Education (2003) and Homeland Security (2008) offer guidance and direction around the four levels of crisis response: (a) *mitigation and prevention* addresses what schools can do reduce or eliminate risks within the school environment, (b) *preparedness* focuses on the process of planning for crisis events, (c) *response* highlights the steps that are taken during a crisis, and (d) *recovery* addresses how the school works to restore the learning and social environment after a crisis event. These components are described in more detail below in Table 15.2.

15.6.1   Crisis Prevention and Preparedness

The primary goal of school crisis prevention and preparedness efforts is to develop school crisis plans and crisis teams. It is important not only for crisis teams to have comprehensive school crisis plans but it is also necessary for these plans to be understood by all school members, practiced on a regular basis, continually reviewed and updated, and tailored to meet the unique needs of each school (Valent 2000). The US Department of Homeland Security's (2008) National Incident Management System (NIMS) and its Incident Command Structure (ICS) is required for all schools that seek to obtain federal preparedness assistance. NIMS provides a standardized structure for school crisis teams, as well as a common set of concepts, terminology, organizational processes, and principles. The basic premise of the ICS is that all staff members have specific functions within a crisis team and can easily transition into these roles in the event of a crisis. While the elements of the ICS are beyond the focus of this chapter, additional information in the NIMS structure and ICS can be found at the US Department of Education's Emergency Response and

Table 15.2 Components to consider when establishing and sustaining a school crisis team (Primary source US Department of Education (2007). This document is in the public domain.)

Determine what crisis teams and plans exist in the district, school, and community
Identify all stakeholders involved in crisis planning
Establish a team of qualified individuals to serve on the school crisis team
Secure administrative support for the school crisis team
Identify or develop the necessary policies to assist all school community members in a crisis
Develop procedures for communicating with all school community members and the media for each specific crisis event (e.g., develop the school crisis plan)
Ensure that all crisis team members and staff have appropriate training and professional development opportunities
Establish ongoing team meetings and select dates at the beginning of the school year to review the team infrastructure, maintain team coherence, and update the details of the school crisis plan

Crisis Management Technical Assistance (rems.ed.gov). Additional components to consider when establishing and sustaining a school crisis team are provided in Table 15.2.

15.6.2 Crisis Response and Recovery

The primary goal of almost any school crisis intervention is to help restore individuals' basic coping skills and problem-solving abilities, and restore individuals to precrisis levels of functioning (Sandoval and Brock 2009). Many of the interventions appropriate for students and staff members are active and direct attempts from crisis interveners to facilitate adaptive coping and directly respond to symptoms of traumatic stress. Often referred to as psychological first aid, the immediate needs of individuals impacted by the crisis event within the school community fall to school crisis team members and those trained to respond to crisis events. These immediate crisis response efforts can be managed through *debriefing groups* (Mitchell and Everly 1996), *group crisis interventions* (Young 1998), and through *individual and classroom crisis interventions* described in the NASP PREPaRE curriculum (Brock et al. 2009). These services typically provide support to students and staff exposed to the crisis event. While the steps of each intervention vary by program, the primary goals are to help impacted students and staff understand crisis facts, recognize how crisis events have impacted their immediate functioning, appreciate the commonality of crisis experiences among school members, and to identify adaptive coping skills and problem-solving strategies. More intensive interventions for those who are acute trauma victims or have severe psychological injury (Jacobs et al. 2004) often require collaboration with community-based mental health professionals. Crisis responders are cautioned not to overrespond in crisis events, as doing so can often send the message that individuals are not capable of independently coping with the crisis event, and can detract from efforts to promote independent problem solving. NASP has developed an evidence-based school crisis prevention and intervention curriculum designed to help better prepare school crisis teams to respond to such events. More information on this curriculum can be found at www. nasponline.org/prepare.

15.7 Threat and Risk Assessments

Threat assessments involve a process by which a threat and the circumstances surrounding that threat are evaluated to uncover evidence or facts indicating the threat is likely to be carried out (Cornell et al. 2009). Threat assessments have been widely used by the Secret Service and law enforcement to analyze a variety of dangerous situations (e.g., threats on public officials and workplace violence) but have only more recently moved into being used in the public school setting. Student threat assessment is different than profiling, as an investigation is triggered by the student's own threatening behaviors versus some broader combination of student characteristics (Cornell et al. 2009). This could include a student who has made direct threats to another peer, or an adolescent who has made ominous statements about imposing harm on an entire group of students. However, the threat assessment is ultimately concerned with whether a student *poses* a threat, not whether he or she has actually *made* a threat (O'Toole 2000; Randazzo et al. 2006). While many students can make a threat, relatively few have the intent and means to carry out the threat. In fact, 70 % of the cases have been reported to involve verbal threats while 30 % involve a plan or means to carry out a plan (Cornell et al. 2009).

Although the Federal Bureau of Investigation (FBI) and Secret Service have highlighted compelling reasons for schools to adopt a threat assessment approach to prevent targeted acts of violence (Fein et al. 2002; O'Toole 2000), these procedures are still relatively new to the school environment. While threat and risk assessment are terms that are often used interchangeably, they serve different purposes. Risk assessments involve assessing what may happen in the future and answer the question of, *what is this student's potential to harm in the future?* The goal of such assessment is to prevent future harm to persons or property. The intent of threat assessments, however, is to evaluate something that has already happened. For example, when students make direct, indirect, veiled, or conditional threats, the focus is to gather information and evaluate facts to determine if a student poses a threat for targeted violence. The same outcome may result, however, in that risk and threat assessments serve to prevent targeted violence. It is important to remember that targeted violence is not random or spontaneous; it does not occur because someone "just snapped." The research on targeted violence suggests it is the result of an understandable, and an often discernable, pattern of thinking and behavior (Borum et al. 1999; Fein and Vossekuil 1998; Fein et al. 1995).

Schools that undergo threat or risk assessment procedures traditionally utilize a team approach. These teams can include school administrators, SROs, school mental health professionals (e.g., school psychologists and school counselors), and others that have training in understanding how student behavior may pose a threat to the school environment. The process of gathering information about the individual of concern includes investigating facts from multiple sources to establish their validity and veracity. In this case, the threshold for concern is the progression of an individual's behavior on a pathway toward violent activity (Reddy et al. 2001). Threat assessment teams are then called upon to determine the level of risk or threat the student poses to the school environment. High-risk behaviors typically include direct, specific threats that are plausible when concrete plans and steps have been taken. Medium-level threats can be concrete and with detail but no plan or active preparation is detectable; low-level threats are often indirect and with inconsistent detail and implausibility (Twemlow et al. 2002). Schools that utilize these types of formalized procedures have been found to have more positive outcomes. For example, one study investigating the use of the Virginia Threat Assessment Guidelines found that students endorsed more positive perceptions of school climate, less bullying, and a greater willingness to seek help in schools using such assessments than control group schools (Cornell et al. 2009). In addition, these schools had fewer long-term suspensions and overall incidents of violence, suggesting that formalized approaches and increased staff awareness of how to respond to crisis events have the potential to result in positive school climate and student safety outcomes.

15.8 Conclusion

Due to the timing and similarity of instances, as well as media portrayal of such events, many incidents of school violence have been viewed as an "epidemic" (Verlinden et al. 2000). However, school violence is not as widespread as many believe, as schools remain one of the safest places for youth (Jimerson et al. 2005). It is important to shift the focus for educators and policy makers toward an examination of school community norms, goals, and values. This is particularly relevant for the purposes of school violence prevention, because incidents of youth victimization tend to occur in environments where uncivil patterns of behaviors prevail (see Swearer et al. 2012). Clearly, promoting safety at schools should include a consideration of both physical and psychological safety considerations in promoting positive outcomes for youth.

References

Adelman, H. S., & Taylor, L. (2000). Moving prevention from the fringes into the fabric of school improvement. *Journal of Educational and Psychological Consultation, 119*, 736. doi:10.1207/s1532768Xjepc1101_03.

Adler-Baeder, F., Kerpelman, J. L., Schramm, D. G., Higginbotham, B., & Paulk, A. (2007). The impact of relationship education on adolescents of diverse backgrounds. *Family Relations, 56*(3), 291–303.

Advancement Project, Alliance for Educational Justice, Dignity in Schools Campaign, and NAACP Legal Defense Fund. (2013). Police in school are not the answer to the Newtown shooting. http://safequalityschools.org/resources/entry/summary-to-issue-brief-police-in-schools-arenot-the-answer.

American Psychiatric Association. (2000). *Diagnostic and statistical manual of mental disorders* (4th ed., text rev.). Washington, DC: American Psychiatric Association.

Anderson, M., Kaufman, J., Simon, T. R., Barrios, L., Paulozzi, L., Ryan, G., Hammond, R., Modzeleski, W., Feucht, T., Potter, L., & School-Associated Violent Deaths Study Group. (2001). School-associated violent deaths in the United States, 1994–1999. *Journal of the American Medical Association, 286*, 2695–2702. doi:10.1001/jama.286.21.2695.

Antle, B. F., Sullivan, D. J., Dryden, A., Karam, E. A., & Barbee, A. P. (2011). Healthy relationship education for dating violence prevention among high-risk youth. *Children and Youth Services Review, 33*, 173–179. doi:10.1016/j.childyouth.2010.08.031.

Bachman, R., Randolph, A., & Brown, B. L. (2011). Predicting perceptions of fear at school and going to and from school for African American and White students: The effects of school security measures. *Youth & Society, 43*, 705–726.

Barrios, L. C., Baer, K., Bennett, G., Bergan, A., Bryn, S., Callaway, S., et al. (2000). Federal activities addressing violence in schools. *Journal of School Health, 70*, 119–140.

Battistich, V., Schaps, E., Watson, M., Solomon, D., & Lewis, C. (2000). Effects of the child development project on students' drug use and other problem behaviors. *Journal of Primary Prevention, 21*, 75–99.

Bauman, S., Underwood, M. K., & Card, N. A. (2013). Definitions: Another perspective and a proposal for beginning with cyberaggresion. In S. Bauman, D. Cross, & J. Walker (Eds.), *Principles of cyberbullying research: Definitions, measures, and methodology* (pp. 41–46). New York: Routledge.

Bauman, S., Mendez, J., Craig, W., & Mishna, F. (in press). Research on bullying in North America. In P. K. Smith, K. Kwak, & Y. Toda (Eds.), *Reducing bullying and cyberbullying in schools: Eastern and western perspectives*. London: Cambridge University Press.

Baumrind, D. (1996). The discipline controversy revisited. *Family Relations, 45*, 405–414. http://www.jstor.org/stable/585170.

Bonanno, R. A., & Hymel, S. (2013). Cyber bullying and internalizing difficulties: Above and beyond the impact of traditional forms of bullying. *Journal of Youth and Adolescence, 42*, 685–697. doi:10.1007/s10964-013-9937-1.

Borum, R., Fein, R., Vossekuil, B., & Berglund, J. (1999). Threat assessment: Defining an approach for evaluating risk of targeted violence. *Behavioral Sciences and the Law, 17*, 323–337. doi:10.1002/(SICI)1099-0798(199907/09)17:3<323::AID-BSL349>3.0.CO;2-G.

Bracy, N. L. (2010). Student perceptions of high-security school environments. *Youth & Society, 43*, 365–395. doi:10.1177/0044118X10365082.

Brock, S. E. (2002). Crisis theory: A foundation for the comprehensive school crisis response team. In S. E. Brock, P. J. Lazarus, & S. R. Jimerson (Eds.), *Best practices in school crisis prevention and intervention* (pp. 5–17). Bethesda: National Association of School Psychologists.

Brock, S. E. (2006a). Crisis intervention and recovery: The roles of school-based mental health professionals. (Available from National Association of School Psychologists, 4340 East West Highway, Suite 402, Bethesda, MD 20814).

Brock, S. E. (2006b). Crisis intervention and recovery: The roles of school-based mental health professionals. Workshop evaluation/test summaries and workshop modification suggestions. (Available from National Association of School Psychologists, 4340 East West Highway, Suite 402, Bethesda, MD 20814.

Brock, S. E., Nickerson, A. B., Reeves, M. A., Jimerson, S. R., Lieberman, R. A., & Feinberg, T. A. (2009). *School crisis prevention and intervention: The PREPaRE model*. Bethesda: National Association of School Psychologists.

Brown, B. (2006). Understanding and assessing school police officers: A conceptual and methodological comment. *Journal of Criminal Justice, 34*, 591–604.

Bryant, R. A., Salmon, K., Sinclair, E., & Davidson, P. (2007). A prospective study of appraisals in childhood posttraumatic stress disorder. *Behaviour Research and Therapy, 45*, 2502–2507. doi:10.1016/j.brat.2007.04.009.

Casella, R. (2003). Zero tolerance policy in schools: Rationale, consequences, and alternatives. *The Teachers College Record, 105*, 872–892. doi:10.1111/1467- 9620.00271.

Cassidy, W., Brown, K., & Jackson, M. (2012). 'Under the radar': Educators and cyberbullying in schools. *School Psychology International, 33*, 520–532. doi:10.1177/0143034312445245.

Christle, C., Nelson, C. M., & Jolivette, K. (2004). School characteristics related to the use of suspension. *Education and Treatment of Children, 27*, 509–526.

Close, S. M. (2005). Dating violence prevention in middle school and high school youth. *Journal of Child and Adolescent Psychiatric Nursing, 18*, 2–9. doi:10.1111/j.1744–6171.2005.00003.x.

Cohen, J., McCabe, L., Michelli, N. M., & Pickeral, T. (2009). School climate: Research, policy, teacher education, and practice. *Teachers' College Record, 111*, 180–213.

Cole, J. D., Watt, N. E., West, S. G., Hawkins, J. D., Asarnow, J. R., Markman, H. J., et al. (1993). The science of prevention: A conceptual framework and some directions for a national research program. *American Psychologist, 48*, 1013–1022. doi:10.1037/0003-066X.48.10.1013.

Coon, J. K., & Travis, L. F. (2012). The role of police in public schools: A comparison of principal and police reports of activities in schools. *Police Practice and Research, 13*, 15–30.

Cornelius, T. L., & Resseguie, N. (2007). Primary and secondary prevention programs for dating violence: A review of the literature. *Aggression and Violent Behavior, 12*, 364–375. doi:10.1016/j.avb.2006.09.006.

Cornell, D. (2013, June 19). Bullying and school climate. Presentation at the BRNET annual meeting, Santa Barbara, CA

Cornell, D. G., & Mayer, M. J. (2010). Why do school order and safety matter? *Educational Researcher, 39*, 7–15. doi:10.3102/0013189X09357616.

Cornell, D., Sheras, P., Gregory, A., & Fan, X. (2009). A retrospective study of school safety conditions in high schools using the Virginia threat assessment guidelines versus alternative approaches. *School Psychology Quarterly, 24*, 119–129. doi:10.1037/a0016182.

Craig, W., Harel-Fisch, Y., Fogel-Grinvald, H., Dostaler, S., Hetland, J., Simons-Morton, B., Molcho, M., Gaspar de Mato, M., Overpeck, M., Due, P., & Pickett, W. (2009). A cross-national profile of bullying and victimization among adolescents in 40 countries. *International Journal of Public Health, 54*(2), 216–224.

Derzon, J., Jimerson, S. R., & Furlong, M. (2006). How effective are school-based violence prevention programs in preventing and reducing violence and other antisocial behaviors? A meta-analysis. Handbook of school violence and school safety: From research to practice, 429–441.

Dusenbury, L., Falco, M., Lakem, A., Brannigan, R., & Bosworth, K. (1997). Nine critical elements of promising violence prevention programs. *Journal of School Health, 67*, 409–414. doi:10.1111/j.1746-1561.1997.tb01286.x.

Evans, C. B. R., Fraser, M. W., & Cotter, K. L. (2014). The effectiveness of school-based bullying prevention programs. *Aggression and Violent Behavior, 19*, 532–544. doi:10.1016/j.avb.2014.07.004.

Fabelo, T., Thompson, M. D., Plotkin, M., Carmichael, D., Marchbanks, M. P. III, & Booth, E. A. (2011). Breaking school rules: A statewide study of how discipline relates to student's success and juvenile justice involvement.

Fagan, A. A., & Catalano, R. F. (2013). What works in youth violence prevention a review of the literature. *Research on Social Work Practice, 23*, 141–156. doi:10.1177/1049731512465899.

Fein, R. A., & Vossekuil, B. (1998). *Protective intelligence and threat assessment investigations: A guide for state and local law enforcement officials. (NIJ/OJP/DOJ Publication No. 170612).* Washington, DC: U.S. Department of Justice.

Fein, R. A., Vossekuil, B., & Holden, G. A. (1995, July). Threat assessment: An approach to prevent targeted violence. http://www.secretservice.gov/ntac/ntac_threat.pdf. Accessed 25 Sept 2014.

Fein, R. A., Vossekuil, B., Pollack, W. S., Borum, R., Modzeleski, W., & Reddy, M. (2002). Threat assessment in schools: A guide to managing threatening situations and creating safe school climates. United States Secret Service and the United States Department of Education, Washington, DC.

Fenning, P., & Rose, J. (2007). Overrepresentation of African American students in exclusionary discipline the role of school policy. *Urban Education, 42*, 536–559. doi:10.1177/0042085907305039.

Flannery, D. J., Modzeleski, W., & Kretschmar, J. M. (2013). Violence and school shootings. *Current Psychiatry Reports, 15*(1), 1–7. doi:10.1007/s11920-012-0331-6.

Foshee, V. A., Bauman, K. E., Arriaga, X. B., Helms, R. W., Koch, G. G., & Linder, G. F. (1998). An evaluation of Safe Dates, an adolescent dating violence prevention program. *American Journal of Public Health, 88*(1), 45–50.

Foshee, V. A., Bauman, K. E., Ennett, S. T., Linder, G. F., Benefield, T., & Suchindran, C. (2004). Assessing the long-term effects of the Safe Dates program and a booster in preventing and reducing adolescent dating violence victimization and perpetration. *American Journal of Public Health, 94*(4), 619–624.

Foshee, V. A., McNaughton Reyes, H. L., Ennett, S. T., Suchindran, C., Mathias, J. P., Karriker-Jaffe, K. J., Bauman, K. E., & Benefield, T. S. (2011). Risk and protective factors distinguishing profiles of adolescent peer and dating violence perpetration. *Journal of Adolescent Health, 48*, 344–350. doi:10.1016/j.jadohealth.2010.07.030.

Frey, K. S., Nolan, S. B., Van Schoiack Edstrom, L., & Hirschstein, M. K. (2005). Effects of a school-based social–emotional competence program: Linking children's goals, attributions, and behavior. *Journal of Applied Developmental Psychology, 26*, 171–200. doi:10.1016/j.appdev.2004.12.002.

Gastic, B. (2011). Metal detectors and feeling safe at school. *Education and Urban Society, 43*, 486–498.

Girouard, C. (2001, March). *School resource officer training program (FS 200105).* Washington, DC: U.S. Department of justice, office of justice programs. Office of Juvenile justice and delinquency prevention.

Gottfredson, G. D., & Gottfredson, D. C. (2001). What schools do to prevent problem behavior and to promote safe environments. *Journal of Educational and Psychological Consultation, 12*, 313–344.

Gregory, A., Cornell, D., Fan, X., Sheras, P., Shih, T., & Huang, F. (2010). Authoritative school discipline: High school practices associated with lower bullying and victimization. *Journal of Educational Psychology, 102*, 483–496. doi:10.1037/a0018562.

Griggs, M., Glover Gagnon, S., Huelsman, T. J., Kidder-Ashley, P., & Ballard, M. (2009). Student-teacher relationships matter: Moderating influences between temperament and preschool social competence. *Psychology in the Schools, 46*, 553–567. doi:10.1002/pits.20397.

Grossman, D. C., Neckerman, H. J., Koepsell, T. D., Liu, P. Y., Asher, K. N., Beland, K., Fresy, K., & Rivara, F. P. (1997). Effectiveness of a violence prevention curriculum among children in elementary school: A randomized controlled trial. *Journal of the American Medical Academy, 277*, 1605–1611. doi:10.1001/jama.1997.03540440039030.

Hahn, R., Fuqua-Whitley, D., Wethington, H., Lowy, J., Crosby, A., Fullilove, M., Johnson, R., Liberman, A., Moscicki, E., Price, L., Snyder, S., Tuma, F., Cory, S., Stone, G., Mukhopadhaya, K., Chattopadhyay, S., & Dahlberg, L. (2007). Effectiveness of universal school-based programs to prevent violent and aggressive behavior: A systematic review. *American Journal of Preventive Medicine, 33*, S114–S129. doi:10.1016/j.amepre.2007.04.012.

Hattie, J. A. C. (2009). *Visible learning: A synthesis of over 800 meta-analyses relating to achievement.* London: Routledge.

Hawkins, J. D., Catalano, R. F., & Miller, J. Y. (1992). Risk and protective factors for alcohol and other drug problems in adolescence and early adulthood: Implications for substance abuse prevention. *Psychological Bulletin, 112*, 64–105. doi:10.1037/0033-2909.112.1.64.

Jackson, A. (2002). Police-school resource officers' and students' perception of the police and offending. *Policing: An International Journal of Police Strategies and Management, 25*, 631–650.

Jackson, S. M., Cram, F., & Seymour, F. W. (2000). Violence and sexual coercion in high school students' dating relationships. *Journal of Family Violence, 15*, 23–36. doi:10.1023/A:1007545302987.

Jacobs, J., Horne-Moyer, H. L., & Jones, R. (2004). The effectiveness of critical incident stress debriefing with primary and secondary trauma victims. *International Journal of Emergency Mental Health, 6*(1), 5–14.

Jimerson, S. R., Brock, S. E., & Cowan, C. C. (2005). Threat assessment: An essential component of a comprehensive safe school program. *Principal Leadership*, October, 11–15.

Johnson, S. L. (2009). Improving the school environment to reduce school violence: A review of the literature. *Journal of School Health, 79*, 451–465. doi:10.1111/j.1746-1561.2009.00435.x.

Kann, L., Brener, N. D., & Wechsler, H. (2007). Overview and summary: School health policies and programs study 2006. *Journal of School Health, 77*, 385–397. doi:10.1111/j.1746-1561.2007.00226.x.

Kellam, S. G., Brown, C. H., Poduska, J. M., Ialongo, N. S., Wang, W., Toyinbo, P., Petras, H., Ford, C., Windham, A., & Wilcox, H. C. (2008). Effects of a universal classroom behavior management program in first and second grades on young adult behavioral, psychiatric, and social outcomes. *Drug and Alcohol Dependence, 95*, S5–S28. doi:10.1016/j.drugalcdep.2008.01.004.

Kim, C. Y., & Geronimo, I. I. (2009). *Policing in schools: Developing a governance document for school resource officers in K–12 schools.* New York: American Civil Liberties Union.

Leary, M. R., Kowalski, R. M., Smith, L., & Phillips, S. (2003). Teasing, rejection, and violence: Case studies of the school shootings. *Aggressive Behavior, 29*, 202–214. doi:10.1002/ab.10061.

Leiderman, S., & Almo, C. (2001). Interpersonal violence and adolescent pregnancy: Prevalence and implications for practice and policy. Center for Assessment and Policy Development and the National Organization on Adolescent Pregnancy, Parenting, and Prevention.

Limber, S. P., Nation, M., Tracy, A. J., Melton, G. B., & Flerx, V. (2004). Implementation of the Olweus Bullying Prevention programme in the Southeastern United States. In P. K. Smith, D. Pepler, & K. Rigby (Eds.), *Bullying in schools: How successful can interventions be?* (pp. 55–79). New York: Cambridge University Press.

Limbos, M. A., Chan, L. S., Warf, C., Schneir, A., Iverson, E., Shekelle, P., et al. (2007). Effectiveness of interventions to prevent youth violence: A systematic review. *American Journal of Preventive Medicine, 33*, 65–74. doi:10.1016/j.amepre.2007.02.045.

Lochman, J. E., & Wells, K. C. (2004). The coping power program for preadolescent aggressive boys and their parents: Outcome effects at the 1-year follow-up. *Journal of Consulting and Clinical Psychology, 72*, 571–578. doi:10.1037/0022-006X.72.4.571.

Maguire, B., Weatherby, G. A., & Mathers, R. A. (2002). Network news coverage of school shootings. *Social Science Journal, 39*, 465–470.

Mayer, M. J., & Furlong, M. J. (2010). How safe are our schools? *Educational Researcher, 39*, 16–26. doi:10.3102/0013189X09357617.

McCord, J., Widom, C. S., Bamba, M. I., & Crowell, N. A. (Eds.). (2000). *Juvenile crime juvenile justice: Panel on Juvenile Crime: Prevention, treatment, and control*. Washington, DC: National Academy Press.

McNeely, C. A., Nonnemaker, J. M., & Blum, R. W. (2002). Promoting school connectedness: Evidence from the national longitudinal study of adolescent health. *Journal of School Health, 72*, 138–146. doi:10.1111/j.1746-1561.2002.tb06533.x.

Merrell, K. W., Gueldner, B. A., Ross, S. W., & Isava, D. M. (2008). How effective are school bullying intervention programs? A meta-analysis of intervention research. *School Psychology Quarterly, 23*, 26–42. doi:10.1037/1045-3830.23.1.26.

Mitchell, J. T., & Everly, G. S. (1996). *Critical incident stress debriefing: An operations manual for the prevention of traumatic stress among emergency services and disaster workers* (2nd edn.). Ellicott City: Chevron Publishing.

Morgan, E., Salomon, N., Plotkin, M., & Cohen, R. (2014). *The school discipline consensus report: Strategies from the field to keep students engaged in school and out of the juvenile justice system*. New York: The Council of State Governments Justice Center.

Morrison, B. E. (2003). Regulating safe school communities: Being responsive and restorative. *Journal of Educational Administration, 41*, 690–704.

Na, C., & Gottfredson, D. C. (2013). Police officers in schools: Effects on school crime and the processing of offending behaviors. *Justice Quarterly, 30*, 619–650.

Nansel, T. R., Overpeck, M., Pilla, R. S., Ruan, W. J., Simons-Morton, B., & Scheidt, P. (2001). Bullying behaviors among US youth. *The Journal of the American Medical Association, 285*, 2094–2100. doi:10.1001/jama.285.16.2094.

National Association of School Psychologists. (2013). Recommendations for comprehensive school safety policies. http://www.nasponline.org/resources/bullying/Bullying_Brief_12.pdf. Accessed 15 Sept 2014.

National Center for Education Statistics & the Bureau of Justice Statistics. (2009). *Indicators of school crime and safety:2008 (NCES 2009-022, NCJ No. 226343)*. Washington, DC: U.S. Department of Education and the U.S. Department of Justice.

National Crime Prevention Council. (n.d.). www.ncpc.org. Accessed 15 Sept 2014.

No Child Left Behind Act of 2001, P. L. 107–110, 115 U.S.C. § 1425 (2002). http://www2ed.gov/policy/elsec/leg/esea02/index.html. Accessed 15 Sept 2014.

O'Malley, M., & Eklund, K. (2012). Creating safe and supportive learning and working environments. In S. E. Brock & S. R. Jimerson (Eds.), *Best practices in school crisis prevention and intervention* (pp. 151–176). Bethesda: National Association of School Psychologists.

O'Toole, M. E. (2000). The school shooter: A threat assessment perspective. Critical incident response group (CIRG), national center for the analysis of violent crimes (NCAVC). FBI Academy, Quantico, VA 22135.

Olweus, D. (1994). Bullying at school: Basic facts and effects of a school based intervention program. *Journal of Child Psychology and Psychiatry, 35*, 1171–1190. doi:10.1111/j.1469-7610.1994. tb01229.x.

Olweus, D. (2003). A profile of bullying at school. *Educational Leadership; 60*, 12–17.

Orpinas, P., Horne, A. M., & Staniszewski, D. (2003). School bullying: Changing the problem by changing the school. *School Psychology Review, 32*, 431–444. http://www.publichealth.uga. edu/hpb/sites/default/files/2003-Orpinas-SchoolBullying.pdf.

Osher, D., Bear, G. G., Sprague, J. R., & Doyle, W. (2010). How can we improve school discipline? *Educational Researcher, 39*, 48–58. doi:10.3102/0013189X09357618.

Osterman, K. F. (2000). Students' need for belonging in the school community. *Review of Educational Research, 7*, 323–367. doi:10.3102/00346543070003323.

Park-Higgerson, H. K., Perumean-Chaney, S. E., Bartolucci, A. A., Grimley, D. M., & Singh, K. P. (2008). The evaluation of school-based violence prevention programs: A meta-analysis. *Journal of School Health, 78*, 465–479. doi:10.1111/j.1746-1561.2008.00332.x.

Payne, A. A., & Gottfredson, D. C. (2004). Schools and bullying: School factors related to bullying and school-based bullying interventions. In C. E. Sanders & G. D. Phye (Eds.), *Bullying: Implications for the classroom*. London: Elsevier.

Perlus, J. G., Brooks-Russell, A., Wang, J., & Iannotti, R. J. (2014). Trends in bullying, physical fighting, and weapon carrying among 6th-through 10th-grade students from 1998 to 2010: Findings from a national study. *American Journal of Public Health, 104*, 1100–1106. doi:10.2105/AJPH.2013.301761.

Puzzanchera, C., & Adams, B. (2011). Juvenile arrests 2009. Office of Juvenile justice and delinquency prevention.

Raffaele-Mendez, L. M., Knoff, H. M., & Ferron, J. M. (2002). School demographic variables and out-of-school suspension rates: A quantitative and qualitative analysis of a large, ethnically diverse school district. *Psychology in the Schools, 39*, 259–277.

Randazzo, M. R., Borum, R., Vossekuil, B., Fein, R., Modzeleski, W., & Pollack, W. (2006). Threat assessment in schools: Empirical support and comparison with other approaches. In S. R. Jimerson & M. J. Furlong (Eds.), *Handbook of school violence and school safety: From research to practice* (pp. 147–156). Mahwah: Lawrence Erlbaum.

Reddy, M., Borum, R., Berglund, J., Vossekuil, B., Fein, R., & Moszeleski, W. (2001). Evaluating risk of targeted violence in schools: Comparing risk assessment, threat assessment, and other approaches. *Psychology in the Schools, 38*, 157–172.

Reinke, W. M., & Herman, K. C. (2002). Creating school environments that deter antisocial behaviors in youth. *Psychology in the Schools, 39*, 549–559. doi:10.1002/pits.10048.

Robers, S., Zhang, J., & Truman, J. (2012). Indicators of school crime and safety: 2011 (NCES 2012-002/NCJ 236021). Washington, DC: U.S. Department of Education and U.S. Department of Justice. http://bjs.ojp.usdoj.gov/content/pub/pdf/iscs11.pdf.

Rutter, M., Maughan, S., & Smith, A. (1979). *15,000 hours: Secondary schools and their impact upon children*. London: Open Books.

Salmivalli, C., Karna, A., & Poskiparta, E. (2011). Counteracting bullying in Finland: The KiVa program and its effects on different forms of being bullied. *International Journal of Behavioral Development, 35*, 405–411.

Samples, F. L. (2004). Evaluating curriculum-based intervention programs: An examination of preschool, primary, and elementary school intervention programs. In C. E. Sanders & G. D. Phye (Eds.), *Bullying: Implications for the classroom* (pp. 203–228). London: Elsevier.

Sandoval, J., & Brock, S. E. (2009). Managing crisis: Prevention, intervention, and treatment. In C. R. Reynolds & T. B. Gutkin (Eds.), *The handbook of school psychology* (pp. 886–904). New York: Wiley.

Schneider, T., Walker, H., & Sprague, J. (2000). *Safe school design: A handbook for educational leaders: Applying the principles of crime prevention through environmental design*. Eugene: ERIC Clearinghouse on Educational Management.

Schreck, C. J., Miller, J. M., & Gibson, C. L. (2003). Trouble in the school yard: A study of the risk factors of victimization at school. *Crime & Delinquency, 49*, 460–484.

Shaw, J. A. (2003). Children exposed to war/terrorism. *Clinical Child and Family Psychology Review, 6*, 237–246. doi:10.1023/B:CCFP.0000006291.10180.bd.

Silverman, J. G., Raj, A., Mucci, L. A., & Hathaway, J. E. (2001). Dating violence against adolescent girls and associated substance use, unhealthy weight control, sexual risk behavior, pregnancy, and suicidality. *Journal of the American Medical Association, 286*, 572–579. doi:10.1001/jama.286.5.572.

Skiba, R. J., & Knesting, K. (2002). *Zero tolerance, zero evidence: An analysis of school disciplinary practice*. San Francisco: Jossey-Bass.

Skiba, R. J., Michael, R. S., Nardo, A. C., & Peterson, R. L. (2000). The color of discipline: Sources of racial and gender disproportionality in school punishment. *The Urban Review, 34*, 317–342. doi:10.1023/A:1021320817372.

Skiba, R. J., Chung, C. G., Trachok, M., Baker, T. L., Sheya, A., & Hughes, R. L. (2014). Parsing disciplinary disproportionality contributions of infraction, student, and school characteristics to out-of-school suspension and expulsion. *American Educational Research Journal, 51*, 640–670. doi:10.3102/0002831214541670.

Smith, P. K. (2014). *Understanding school bullying: Its nature and prevention strategies*. London: Sage.

Sprague, J., & Horner, R. (2007). School-wide positive behavioral support. In S. R. Jimerson & M. J. Furlong (Eds.), *Handbook of school violence and school safety: From research to practice* (pp. 412–428). Mahwah: Lawrence Erlbaum.

Sprague, J. R., & Walker, H. M. (2005). *Safe and healthy schools: Practical prevention strategies*. New York: Guildford Press.

Steinberg, M. P., Allensworth, E., & Johnson, D. W. (2013). *What conditions jeopardize and support safety in urban schools? The influence of community characteristics, school composition and school organizational practices on student and teacher reports of safety in Chicago*. In UCLA Center for Civil Rights Remedies Closing the Discipline Gap: Research to Practice Conference, Washington, DC.

Sugai, G., Sprague, J. R., Horner, R. H., & Walker, H. M. (2000). Preventing school violence the use of office discipline referrals to assess and monitor school-wide discipline interventions. *Journal of Emotional and Behavioral Disorders, 8*, 9–101. doi:10.1177/106342660000800205.

Sugimoto-Matsuda, J. J., & Braun, K. L. (2014). The role of collaboration in facilitating policy change in youth violence prevention: A review of the literature. *Prevention Science, 15*, 194–204. doi:10.1007/s11121-013-0369-7.

Swearer, S., Espelage, D., Koenig, B., Berry, B., Collins, A., & Lembeck, P. (2012). A social–ecological model for bullying prevention and intervention in early adolescence. In S. R. Jimerson, A. B. Nickerson, M. J. Mayer, & M. J. Furlong (Eds.), *Handbook of school violence and school safety* (2nd edn., pp. 333–355). New York: Routledge.

Task Force on Community Preventive Services. (2007). A recommendation to reduce rates of violence among school-aged children and youth by means of universal school-based violence prevention programs. *American Journal of Preventive Medicine, 33*, S112–S113.

Thapa, A., Cohen, J., Guffey, S., & Higgins-D'Alessandro, A. (2013). A review of school climate research. *Review of Educational Research, 83*, 357–385. doi:10.3102/0034654313483907.

Theriot, M. T. (2009). School resource officers and the criminalization of student behavior. *Journal of Criminal Justice, 37*, 280–287.

Thomas, D. E., & Bierman, K. L. (2006). The impact of classroom aggression on the development of aggressive behavior problems in children. *Development and psychopathology, 18*, 471–487.

Tokunaga, R. S. (2010). Following you home from school: A critical review and synthesis of research on cyberbullying victimization. *Computers in Human Behavior, 26*, 277–287. doi:10.1016/j.chb.2009.11.014.

Ttofi, M., & Farrington, D. (2009). What works in preventing bullying: Effective elements of anti-bullying programmes. *Journal of Aggression, Conflict, and Peace Research, 1*, 13–24.

Ttofi, M. M., & Farrington, D. P. (2011). Effectiveness of school-based programs to reduce bullying: A systematic and meta-analytic review. *Journal of Experimental Criminology, 7*, 27–56. doi:10.1007/s11292-010-9109-1.

Twemlow, S. W., Fonagy, P., Sacco, F. C., O'Toole, M. E., & Vernberg, E. (2002). *Premeditated mass shootings in schools: Threat assessment. American Academy of Child and Adolescent Psychiatry, 41, 475–477. U.S. Department of Education. (2003). Practical information on crisis planning: A guide for schools and communities.* Washington, DC: Author.

US Department of Education's Emergency Response and Crisis Management Technical Assistance Center. (2007). Steps for developing a school emergency management plan. Retrieved online at rems.ed.gov/

U.S. Department of Homeland Security. (2008, December). National incident management system. https://www.fema.gov/pdf/emergency/nims/NIMS_core.pdf. Accessed 25 Sept 2014.

Vagi, K. J., Rothman, E. F., Latzman, N. E., Tharp, A. T., Hall, D. M., & Breiding, M. J. (2013). Beyond correlates: A review of risk and protective factors for adolescent dating violence perpetration. *Journal of youth and adolescence, 42*, 633–649. doi:10.1007/s10964-013-9907-7.

Vaillancourt, R., Hymel, S., & McDougall, P. (2013). The biological underpinnings of peer victimization: Understanding why and how the effects of bullying can last a lifetime. *Theory Into Practice, 52*, 214–248. doi:10.1080/00405841.2013.829726.

Valent, P. (2000). Disaster syndromes. In G. Fink (Ed.), *Encyclopedia of stress* (Vol. 1, pp. 706–709). San Diego: Academic Press.

Verlinden, S., Hersen, M., & Thomas, J. (2000). Risk factors in school shootings. *Clinical Psychology Review, 20*, 3–56.

Vossekuil, B., Fein, R. A., Reddy, M., Borum, R., & Modzeleski, W. (2002). The final report and findings of the Safe School Initiative: Implications for the prevention of school attacks in the United States. DIANE Publishing.

Walker, J. M. (2009). Authoritative classroom management: How control and nurturance work together. *Theory into Practice, 48*, 122–129.

Wang, J., Nansel, T. R., & Iannotti, R. J. (2011). Cyber bullying and traditional bullying: Differential association with depression. *Journal of Adolescent Health, 45*, 368–375. doi:10.1016/j.jadohealth.2009.03.021.

Welsh, B. C., Braga, A. A., & Sullivan, C. J. (2014). Serious youth violence and innovative prevention: On the emerging link between public health and criminology. *Justice Quarterly, 31*, 500–523. doi:10.1080/07418825.2012.690441.

Wienke, D., Anthonijsz, I., Abrahamse, S., Daamen, W., & Nieuwboer, A. (2014). *Beoordeling anti-pestprogramma's: Rapportage van de commissie voor het Ministerie Onderwijs, Cultuur en Wetenschap (OCW)*. Utrecht: Nederlands Jeugdinstituut.

Wilson, D. (2004). The interface of school climate and school connectedness and relationships with aggression and victimization. *Journal of School Health, 74*, 293–299. doi:10.1111/j.1746-1561.2004.tb08286.x.

Wilson, S. J., & Lipsey, M. W. (2007). School-based interventions for aggressive and disruptive behavior: Update of a meta-analysis. *American journal of preventive medicine, 33*, S130–S143. doi:10.1016/j.amepre.2007.04.011.

Wolfe, D. A. (2006). Preventing violence in relationships: Psychological science addressing complex social issues. *Canadian Psychology/Psychologie canadienne, 47*, 44–50. doi:10.1037/h0087043.

Yoon, J., & Bauman, S. (2014). Teachers: A critical but overlooked component of bullying prevention and intervention. *Theory into Practice, 53*(4). 308–314. doi:10.1080/00405841.2014.947226.

Young, M. A. (1998). *The community crisis response team training manual* (2nd edn.). Washington, DC: National Organization for Victim Assistance.

Chapter 16
School-Based Adolescent Suicide Prevention

Teresa D. LaFromboise and Shadab Hussain

16.1 Introduction and Prevalence

Suicidal behavior among school age youth has been a national challenge since the mid-1950s when a dramatic increase in "aggressive and hostile acts directed against the self and the body" was first noted (Berman 2009, p. 237). According to the Centers for Disease Control and Prevention (CDC), suicide is third among the leading causes of death for youth and young adults between 10 and 24 years of age in the USA. Data from the 2013 Youth Risk Behavior Survey (YRBS) reveal that—in the year before the survey was distributed—17% of the high school (9th–12th-grade) students who responded had seriously considered their own suicide. Thirteen percent planned how they would attempt suicide, and 8.0% made a suicide attempt within their lifetime. Female and Hispanic respondents were more likely to be involved in suicidal behavior (i.e., suicidal thoughts, suicide attempts, and death by suicide) than Black and White respondents, respectively.

Furthermore, the younger the respondents, the more likely they were to take part in suicide-related activities, with 9th-grade students most at risk (CDC 2014). Findings of the National Comorbidity Survey Replication Adolescent Supplement (NCS-A), the first national survey of US adolescents to assess Diagnostic and Statistical Manual of Mental Disorders, Fourth Edition (DSM-IV) mental disorders and suicidal behavior using structured diagnostic interviews, indicate that 12.1% of adolescent respondents engaged in suicidal ideation, 4.0% created a suicide plan, and 4.1% actually tried to die by suicide. Furthermore, most NCS-A respondents who went on to design a suicide plan reported that they did so within the first year

T. D. LaFromboise (✉)
Graduate School of Education, Stanford University, 485 Lasuen Mall, Stanford, CA 97305-3096, USA
e-mail: lafrom@stanford.edu

S. Hussain
Graduate School of Education, Stanford University, 5 Comstock Circle Apt 422B, Stanford, CA 94305, USA
e-mail: shadabh1@stanford.edu

© Springer Science+Business Media New York 2015
K. Bosworth (ed.), *Prevention Science in School Settings,*
Advances in Prevention Science, DOI 10.1007/978-1-4939-3155-2_16

of onset of suicidal ideation (Nock et al. 2013). Although the extent of suicide plans and attempts differ considerably in these two self-report studies, both emphasize the US public health hazard of unrelenting adolescent suicidal behavior.

In 1984, school-based suicide prevention programs were implemented in reaction to a significant escalating trend in suicidal behavior among adolescents in many Western industrialized countries (Garland et al. 1989; White and Morris 2010). Since 2000, these programs have been conducted in 77% of US public schools (Brener et al. 2001). The rationale for schools adopting them hinges upon recognition that a significant amount of suicidal behavior occurs among ostensibly, well-functioning students. School suicide prevention programs try to reach the greatest number of students through population-based strategies to identify and assist the smaller number of students who are at risk. The ultimate goal is to help at-risk students receive psychological treatment before they become acutely suicidal.

The purpose of this chapter is to examine an often overlooked issue in school-based prevention: the relevance of culture for suicidal behavior and suicide prevention. We review research on risk factors for adolescent suicide including research studies that included adolescents from nondominant racial and ethnic groups as study participants. We feature evidence-based prevention interventions found to affect desired outcomes for suicide prevention and critique them in terms of the inclusion of cultural considerations in the intervention development and outcome study design. Finally, we recommend strategies for school-based suicide prevention going forward with culture and nondominant racial and ethnic group diversity in mind.

16.2   Risk Factors Associated with Adolescent Suicide

Suicide is a complex phenomenon controlled by cultural as well as social determinants of behavior (Joe et al. 2008). An ecological model (Brofenbrenner 1977) that accentuates the salience of environmental, contextual, and sociohistorical influences on student development provides an effective framework with which to consider both cultural and social determinants of suicidal behavior. This approach positions an adolescent at the center of complex systems: the microsystem, the exosystem, and the macrosystem. The centrality of an adolescent's direct interactions upon and within the environment, as well as reciprocal interactions of the adolescent within ever-widening systems of influence, is the structure of this model. According to the ecological perspective, mental health problems such as suicide display differently and at differential rates depending upon the multitude of contexts in which an adolescent engages (Ayyash-Abdo 2002; Baber and Bean 2009; King and Merchant 2008). The conditions where an adolescent lives, studies, and plays as well as the clean air and water, adequate housing, public safety, health-care services, and societal factors such as institutional racism or bias against immigrants are but a few of the social determinants (Jackson 2015) of suicide that can be accommodated in the outer layer of this model.

16.2.1   Individual Level

Psychological characteristics of the adolescent well-known for suicide risk include depression, hopelessness, anxiety, and substance abuse. In its mild form, depression is probably the most common psychological disturbance among adolescents (Graber and Sontag 2004). Indeed, all individuals experience periods of sadness or depressed mood at some time or another in their lives. However, depression during adolescence may be particularly problematic. Adolescents often report a pattern of depressive symptoms that includes a wider range of symptoms than sadness alone (e.g., anger, anxiety). Estimates of the lifetime prevalence of major depressive disorder (MDD) in adolescence range from 15 to 20 % (Lewinsohn and Essau 2002). Waldrop et al. (2007) report that adolescents who met the criteria for major depressive episodes were four times more likely to report suicidal ideation and six times more likely to report suicide attempts. About 36.8 % of Hispanics, 27.5 % of Black, and 27.3 % of White adolescents stated on the 2013 YRBS that they felt sad or hopeless almost every day for 2 or more weeks at a time (CDC 2014). High rates of depression may occur during adolescence in part because of the increasing prevalence of stressful events and in part because of the cognitive changes during this life stage that require introspection (Avenevoli and Steinberg 2001). According to the NCS-A, disorders that predict the transition from suicidal ideation to a planned suicide attempt are MDD/dysthymia, eating disorders, attention-deficit/hyperactivity disorder, conduct disorder, and intermittent explosive disorder (Nock et al. 2013). Depression is a critical risk factor in school-based suicide prevention since depression proliferates, and the likelihood of suicidal behavior increases during adolescence.

Adolescents who are distressed are often susceptible to negative and/or rigid thoughts. Hopelessness, a cognitive vulnerability that often accompanies depression, has been defined as a lowered expectation of obtaining certain goals or achieving success (Beck 1986). Empirical research links adolescent hopelessness to depression, psychopathology, high-risk practices, violent behavior, and suicide (Gillham and Reivich 2004). Goldston et al. (2008) contend that, among adolescents who attempt suicide, higher levels of hopelessness increase the risk for repeated suicide attempts. Thompson et al. (2005) found direct effects of depression and hopelessness on suicidal behavior for males and direct effects of hopelessness, but not depression, for females. Importantly, Chioqueta and Stiles (2007) reveal that factors, such as self-esteem and life satisfaction, protect against the detrimental effects of hopelessness on suicidal ideation.

Anxiety is a risk factor linked to depression, hopelessness, and suicide. Those diagnosed as anxious and subthreshold anxious (did not meet the criteria for being anxious but had significant functional impairment) were found to be almost twice as likely to have suicidal ideation when compared with their non-anxious peers (Balazs et al. 2013). In a study by Thompson et al. (2005), anxiety was directly associated with depression and hopelessness for both males and females. Cougle et al. (2009) established that adolescent anxiety, along with depression and substance abuse, significantly contributes to increased suicide attempts and completions. The relationship between anxiety and suicidal ideation may be linked to the importance of belongingness and peer approval during adolescence. Social anxiety is associated with a thwarted sense of belongingness, which can lead to suicidal ideation (Davidson et al. 2011). However, symptoms of anxiety can be triggered by many other issues adolescents face such as complications associated with academic competition, peer pressure, and other forms of interpersonal conflict.

Substance abuse is a robust risk factor for suicide. A drug or alcohol-induced predisposition to impulsivity and emotional volatility can enhance a youth's predisposition to suicidal behavior by 25 % (Gould et al. 1998). There is increasing indication that the problems of substance use, violent aggression, and depressive symptoms co-occur in a substantial proportion of youth who attempt or who die by suicide (Pena et al. 2012). Among adolescents with low levels of depressed mood, alcohol use has been found to accelerate the transition from suicidal ideation to suicide attempt (McManama O'Brien et al. 2013). A national study of 8th, 10th, and 12th graders verified that boys engage in marijuana and stimulant use more frequently than girls and that alcohol and cigarette use rates of girls and boys at each grade level were identical (Wallace et al. 2003). The strength of the relationship between drug use and suicide among high school students in the USA dramatically increases with particular illicit drugs. A strong association between suicide and heroin use, methamphetamines, and steroids, and a moderate association between suicide and cocaine, ecstasy, hallucinogens, and inhalant use were found by Wong et al. (2013).

According to the NCS-A, the great majority of adolescents who engage in suicidal behaviors also experience mental illness. However, mental disorders that most powerfully predict suicidal thoughts are different from those that most powerfully predict the transition from suicidal ideation to suicide plans or that predict the transition from suicide plans to suicide attempts (Nock et al. 2013). Differentiating among those disorders usually occurs at the point of screening and referral for further psychological treatment. Other leading risk factors for adolescent suicide include previous suicide attempts and family history of suicide (CDC 2014).

16.2.2 Microsystem Level

King and Merchant (2008) reviewed psychological autopsy studies, community-based prospective studies, and clinical studies conducted within the last two decades to better understand microsystem-level influences on adolescent suicide risk. They summarized a number of studies across diverse samples that point to the influential role of family support on severe suicidal behavior. When controlling for the presence of a mood, anxiety, or disruptive disorder, there was still an association between suicidal ideation/attempts and family variables such as poor family environment and limited parental monitoring. O'Donnell et al. (2003) established an association between family support and suicide in a study of adolescents from economically disadvantaged communities of primarily African American and Latino/a heritage living in Brooklyn, New York. Early childhood neglect or abuse has been found to predict suicidal thoughts and behaviors into early adulthood (Johnson et al. 2002). Family economic pressure and parental depression symptoms were reported by Yoder and Hoyt (2005) to be indirectly related to adolescent suicidal ideation. Family structure also impacts suicidality. Gould et al. (1998) reported that adolescent suicide completers were significantly more likely to come from a non-intact family of origin. Rubenstein et al. (1998) bolstered the claim that students in intact families were least likely to be suicidal. They found that youth in separated/divorced families were at intermediate risk, and those living in remarried families were at the highest risk.

Adolescents typically spend more time with their peers than with their families. Those with supportive friends face fewer psychological problems and experience higher perceived social acceptance (Lagana 2004). Those who are negotiating romantic relationships may be especially vulnerable when a relationship ends, especially if they do not have support elsewhere in their lives. As previously stated, a thwarted sense of belongingness can contribute to social anxiety and thus may be related to suicidal ideation (Davidson et al. 2011). In a study of friendships and suicide among 13,465 male and female adolescents from the National Longitudinal Survey of Adolescent Health (Add Health Study), Bearman and Moody (2004) found that female adolescents' suicidal thoughts are significantly increased by social isolation and friendship patterns in which friends were not friends with each other, that is, their companionship circle traversed multiple, disconnected individuals. Winterrowd et al. (2010) indicate that Mexican American adolescent girls and boys who indicated high suicidal behavior also felt detached from their friends. For girls in good academic standing, this disconnection increased suicidality by 13%.

Peer support can be both a risk factor and a protective factor for suicide. There is some research which finds support for linking deviant friends (e.g., high delinquency, disconnected from school) with suicidality (South et al. 2005). Winterrowd and Canetto (2013) found group differences in the association between peer support and suicidal behavior among Mexican American and European American adolescents. More specifically, European American adolescents who had friends who were disconnected from school at the age of 17 had increased suicidality 3 years later; however, Mexican American adolescents with disconnected friends were less likely to exhibit suicidal behavior 3 years later. Matlin et al. (2011) established the direct and moderating effect of peer support on suicidality for African American adolescents. Participants who reported having low depression had decreased suicidality as their peer support increased. Overall, these studies emphasize the differential role peer support can play between gender and ethnic groups.

Feelings of belongingness can also be undermined by peer rejection and peer violence. Children who are bullied are more than twice as likely to engage in suicidal behaviors as their peers who are not bullied (van Geel et al. 2014). Moderate and frequent peer victimization (e.g., belittling race/religion, physical hits, and spreading false rumors about the victim) is reported by 10–20% of high school students in Nassau, Suffolk, and Westchester counties in New York (Brunstein Klomek et al. (2008). When Russell and Joyner (2001) analyzed cross-sectional data from the

Add Health Study, they found that, after controlling for the effects of sexual orientation, hopelessness, depression, alcohol abuse, family and friend suicidality, adolescents who reported being bullied were more likely to engage in suicidal thoughts and suicide attempts. This study strongly suggests that, regardless of gender, the experiences of victimization and the act of bullying another person place both the perpetrator and the victim at risk for suicide. Furthermore, they indicate that increased peer victimization is related to increased depression and suicidality for both genders. However, females who were belittled about their appearance and speech were more likely to be at risk for depression than males, highlighting another gender difference among adolescents. A group that is particularly at increased risk for suicide are lesbian, gay, bisexual, transgender, and queer (LGBTQ) students due to verbal and physical victimization based upon their sexual orientation (D'Augelli et al. 2002; Ybarra et al. 2014).

Educators at school sites who take the health of their students seriously are aware of the interplay between suicide risk and protective factors. To date, research findings on the relation between school performance and suicide are mixed (Hooven et al. 2012). Lower levels of academic achievement may co-occur with depression or anxiety associated with failure, which increases the risk of suicidal behavior. Being held back one grade in school is a risk factor for suicide attempts (Borowsky et al. 2001). Other signs of failure such as significant decline in academic performance or thwarted achievement goals (e.g., not being accepted into one's first choice university) may erode self-confidence and lead to suicidal behavior (Borowsky et al. 2013; Lyon et al. 2000; Watt and Sharp 2001).

16.2.3   Exosystem Level

The way media portrays suicide provides an example of a pervasive influence at the exosystem level. Previous research on the impact media has on adolescent suicidality reveals that fictional stories and the reporting of suicides of both celebrities and noncelebrities have had an increasing effect on suicide rates (Stack 2003). These accounts may strongly impact adolescents with high psychopathology, and they may encourage "copycat suicides" in which a victim commits suicide in a similar method as that reported in news articles or books. The media tends to sensationalize suicide with dramatic headlines (e.g., "JD commits suicide by hanging at the young age of 24") or describe the lethal method in detail (e.g., "JD hung himself with a belt in his bedroom"). Research by Jamieson et al. (2003) emphasize the importance of responsible reporting of suicide to reduce the risk of suicidality in vulnerable individuals. Some of these practices include brevity in headlines (e.g., "JD died at 24"), emphasis on suicide as a public health issue, and inclusion of information about suicide prevention strategies through listing warning signs and/or numbers for suicide prevention hotlines (Jamieson et al. 2003; Pirkis et al. 2006). In the past decade, social media has emerged as a dominant mode of communication by adolescents through websites like Facebook, Instagram, Tumblr, message boards, and gaming sites. It is relatively simple to search for suicide methods on Google and to find websites in which members who are pro-suicide encourage that behavior (Luxton et al. 2012). Cyberbullying—spreading false or hostile information about a victim—is a common occurrence on social media sites and has been linked to depression, isolation, and suicidality (O'Keeffe and Clarke-Pearson 2011).

16.2.4   Macrosystem Level

Ethnic/racial and gender differences operating at the macrosystem level are too often ignored in school-based suicide prevention. However, burgeoning diversity within US schools can no longer be overlooked. The population of first-generation immigrants from Latin America, which was less than 1% in 1980, increased from 19.0% in 1970 to 43.7% in 1990 and further expanded to 53.3% in 2003 (Portes and Rumbaut 2006). Today within public schools, students encounter diversity in languages, beliefs, and practices. Non-Hispanic White students are the new minority, and students from ethnically diverse backgrounds, often referred to as "students of color," are the new mainstream in the states/districts of Hawaii, Washington, DC, California, New Mexico, and Texas (Hussar and Bailey 2013). Thus, increasingly students need access to culturally responsive prevention interventions.

The range of beliefs about a group's existence and what makes for a meaningful life within that group inform an adolescent's understanding of the virtues and vices of suicide. Nondominant racial and ethnic groups differ in rates of suicide and reasons for engaging in suicidal behavior. In 2000, the rates of death by suicide were 4.7 times higher for boys than for girls ages 15–19 (National Center for Injury Prevention and Control 2005). There was a 3:1 estimated adolescent suicide attempt ratio among girls to boys between 2005 and 2009 (CDC 2014). The reasons for this high male to female suicide ratio include the fact that males engage in higher rates of suicide risk factors and also are less likely to engage in protective practices such as seeking help and building social support systems. Males also use more lethal means (e.g., firearms or suffocation) than girls who tend to poison themselves with prescription drugs.

According to Goldston et al. (2008), the rate of death by suicide among adolescents differs by a factor of 20 between the highest risk ethnic group (American Indian/Alaska Native (AI/AN) males) and the lowest risk ethnic group (African American females). The group with the highest rate of suicide attempts is AI/AN females, followed by Latinas, AI/AN males, and Asian American/Pacific Islander (AA/PI) females. The groups with the lowest rate of suicide attempts are White and African American males. However, the rate of increase in suicide is increasing faster for African Americans than the rate for age-matched Whites (McKenzie 2012). AA/PI are one of the most rapidly growing ethnic groups in the USA. AA/PI adolescents have among the lowest rates of suicide in the USA; however, this group is extremely heterogeneous with significant intergroup differences in suicidal behavior. For example, suicide is the leading cause of death for South Asian youth 15–24 years of age (Hoyert and Kung 1997).

The high rate of suicide among AI/AN adolescent males is often attributed to perceived discrimination and acculturation stress (Yoder et al. 2006). Furthermore, suicide clustering in reservations/villages already affected by historical trauma leads to repeated trauma and fractured communities (Goldston et al. 2008). Latina adolescents are known to struggle with conflict between the developmental desire for autonomy and the cultural value of *familismo,* a belief in the utmost importance of family unity including getting along with and providing for the well-being of one's family and extended family. This belief supports traditional Latina gender roles. Conflicting cultural expectations such as this one exacerbate parent–adolescent conflict, lower self-esteem, and internalizing behaviors and suicide attempts (Kuhlberg et al. 2010; Zayas et al. 2005). Recently, Castle et al. (2011) found an association between acculturation and suicidal ideation among African American youth 18–24 years of age, leading to speculation about the cost of affiliation with other American youth who may adhere to a greater acceptance of suicide. These selected examples of behavior patterns impelled by culture change shed light upon the differential dynamics of suicidal behavior within and between nondominant racial/ethnic groups.

16.3   School-Based Suicide Prevention Interventions

The review of research on risk factors above suggests that school-based interventions for adolescents would be most effective if they reflect the culture of the population(s) served. Service providers (e.g., teachers, counselors, nurses) should represent the diverse backgrounds of students in order that they relate more readily to the intervention and act to support the intervention goals. Furthermore, it is important that all nondominant racial/ethnic groups be included in the planning and delivery of prevention interventions. An excellent application of this principle applied to substance abuse prevention with Mexican/Mexican American, African American, and European American adolescents is available (Kulis et al. 2005).

Systematic reviews of research on school-based suicide prevention interventions reveal a growing number of potentially effective programs (Balaguru et al. 2013; Katz et al. 2013; Robinson et al. 2013). Presently, five main types of suicide prevention interventions in schools have been identified: (a) awareness/education curricula, (b) peer leadership training, (c) skills training, (d) gatekeeper training, and (e) screening. *Awareness/education curricula* focus on increasing accurate knowledge about suicide and encourage self-disclosure among peers to develop positive attitudes toward seeking help. *Peer leadership training* assists student leaders in learning to respond to suicidal peers and then to refer them to a "trusted adult" for further referral to treatment. *Skills training* fosters the growth of skills to support protective factors in the prevention of suicide (e.g., problem solving, self-regulation). Emphasis is also placed on the reduction of risk factors to prevent the development of suicidal behavior (e.g., depression management, anger regulation). *Gatekeeper training* teaches school staff, students, and their parents about symptoms of suicide and additionally provides information regarding risk and protective factors to improve identification and referral of at-risk students to available resources. Lastly, *screening* programs assess suicidal ideation, depression symptoms, and other clinical mental health disorders (including multiple problems such as depression along with disturbed eating or binge drinking) and refer students displaying disorders to psychological services.

We selected evidence-based interventions to review in this section based upon two criteria: whether they were found to yield outcomes associated with the prevention of adolescent suicide and whether they recruited study samples that included nondominant racial and ethnic group participants in their effectiveness studies. Within each brief description of the following interventions, the standard class of prevention—universal, selected, or indicated—is designated (Goldsmith et al. 2002). *Universal* prevention focuses on an entire school population regardless of status; in this case, all students in a school would receive suicide prevention. Universal programs often aim to increase knowledge about suicide and suicide prevention and to improve attitudes concerning help seeking. Additionally, these programs teach students responsive strategies to help troubled peers. *Selected* prevention targets at-risk students who are in danger of becoming suicidal and attempts to reduce risk factors while increasing protective factors. *Indicated* prevention targets students who show early signs of suicidal behavior and refers them to psychological services. Ideally, delivery of services for suicidal adolescents would occur in school settings such as school-based health clinics.

Sources of Strength (SOS)   SOS is a universal program that emphasizes awareness/education and peer leadership to reduce suicidal behaviors (LoMurray 2005). This intervention was originally designed for youth living in rural areas to tackle issues related to youth suicide, such as violence and substance use. SOS was then modified for widespread use with students across the USA. Its curriculum includes suicide awareness, positive messaging, empowering activities, and screening strategies. Peer leaders are trained in responding to students who display risk factors for suicide, directing them to a trusted adult for further support. At a 3-month follow-up, participants in the program reported reduced suicide attempts and increased knowledge about suicide. Additionally, trained peer leaders reported increased adaptability in attitudes toward suicide and other types of mental illness, and enhanced ability when referring a suicidal friend to an adult (Aseltine and DeMartino 2004; Aseltine et al. 2007).

SOS strongly emphasizes suicide as an action and behavior rather than the result of mental illness. It also fosters positive youth development and personal growth. While SOS evaluations reveal decreases in students' suicidal behavior, there were no effects on suicidal ideation. SOS does not appear to explicitly address culture-specific issues that may influence risk behavior, yet positive effects of SOS were observed among participants from diverse racial and ethnic backgrounds. Finally, an evaluation of the program conducted by Aseltine and DeMartino (2004) revealed that the help-seeking behaviors of youth in urban communities were generally low following this intervention.

American Indian Life Skills Development (AILS) AILS is a universal, culturally supported suicide prevention intervention emphasizing social cognitive skills training to reduce high rates of AI/AN adolescent suicidal behaviors (LaFromboise 1996). The intervention focuses on seven main themes: (1) building self-esteem, (2) identifying emotions and stress, (3) increasing communication and problem-solving skills, (4) recognizing self-destructive behavior and finding ways to eliminate it, (5) learning information about suicide, (6) helping a suicidal friend go for help, and (7) planning ahead for a great future. AILS accommodate between 13 and 56 lessons depending upon implementation opportunities. Students are taught an array of psychosocial skills necessary for effectively dealing with the challenges of everyday life (e.g., emotional identification, problem solving, and anger regulation) with the aim to decrease depression, hopelessness, anger, and anxiety. Ideally, AILS would be offered as a required course in a tribal or Bureau of Indian Education school serving AI/AN reservation students. AILS also has been adapted for AI/AN adolescents in urban and suburban settings.

Immediately following AILS, participants reported less hopelessness, less suicidal ideation and attempts, greater self-efficacy to manage anger, and they demonstrated greater effectiveness in helping a friend solve problems and go for help than those in the no-treatment comparison group (LaFromboise and Howard-Pitney 1995). While evaluations of AILS reveal reduced suicidal ideation in students, the curriculum is lengthy, and proper AILS implementation requires a large time commitment (LaFromboise and Lewis 2008). A 30-, 35-min version of AILS, entitled AILS-M, has been created to include relevant developmental issues of concern to early adolescents.

Reconnecting Youth (RY) RY is a selected intervention utilizing a skills training approach which targets high school students 14–19 years of age who demonstrate poor academic achievement, are at risk for dropping out of school, and exhibit maladaptive symptoms such as aggressive behavior (Eggert and Nicholas 2004). RY emphasizes the prevention of substance use and emotional distress while fostering resilience. Additionally, opportunity for social bonding is achieved through intervention activities which form connections within the school and encourage parent involvement. RY participants have reported reduced depression, hopelessness and suicidal behaviors, and increased self-esteem and social support (Eggert et al. 1995; Eggert et al. 2002). RY has been associated with participants' increased school attendance (Castro-Villareal 2013) and also was found to reduce hopelessness and suicidal ideation among AI/AN early adolescents immediately following the intervention and at 1-year follow-up (LaFromboise and Malik 2012).

Coping and Support Training (CAST) CAST is a selected prevention program adapted from RY that uses a skills training approach with high school students 14–19 years of age following their referral to the program based upon initial screening. CAST consists of 12 sessions given over 6 weeks administered by service providers (e.g., teachers, nurses). The goal of CAST is to decrease suicidal behavior and increase social and emotional development by focusing on mood management and school performance and by decreasing involvement with illicit substances. Participants of CAST have demonstrated increased problem-solving skills, perceived family support and self-control, and decreased symptoms of depression and hopelessness (Thompson et al. 2001).

RY and CAST may lead to iatrogenic effects since already at-risk students may form stronger connections with deviant classmates during the intervention (Katz et al. 2013). Furthermore, while there is improvement for students who are at risk of dropping out and who display aggression, students living in rural and underserved communities may not have access to the mental health services that screening implies. Neither RY nor CAST explicitly attends to cultural factors that may influence risk behavior.

Good Behavior Game (GBG) GBG is a behavior management approach that has evolved into a universal, primary prevention program for elementary school students to teach self-regulation skills (Barrish et al. 1969). The GBG socializes children into displaying cooperative rather than disruptive or aggressive behavior, both of which are risk factors for substance abuse and suicide. To play the GBG, a teacher splits the classroom into two or more teams which are rewarded for being adaptive to academic social expectations (e.g., being on task for brief periods of time, not talking out of turn). Eventually, they are expected to be cooperative for longer periods of time. The winner of the GBG is the team with the least amount of infractions. GBG has demonstrated long-term effects (following elementary school-age participants on into adolescence) on decreased impulsive/disruptive behavior, substance use, drug addictions, and lower rates of suicidal ideation and suicide attempts (Kellam et al. 2008). GBG was found to be particularly effective with male students; however, a strong effect was not found for reducing maladaptive behaviors in female students. There may be other factors which explain why girls develop aggressive behavior and use drugs later in adolescence (Kellam et al. 2008). By incorporating the program into the classroom at an early age, there is a high cost to effectiveness ratio.

GBG has been implemented in a number of culturally distinct sites in the USA with Latina/o, AI/AN, and African American children (Storr et al. 2002). It has also been put into practice in inner-city and suburban sites in Manitoba, Canada, with recent immigrants from war-torn North Africa (Saigh and Umar 1983), First Nations and Metis children, and children attending Huttrite Colony Schools (Embry, personal communication, February 29, 2012). Despite its widespread implementation, some groups may not respond readily to the GBG because a "bad behavior" in a classroom context contradicts behavior encouraged in a family or community context. For example, sharing answers among peers could be construed as talking out of turn. Discrepant contingencies emanating from cultural beliefs about proper behavior may be confusing to young students. Additionally, the GBG creates a competitive classroom atmosphere, which could be maladaptive for students from cultures that promote collectivism over individualism.

Gatekeeper Training The Question, Persuade, Refer (QPR) intervention is a universal program designed to teach gatekeepers strategies to recognize warning signs of suicide and to respond effectively to a suicidal individual (Quinnett 1995). Participants learn to respond to a suicidal person through questioning the individual's suicidal intent, persuading the individual to seek help, and referring the individual to an appropriate resource. In schools, gatekeepers are usually school staff and students. When implementing this program, it is important for schools to organize professional assessment and treatment for suicidal students. Gatekeepers participating in QPR report increased knowledge and a more positive attitude toward suicide prevention. They also gain useful skills when responding to a suicidal individual (Tompkins et al. 2010; Wyman et al. 2008).

While gatekeepers have reported increased knowledge in communicating with students about suicide, student queries related to suicidality increased only for those gatekeepers—in this case, staff members—who already had previous experience talking to students about suicide. Additionally, staff members' communication style with students did not change, suggesting a reason for students' reluctance to speak with adults about suicide. The sample for this outcome study consisted of White, non-Hispanic staff members, so whether the training is relevant and effective across nondominant racial and ethnic groups (Wyman et al. 2008) or whether gatekeeper skills are retained overtime (Cross et al. 2011) is an area for further study. Lipson's 2014 review of 21 gatekeeper training studies conducted in schools around the world suggests that positive training effects tend to diminish over time.

Each evidence-based, school suicide prevention intervention featured above aims to train peers and school staff to become more responsive to suicidal individuals. Each also goes far beyond suicide prevention: They encourage relationship development and introduce socially responsible alternatives to risk behaviors. GBG has been touted as a "behavioral vaccine" because of its usefulness in targeting problem behaviors early in elementary school to prevent later maladaptive behavior such as adolescent aggression and suicidal behavior (Embry 2002). SOS, AILS, RY, and CAST help students develop essential social and emotional skills and practice safe and healthy behaviors. AILS is an example of a culturally supported intervention that highlights the integral role culture plays in AI/AN suicide and suicide prevention.

Research on school-based suicide prevention is at a preliminary stage of development with respect to cultural competence. Few developers of the interventions reviewed above recommend that service providers represent the racial and ethnic backgrounds of their students. Perhaps this is because most potential service providers who work in schools within the USA come from predominately European American backgrounds, thus prohibiting requirements for cultural matching.

All of the intervention evaluations noted above included nondominant racial or ethnic group participants in their samples. However, few actually incorporated cultural factors into the research designs assessing the effectiveness of the intervention or into the evaluations of service delivery procedures employed in the intervention. None of the evaluation studies cited in this section paid attention to the conceptual, linguistic, or psychometric equivalence of the psychological measures to determine outcome (see Helms 2015).

LaFromboise and Howard-Pitney (1994; 1995) described cultural attributes of the service providers (e.g., language spoken during intervention delivery, heritage of the interventionists) in their 1995 intervention study. They also accommodated cultural considerations in the design of AILS (e.g., emphasized realistic situational contexts in which behaviors occur; encouraged culturally appropriate ways that students can express grief and anger) and its evaluation (e.g., included tribal members in the intervention service provider team; provided confederate clients from tribes other than the tribe of the study participants in role plays in the behavioral portion of the study due to a cultural taboo against tribal members enacting the role of a suicidal person).

Although the interventions detailed above have been described to be effective in suicide prevention programs with diverse students, none of the studies which support their effectiveness considered the differential impact of the intervention on multiple ethnic groups simultaneously or analyzed within ethnic group differences depending upon, for example, varying levels of student reactions to acculturation stress or language barriers.

16.4   Conclusion

The unexpected and dramatic increase in psychopathology among our youth and specifically within the educational system has resulted in an immediate challenge. However, that challenge has lagged significantly behind in terms of both chronological time and impact. School-based suicide prevention programs have only been in existence since 1984, and the statistics indicate that much more needs to be done to eradicate this modern day phenomena within our educational system.

One initial and critical step is to deconstruct the situation at multiple levels, including individual, microsystem, exosystem, and macrosystem levels. Historically, suicide prevention has focused on the treatment of the individual, and this type of intervention should continue but not at the cost of ignoring the gestalt of the disorder. Specific efforts have evolved for the last decades or two on economically viable, rapidly deployed, and clinically efficacious efforts to target not only the individual but the larger system —from social media to society and everything in between. Considering the relatively new introduction to this complicated problem, issues with customized delivery that target specific variables (e.g., ethnicity) still need significant innovation and evaluation.

Clearly, however, the problem of adolescent suicide has now been identified, and its manifestations at different levels have become understood. The focus remains on understanding how to customize and deliver specific programs to specific disorder processes and community situations. Much has to be done, but the issues have been addressed and intervention programs have started. The next generation of school/community-based suicide prevention interventions will undoubtedly occur soon and with greater impact.

References

Aseltine, R. H. Jr., & DeMartino, R. (2004). An outcome evaluation of the SOS suicide prevention program. *American Journal of Public Health, 94,* 446–451. doi:10.2105/AJPH.94.3.446.

Aseltine, R. H. Jr., James, A., Schilling, E. A., & Glanovsky, J. (2007). Evaluating the SOS suicide prevention program: A replication and extension. *BMC Public Health, 7,* 161. doi:10.1186/1471-2458-7-161.

Avenevoli, S., & Steinberg, L. (2001). *The continuity of depression across the adolescent transition. Advances in child development and behavior* (pp. 139–173). San Diego: Academic. doi:10.1016/S0065-2407(02)80064-7.

Ayyash-Abdo, H. (2002). Adolescent suicide: An ecological approach. *Psychology in the Schools, 39,* 459–475. doi:10.1002/pits.10042.

Baber, K., & Bean, G. (2009). Frameworks: A community-based approach to preventing youth suicide. *Journal of Community Psychology, 37,* 684–696.

Balaguru, V., Sharma, J., & Waheed, W. (2013). Understanding the effectiveness of school-based interventions to prevent suicide: A realist review. *Child and Adolescent Mental Health, 18*(3), 131–139. doi:10.1111/j.1475-3588.2012.00668.x.

Balazs, J., Miklósi, M., Kereszteny, A., Hoven, C. W., Carli, V., Wasserman, C., & Wasserman, D. (2013). Adolescent subthreshold-depression and anxiety: Psychopathology, functional impairment and increased suicide risk. *Journal of Child Psychology and Psychiatry, 54,* 670–677. doi:10.1111/jcpp.12016.

Barrish, H. H., Saunders, M., & Wolf, M. M. (1969). Good behavior game: Effects of individual contingencies for group consequences on disruptive behavior in a classroom. *Journal of Applied Behavior Analysis, 2,* 119–124. http://www.search.proquest.com/docview/615628148?accountid=14026.

Bearman, P. S., & Moody, J. (2004). Suicide and friendships among American adolescents. *American Journal of Public Health, 94*(1), 89–95. doi:10.2105/AJPH.94.1.89.

Beck, A. T. (1986). Hopelessness as a predictor of eventual suicide. *Annals of the New York Academy of Sciences, 487,* 90–96. doi:10.1111/j.1749-6632.1986.tb27888.x.

Berman, A. L. (2009). School-based suicide prevention: Research advances and practice implications. *School Psychology Review, 38,* 233–238. http://wearch.proquest.com/docview/622040142?accountid=14026.

Borowsky, I. W., Ireland, M., & Resnick, M. D. (2001). Adolescent suicide attempts: Risks and practices. *Pediatrics, 107,* 485–493.

Borowsky, I. W., Taliaferro, L. A., & McMorris, B. J. (2013). Suicidal thinking and behavior among youth involved in verbal and social bullying: Risk and protective factors. *Journal of Adolescent Health, 53,* S4–S12. doi:10.1016/j.jadohealth.2012.10.280.

Brener, N. D., Martindale, J., & Weist, M. D. (2001). Mental health and social services: Results from the school health policies and programs study 2000. *Journal of School Health, 71,* 305–312. doi:10.1111/j.1746-1561.2001.tb03507.x.

Brofenbrenner, U. (1977). Toward an experimental ecology of human development. *American Psychologist, 32,* 513–531. doi:10.1037/0003-066X.32.7.513.

Brunstein Klomek, A., Marrocco, F., Kleinman, M., Schonfeld, I. S., & Gould, M. (2008). Peer victimization, depression, and suicidiality in adolescents. *Suicide and Life-Threatening Behavior, 38,* 166–180. doi:10.1521/suli.2008.38.2.166.

Castle, K., Conner, K., Kaukeinen, K., & Tu, X. (2011). Perceived racism, discrimination, and acculturation in suicidal ideation and suicide attempts among Black young adults. *Suicide and Life-Threatening Behavior, 41,* 342–351. doi:10.1111/j.1943-278X.2011.00033.x.

Castro-Villareal, F. (2013). The effects of a school-based intervention program on academic outcomes. (Order No. AAI3498662, Dissertation Abstracts International Section A: Humanities and Social Sciences).

Centers for Disease Control and Prevention. (2014). *Youth risk behavior surveillance—United States, 2013.* Atlanta: U.S. Department of Health and Human Services. http://www.cdc.gov/mmwr/pdf/ss/ss6304.pdf.

Chioqueta, A. P., & Stiles, T. C. (2007). The relationship between psychological buffers, hopelessness, and suicidal ideation: Identification of protective factors. *Crisis: The Journal of Crisis Intervention and Suicide Prevention, 28*, 67. doi:10.1027/0227-5910.28.2.67.

Cougle, J. R., Keough, M. E., Riccardi, C. J., & Sachs-Ericsson, N. (2009). Anxiety disorders and suicidality in the National Comorbidity Survey-Replication. *Journal of Psychiatric Research, 43*, 825–829. doi:10.1016/j.jpsychires.2008.12.004.

Cross, W. F., Seaburn, D., Gibbs, D., Schmeelk-Cone, K., White, A. M., & Cane, E. D. (2011). Does practice make perfect? A randomized control trial of behavioral rehearsal on suicide prevention gatekeeper skills. *The Journal of Primary Prevention, 32*, 195–211.

D'Augelli, A. R., Pilkington, N. W., & Hershberger, S. L. (2002). Incidence and mental health impact of sexual orientation victimization of lesbian, gay, and bisexual youths in high school. *School Psychology Quarterly, 17*, 148–167. doi:10.1521/scpq.17.2.148.20854.

Davidson, C. L., Wingate, L. R., Grant, D. M., Judah, M. R., & Mills, A. C. (2011). Interpersonal suicide risk and ideation: The influence of depression and social anxiety. *Journal of Social and Clinical Psychology, 30*, 842–855. doi:10.1521/jscp.2011.30.8.842.

Eggert, L. L., & Nicholas, L. J. (2004). *Reconnecting youth*. Bloomington: National Educational Service.

Eggert, L. L., Thompson, E. A., Herting, J. R., & Nicholas, L. J. (1995). Reducing suicide potential among high-risk youth: Tests of a school-based prevention program. *Suicide and Life-Threatening Behavior, 25*, 276–296. doi:10.1111/j.1943-278X.1995.tb00926.x.

Eggert, L. L., Thompson, E. A., Randell, B. P., & Pike, K. C. (2002). Preliminary effects of brief school-based prevention approaches for reducing youth suicide—risk behaviors, depression, and drug involvement. *Journal of Child and Adolescent Psychiatric Nursing, 15*, 48–64. doi:10.1111/j.1744-6171.2002.tb00326.x.

Embry, D. D. (2002). The good behavior game: A best practice candidate as a universal behavioral vaccine. *Clinical Child and Family Psychology Review, 5*, 273–297. doi:10.1023/A:1020977107086.

Garland, A., Shaffer, D., & Whittle, B. (1989). A national survey of school-based, adolescent suicide prevention programs. *Journal of the American Academy of Child and Adolescent Psychiatry, 28*, 931–934.

Gillham, J., & Reivich, K. (2004). Cultivating optimism in childhood and adolescence. *The Annals of the American Academy of Political and Social Science, 591*, 146–163. doi:10.1177/0002716203260095.

Goldsmith, S. K., Pellmar, T. C., Kleinman, A. M., & Bunney, W. E. (Eds.). (2002). *Reducing suicide: A national imperative*. Washington DC: National Academies Press.

Goldston, D. B., Molock, S. D., Whitbeck, L. B., Murakami, J. L., Zayas, L. H., & Hall, G. C. N. (2008). Cultural considerations in adolescent suicide prevention in psychosocial treatment. *American Psychologist, 63*, 14–31. doi:10.1037/0003-066X.63.1.14.

Gould, M. S., King, R., Greenwald, S., Fisher, P., Schwab-Stone, M., Kramer, R., & Shaffer, D. (1998). Psychopathology associated with suicidal ideation and attempts among children and adolescents. *Journal of the American Academy of Child and Adolescent Psychiatry, 37*, 915–923. doi:10.1097/00004583-199809000-00011.

Graber, J. A., & Sontag, L. M. (2004). *Internalizing problems during adolescence. Handbook of adolescent psychology* (pp. 642–682). Hoboken: Wiley.

Helms, J. E. (2015). An examination of the evidence in culturally adapted evidence-based or empirically supported interventions. *Transcultural Psychiatry, 52*, 174–197.

Hooven, C., Walsh, E., Pike, K. C., & Herting, J. R. (2012). Promoting CARE: Including parents in youth suicide prevention. *Family & Community Health, 35*, 225–234. doi:10.1097/FCH.0b013e318250bcf9.

Hoyert, D., & Kung, H. (1997). Asian or Pacific Islander mortality, selected states. *Monthly Vital Statistics Report, 46*, 1–63. http://www.cdc.gov/nchs/data/mvsr/supp/mv4601s.pdf.

Hussar, W. J., & Bailey, T. M. (2013). *Projections of education statistics to 2022 (NCES2014-051). U. S. Department of Education, National Center for Education Statistics.* Washington, DC: U. S. Government Printing Office.

Jackson, V. H. (2015). Practitioner characteristics and organizational contexts as essential elements in the evidence-based practice versus cultural competence debate. *Transcultural Psychiatry, 52*, 150–173.

Jamieson, P., Jamieson, K. H., & Romer, D. (2003). The responsible reporting of suicide in print journalism. *American Behavioral Scientist, 46*, 1643–1660. doi:10.1177/0002764203254620.

Joe, S., Canetto, S. S., & Romer, D. (2008). Advancing prevention research on the role of culture in suicide prevention. *Suicide and Life-Threatening Behavior, 38*, 354–362.

Johnson, J. G., Cohen, P., Gould, M. S., Kasen, S., Brown, J., & Brook, J. S. (2002). Childhood adversities, interpersonal difficulties, and risk for suicide attempts during late adolescence and early adulthood. *Archives of General Psychiatry, 59*, 741–749. doi:10.1001/archpsyc.59.8.741.

Katz, C., Bolton, S.-L., Katz, L. Y., Isaak, C., Tilston-Jones, T., & Sareen, J. (2013). A systematic review of school-based suicide prevention programs. *Depression and Anxiety, 30*, 1030–1045. doi:10.1002/da.22114.

Kellam, S. G., Brown, H. C., Poduska, J. M., Ialongo, N. S., Wang, W., Toyinbo, P., & Wilcox, H. C. (2008). Effects of a universal classroom behavior management program in first and second grades on young adult behavioral, psychiatric, and social outcomes. *Drug and Alcohol Dependence, 95*, S5–S28. doi:10.1016/j.drugalcdep.2008.01.004.

King, C. A., & Merchant, C. R. (2008). Social and interpersonal factors relating to adolescent suicidality: A review of the literature. *Suicide and Life-Threatening Behavior, 12*, 181–196. doi:10.1080/13811110802101203.

Kuhlberg, J. A., Pena, J. B., & Zayas, L. H. (2010). Familism, parent-adolescent conflict, self-esteem, internalizing behaviors and suicide attempts among adolescent Latinas. *Child Psychiatry and Human Development, 41*, 425–440. doi:10.1007/s10578-010-0179-0.

Kulis, S., Marsiglia, F. F., Elek, E., Dustman, P., Wagstaff, D. A., & Hecht, M. L. (2005). Mexican/Mexican American adolescents and keepin' it REAL: An evidence-based substance use prevention program. *Children and Schools, 27*, 133–145.

LaFromboise, T. (1996). *American Indian life skills development curriculum*. Madison: University of Wisconsin Press.

LaFromboise, T. D., & Howard-Pitney, B. (1994). The Zuni life skills development curriculum: A collaborative approach to curriculum development. *American Indian and Alaska Native Mental Health Research, 4*, 98–121. http://search.proquest.com/docview/618528491?accountid=14026.

LaFromboise, T. D., & Howard-Pitney, B. (1995). The Zuni life skills development curriculum: Description and evaluation of a suicide prevention program. *Journal of Counseling Psychology, 42*, 479–486. doi:10.1037/0022-0167.42.4.479.

LaFromboise, T. D., & Lewis, H. A. (2008). The Zuni life skills development program: A school/community-based suicide prevention intervention. *Suicide and Life-Threatening Behavior, 38*, 343–353. doi:10.1521/suli.2008.38.3.343.

LaFromboise, T. D., & Malik, S. S. (2012, May). *Development of the American Indian Life Skills Curriculum: Middle School Version*. Poster presentation, Second Biennial conference of the society for the psychological study of ethnic minority issues. Ann Arbor, MI.

Lagana, M. T. (2004). Protective factors for inner-city adolescents at risk of school dropout: Family factors and social support. *Children & Schools, 26*, 211–220. doi:10.1093/cs/26.4.211.

Lewinsohn, P. M., & Essau, C. A. (2002). Depression in adolescents. In I. H. Gotlib & C. L. Hammen (Eds.), *Handbook of depression* (pp. 541–559). New York: Guilford.

Lipson, S. K. (2014). A comprehensive review of mental health gatekeeper-trainings for adolescents and young adults. *International Journal of Adolescent Medicine and Health, 26*, 309–320. doi:10.1515/ijamh-2013-0320.

LoMurray, M. (2005). *Sources of strength facilitators guide: Suicide prevention peer gatekeeper training*. Bismarck: The North Dakota Suicide Prevention Project.

Luxton, D. D., June, J. D., & Fairall, J. M. (2012). Social media and suicide: A public health perspective. *American Journal of Public Health, 102*, S195–S200. doi:10.2105/AJPH.2011.300608.

Lyon, M. E., Benoit, M., O'Donnell, R. M., Getson, P. R., Silber, T., & Walsh, T. (2000). Assessing African American adolescents risk for suicide attempts: Attachment theory. *Adolescence, 35,* 121–134. http://search.proquest.com/docview/619481509?accountid=14026.

Matlin, S. L., Molock, S. D., & Tebes, J. K. (2011). Suicidality and depression among African American adolescents: The role of family and peer support and community connectedness. *American Journal of Orthopsychiatry, 81,* 108–117. doi:10.1111/j.1939-0025.2010.01078.x.

McKenzie, K. (2012). Suicide studies in ethnic minorities: Improving the science to help develop policy. *Ethnicity & Health, 17,* 7–11. doi:10.1080/13557858.2012.678306.

McManama O'Brien, K. H., Becker, S. J., Spirito, A., Simon, V., & Prinstein, M. J. (2013). Differentiating adolescent suicide attempters from ideators: Examining the interaction between depression severity and alcohol use. *Suicide and Life-Threatening Behavior, 44,* 23–33. doi:10.1111/sltb.12050.

National Center for Injury Prevention and Control. (2005). WISQARS fatal injuries: Mortality reports. http://webapp.cdc.gov/sasweb/ncipc/mortrat.html. Accessed 16 June 2005.

Nock, M. K., Green, J. G., Hwang, I., McLaughlin, K. A., Sampson, N. A., Zaslavsky, A. M., & Kessler, R. C. (2013). Prevalence, correlates, and treatment of lifetime suicidal behavior among adolescents. *JAMA Psychiatry, 70,* 300–310. doi:10.1001/2013.jamapsychiatry.55.

O'Donnell, L., Stueve, A., Wardlaw, D., & O'Donnell, C. (2003). Adolescent suicidality and adult support: The reach for health study of urban youth. *American Journal of Health Behavior, 27,* 633–644.

O'Keeffe, G. S., & Clarke-Pearson, K. (2011). The impact of social media on children, adolescents, and families. *Pediatrics, 127,* 800–804. doi:10.1542/peds.2011-0054.

Pena, J. B., Matthieu, M. M., Zayas, L. H., Masyn, K. E., & Caisne, E. D. (2012). Co-occurring risk behaviors among White, Black, and Hispanic US high school adolescents with suicide attempts requiring medical attention, 1999–2007: Implications for future prevention initiatives. *Social Psychiatry and Epidemiology, 47,* 29–42.

Pirkis, J., Blood, R. W., Beautrais, A., Burgess, P., & Skehan, J. (2006). Media guidelines on the reporting of suicide. *Crisis: The Journal of Crisis Intervention and Suicide Prevention, 27,* 82–87. doi:10.1027/0227-5910.27.2.82.

Portes, A., & Rumbaut, R. G. (2006). *Immigrant America: A portait* (3rd ed.). Berkeley: University of California Press.

Quinnett, P. (1995). *QPR: Ask a question, save a life.* Spokane: The QPR Institute at www.qprinsitute.com.

Robinson, J., Cox, G., Malone, A., Williamson, M., Baldwin, G., Fletcher, K., & O'Brien, M. (2013). A systematic review of school-based interventions aimed at preventing, treating, and responding to suicide-related behavior in young people. *Crisis: The Journal of Crisis Intervention and Suicide Prevention, 34,* 164–182. doi:10.1027/0227-5910/a000168.

Rubenstein, J. L., Halton, A., Kasten, L., Rubin, C., & Stechler, G. (1998). Suicidal behavior in adolescents: Stress and protection in different family contexts. *American Journal of Orthopsychiatry, 68,* 274–284. doi:10.1037/h0080336.

Russell, S. T., & Joyner, K. (2001). Adolescent sexual orientation and suicide risk: Evidence from a national study. *American Journal of Public Health, 91,* 1276–1281. doi:10.2105/AJPH.91.8.1276.

Saigh, P. A., & Umar, A. M. (1983). The effects of a good behavior game on the disruptive behavior of Sudanese elementary school students. *Journal of Applied Behavior Analysis, 16,* 339–344. doi:10.1901/jaba.1983.16-339.

South, S. J., Haynie, D. L., & Bose, S. (2005). Residential mobility and the onset of adolescent sexual activity. *Journal of Marriage and Family, 67,* 499–514. doi:10.1111/j.0022-2445.2005.00131.x.

Stack, S. (2003). Media coverage as a risk factor in suicide. *Journal of Epidemiology and Community Health, 57,* 238–240. doi:10.1136/jech.57.4.238.

Storr, C. L., Ialongo, N. S., Kellam, S. G., & Anthony, J. C. (2002). A randomized controlled trial of two primary school intervention strategies to prevent early onset tobacco smoking. *Drug and Alcohol Dependence, 66,* 51–60. doi:10.1016/S0376-8716(01)00184-3.

Thompson, E. A., Eggert, L. L., Randell, B. P., & Pike, K. C. (2001). Evaluation of indicated suicide risk prevention approaches for potential high school dropouts. *American Journal of Public Health, 91*, 742–752. doi:0.2105/AJPH.91.5.742.

Thompson, E. A., Mazza, J. J., Herting, J. R., Randell, B. P., & Eggert, L. (2005). The mediating roles of anxiety, depression, and hopelessness on adolescent suicidal behaviors. *Suicide and Life-Threatening Behavior, 35*, 14–34. doi:10.1521/suli.35.1.14.59266.

Tompkins, T. L., Witt, J., & Abraibesh, N. (2010). Does a gatekeeper suicide prevention program work in a school setting? Evaluating training outcome and moderators of effectiveness. *Suicide and Life-Threatening Behavior, 40*, 506–515. doi:10.1521/suli.2010.40.5.506.

van Geel, M., Vedder, P., & Tanilon, J. (2014). Relationship between peer victimization, cyberbullying, and suicide in children and adolescents: A meta-analysis. *JAMA Pediatrics, 168*, 435–442. doi:10.1001/jamapediatrics.2013.4143.

Waldrop, A. E., Hanson, R. F., Resnick, H. S., Kilpatrick, D. G., Naugle, A. E., & Saunders, B. E. (2007). Risk factors for suicidal behavior among a national sample of adolescents: Implications for prevention. *Journal of Traumatic Stress, 20*, 869–879.

Wallace, J. M., Bachman, P. M., O'Malley, P. M., Schulenberg, J. E., Cooper, S. M., & Johnston, L. D. (2003). Gender and ethnic differences in smoking, drinking, and illicit drug use among American 8th, 10th, and 12th grade students, 1976–2000. *Addiction, 98*, 225–234.

Watt, T. T., & Sharp, S. F. (2001). Gender differences in strains associated with suicidal behavior among adolescents. *Journal of Youth and Adolescence, 30*, 333–348. doi:10.1023/A:1010444212607.

White, J., & Morris, J. (2010). Precarious spaces: Risk, responsibility and uncertainty in school-based suicide prevention programs. *Social Science & Medicine, 71*, 2187–2194.

Winterrowd, E., & Canetto, S. S. (2013). The long-lasting impact of adolescents' deviant friends on suicidality: A 3-year follow-up perspective. *Social Psychiatry and Psychiatric Epidemiology, 48*, 245–255. doi:10.1007/s00127-012-0529-2.

Winterrowd, E., Canetto, S. S., & Chavez, E. L. (2010). Friendships and suicidality among Mexican American adolescent girls and boys. *Death Studies, 34*, 641–660. doi:10.1080/07481181003765527.

Wong, S. S., Zhou, B., Goebert, D., & Hishenuma, S. (2013). The risk of adolescent suicide across patterns of drug use: A national representative study of high school students in the United States from 1999 to 2009. *Social Psychiatry and Psychiatric Epidemiology, 48*, 1611–1620. doi:10.1007/s00127-013-0721-z.

Wyman, P. A., Brown, C. H., Inman, J., Cross, W., Schmeelk-Cone, K., Guo, J., & Pena, J. B. (2008). Randomized trial of a gatekeeper program for suicide prevention: 1-year impact on secondary school staff. *Journal of Consulting and Clinical Psychology, 76*, 104–115. doi:10.1037/0022-006X.76.1.104.

Ybarra, M. L., Espelage, D. L., & Mitchell, K. J. (2014). Differentiating youth who are bullied from other victims of peer-aggression: The importance of differential power and repetition. *Journal of Adolescent Health, 55*, 293–300. doi:10.1016/j.jadohealth.2014.02.009.

Yoder, K. A., & Hoyt, D. R. (2005). Family economic pressure and adolescent suicidal ideation: Application of the family stress model. *Suicide and Life-Threatening Behavior, 35*, 251–264. doi:10.1521/suli.2005.35.3.251.

Yoder, K. A., Whitbeck, L. B., Hoyt, D. R., & LaFromboise, T. (2006). Suicidal ideation among American Indian youths. *Archives of Suicide Research, 10*, 177–190.

Zayas, L., Lester, R., Cabassa, L., & Fortuna, L. (2005). Why do so many Latina teens attempt suicide? A conceptual model for research. *American Journal of Orthopsychiatry, 75*, 275–287. doi:10.1037/0002-9432.75.2.275.

Chapter 17
Dropout Prevention: A Previously Intractable Problem Addressed Through Systems for Monitoring and Supporting Students

Elaine Allensworth

Students who fail to graduate from high school have substantially worse long-term health, social, and economic outcomes in life than students who obtain a high school degree (Belfield and Levin 2007). The economic costs of dropping out are severe and have become worse over the last 30 years, with dropouts earning dramatically less income and being more likely to experience unemployment than ever before compared to high school graduates (Day and Newburger 2002; Heckman and LaFontaine 2007; Sum et al. 2009; US Department of Labor, Bureau of Labor Statistics 2013a). Following the recession of 2008, the unemployment rate of high school graduates was more than double that of college graduates (US Department of Labor, Bureau of Labor Statistics 2013b). Dropouts also have a much higher risk of incarceration than high school graduates (Harlow 2003; Sum et al. 2009). Dropouts are less likely than graduates to have health insurance and more likely to make poor health decisions; they are less likely to exercise regularly, more likely to be obese, more likely to smoke, more likely to become teenage parents, and less likely to wear seat belts or engage in preventative care, such as flu shots or cancer screenings (Centers for Disease Control and Prevention 2008; Cutler and Lleras-Muney 2006; Manlove 1998; McLanahan 2009; Pleis and Lucas 2009). As a result, high school graduates tend to be healthier and live longer than dropouts (Currie 2009; Cutler and Lleras-Muney 2006; Wong et al. 2002). Thus, dropout prevention is at the intersection between issues that public school educators and prevention scientists care deeply about. It is also a problem for which preventative measures can pay big dividends.

The scope of the problem is large. More than one fifth of US students fail to graduate from high school. Despite increasingly negative life outcomes for high school dropouts, trends in graduation rates had been mostly flat or declining for 40 years, declining since the 1960s and picking up only in the last few years (Heckman and LaFontaine 2007; Murnane 2013; US Department of Education (USDE),

E. Allensworth (✉)
University of Chicago Consortium on Chicago School Research,
1313 E. 60th St., Chicago, IL 60637, USA
e-mail: elainea@ccsr.uchicago.edu

© Springer Science+Business Media New York 2015
K. Bosworth (ed.), *Prevention Science in School Settings*,
Advances in Prevention Science, DOI 10.1007/978-1-4939-3155-2_17

National Center for Education Statistics 2013; Warren and Halpern-Manners 2007). Racial-ethnic minority students are particularly unlikely to graduate; nationally, graduation rates for Black and Hispanic students were 64 and 67%, respectively, in 2010 compared to 81% for white students, and boys are less likely to graduate than girls (US Department of Education (USDE), National Center for Education Statistics n.d.). Graduation rates for African American and Latino boys are at about 57 and 63%, respectively. Graduation rates are so low in some high schools that they were deemed "dropout factories" in an influential 2004 report on the dropout crisis. In these schools, students were more likely to drop out than to graduate. Located primarily in urban school districts and in the South, these schools served half of the nation's African American students and nearly 40% of Latino students in the country (Balfanz and Legters 2004).

The good news is that graduation rates have been improving in the last several years. While graduation rates had been fairly flat for many years—hovering between 71 and 74% since 1990—the last 2 years for which the Department of Education has put out statistics (2009 and 2010) have shown an improvement to 78% (US Department of Education 2013). The number of "dropout factories" declined from about 2000 schools in 2002 to about 1500 in 2010, and about 200,000 fewer students are enrolled in these schools (Balfanz et al. 2012). However, these improvements have been uneven. Some states and school districts have shown double-digit improvements in graduation rates, while others have barely changed.

Chicago is one place that has seen substantial improvements. In 1992, with district graduation rates at about 48%, Chicago students were about as likely to drop out as to graduate (Luppescu et al. 2011). Now, students in Chicago are twice as likely to graduate as to drop out, with graduation rates at 69% in 2014. Improvements in graduation rates have particularly accelerated over the last 5 years, and they are forecast to reach 80% in the next 5 years, based on the academic performance of current Chicago high school students (Emanuel and Byrd-Bennett 2013). These improvements in graduation rates occurred despite no improvements in students' tested skills upon entering high school and occurred among all races/ethnicities and income groups, and in both boys and girls. High school educators in many Chicago schools have transformed their approach to the problem of student dropout. The district is one of many using data to systematically drive improvements in students' educational attainment, by identifying students who need support and providing the right type of support when they need it.

17.1 High School Dropout Used to Be Viewed as a Problem That Was Almost Impossible to Address

A decade ago, little was known about how to reduce dropout rates. The causes of the problem were attributed to myriad factors affecting students outside of school and in the years prior to high school. Family history, peers, health, mobility, neighborhood crime, and resources all played a role, as did students' academic skills, success, and engagement throughout the primary, elementary, and middle-grade years (Alexander et al. 2003; Finn 1989; Rumberger 2004; Rumberger and Larson 1998). Though it is informative to know all of the different factors associated with high school dropout, such a broad perspective makes the problem of dropping out impossible for high schools to address. If its causes are located in so many factors that are outside of school, or occur many years prior to high school, there seems to be little that high schools can do.

Furthermore, there was no clear way to identify students who should be targeted for interventions. Even though many variables were related to dropout, none was a precise predictor of who would drop out, making it difficult to target intervention. Even models that considered multiple risk factors together resulted in poor prediction with much misclassification. Research highlighted the fact that intervention was difficult because it was not possible to accurately predict who was at risk (Gleason and Dynarski 2002). For example, statistical models that try to predict graduation status using some of the variables identified as having significant relationships with dropout—students' eighth-grade reading and math test scores, gender, race, age on entering high school (a marker of grade retention), socioeconomic status, neighborhood poverty, and school mobility—correctly classify only 65 % of students as dropouts or graduates, and such models identify only a quarter of eventual dropouts as being at greater than a 50 % chance of dropping out (Allensworth and Easton 2007). Such identification challenges made intervention problematic.

As a result, intervention programs often focused on students who were very likely to drop out. Nobody wants to spend money on interventions for students who would do fine without intervention. Dropout prevention programs often targeted students who failed half of their classes or missed large numbers of days of school. Yet, by the time students are failing half of their classes or showing frequent absences, their probability of graduating is less than 5 % (Allensworth and Easton 2007). Even if an intervention could double or triple students' likelihood of graduating, they would still be extremely unlikely to graduate. At the same time, many students at risk of dropping out were not correctly identified for intervention. Consider this—in schools with dropout rates at 50 % or higher, the *typical* student is at risk of not graduating. On average in this country, a *quarter* of students are at risk of not graduating—not just a small group of students who are extremely different from others. Yet, dropout prevention programs are often designed as add-on programs to be implemented with small groups of students. In schools where very few students fail to graduate, this approach makes sense. But in typical schools, and particularly in schools with very high dropout rates, schools need much more systematic approaches to improving graduation rates.

17.1.1 Early Identification Is Possible, Based on Students' Course Performance

In recent years, research has shown that early identification is possible (Allensworth and Easton 2005, 2007; Bruce et al. 2011; Gwynne et al. 2009; Neild et al. 2007). The availability of longitudinal student-level data systems and research on student course performance tied to dropout have shown that early identification can be done accurately by monitoring students' attendance and course grades in the first year of high school. A study in Chicago showed that each semester "F" grade a student received in ninth grade lowered the probability of graduating by 15 percentage points; and each week of absence per semester in the ninth-grade year lowered the probability of graduating by 25 percentage points (Allensworth and Easton 2007). Some students can even be identified as at high risk much earlier than ninth grade; these are students who are absent 20 % of school days or more, or receiving failing course grades in English or math, at any time in the middle grades (Allensworth et al. 2014; Balfanz et al. 2007; Neild and Balfanz 2006). It is rare for a student to drop out without first showing other signs of disengagement, such as increasing absences or failing classes over multiple years. Almost all dropouts begin the process of dropping out through absences and failure to complete assignments. Yet, because the process is slow and occasional absences or missed assignments seem insignificant, there is often little attempt to intervene before students fall too far behind to catch up.

In their first year in high school, Chicago students' graduation status can be predicted with 80 % accuracy, based on their attendance, course grades, or pass rates (Allensworth and Easton 2007). Any of those indicators is vastly better at predicting graduation than students' test scores, economic status, race/ethnicity, gender, mobility, and age-for-grade, variables which together correctly predict graduation status only 65 % of the time. By combining all of this background information with students' course grades into one model, the prediction of who will graduate improves by just 1 percentage point—from 80 to 81 %. In other words, once school personnel know whether a student is passing his or her classes in ninth grade, all the other background information about that student does not give substantially more information about whether he or she will graduate. This does not mean that background factors do not matter. Instead, it suggests that these background factors influence high school graduation by affecting students' performance in their classes. Graduation requires accumulating enough course credits to obtain a diploma. Most students drop out after failing too many classes to obtain sufficient credits; this happens after spending several years in high school.

While myriad factors in students' lives—from their academic skills to their health, income, and family background—affect their persistence in school, these factors affect persistence indirectly, through students' performance in their classes. Rather than having to monitor and address all the factors that could potentially interfere with students' performance in school, school personnel just need to know when these factors are interfering with students' course performance—and that is something they can easily monitor. This takes the problem from one that is outside of the realm of schools to one that is fully tied to their core mission.

17.1.2   Students Often Fall Off-Track to Graduation During School Transitions

Some students can be identified as at high risk for dropping out very early, by sixth grade (Allensworth et al. 2014; Balfanz et al. 2007). These are largely students with chronic absences in the middle grades and before as well as those with course failures or suspensions in the middle-grade years. Yet, many future dropouts do not show signs of trouble until high school. The ninth-grade year is a crucial transition. Studies from across the country have documented large declines in student engagement and grades during the high school transition (Benner and Graham 2009; Roderick and Camburn 1999; Seidman et al. 1996; Simmons and Blyth 1987). In Chicago, students' grades decline, on average, by half of a grade point average (GPA) point between eighth and ninth grades (Rosenkranz et al. 2014). Chicago is a district with many schools serving grades K–8, meaning there is no middle school transition. In districts with middle schools or junior high schools, many students also show a decline with that transition. For vulnerable students, this can mean an earlier decline in grades, attendance, and course pass rates. In Philadelphia, for example, about half of eventual dropouts could be identified during middle school through early warning indicators (less than 80 % attendance, failing grades in math or English, an out-of-school suspension; Balfanz et al. 2007; Neild and Balfanz 2006). In Chicago, only 5 % of eventual dropouts show such poor course performance before the ninth grade (Allensworth et al. 2014).

School transitions are challenging for students. On average, students' grades, attendance, and attitudes toward school decline in the transition to middle school, junior high school, or high school (Crockett et al. 1989; Eccles et al. 1991; Feldlaufer et al. 1988; Felner et al. 1982; Schulenberg et al. 1984; Seidman et al. 1994; Simmons et al. 1991). Urban and minority students are particularly vulnerable to large declines in school engagement, with many experiencing large increases in absenteeism and course failure during school transition years (Reyes et al. 1994; Roderick 1993; Seidman et al. 1994; Simmons et al. 1991). Once students start failing courses, they get further and further behind, until they realize they will not graduate. Most dropouts spend several years in high school, but never succeed in earning sufficient credits to graduate; many never even earn enough credits to move out of the ninth grade. Again, in Philadelphia, one third of dropouts were found never to have accumulated enough credits to move to sophomore standing, even though they had been enrolled in high school for several years (Neild 2009). In Chicago, nearly half (46 %) of students who left high school at age 17 or older had fewer than 5 credits (never having completed ninth grade) after being enrolled for approximately 3 years and 70 % had fewer than ten credits (Roderick and Camburn 1996). Course failure not only prevents students from accumulating the credits they need to eventually graduate, it also can undermine students' sense of self-efficacy and belonging in school. These negative mindsets, in turn, lead to further withdrawal of academic effort, contributing to a downward spiral in performance (Kaplan et al. 1995; Roderick and Camburn 1996). Without adult intervention, there is little recovery from failure (Roderick and Camburn 1999).

17.1.3   School Practices Affect Individual Students' Likelihood of Withdrawal

What is it about the high school environment that leads students to demonstrate dramatically worse academic performance compared to the prior year? A number of changes occur in the school environment, but one striking difference is the change in the degree to which teachers have strong relationships with their students and take responsibility for their success. High schools are usually larger than elementary or middle schools, with new academic and social expectations and less personal attention or adult support (Lee et al. 1993). The typical high school teacher sees more than 100 students a day, for only about 40 minutes at a time, with no knowledge of where those students are for the remainder of the school day. As a result, there are very large drops in the degree to which students say they trust their teachers and receive personal support or attention (Farrington et al. 2012). Students are able to fall progressively further behind without any significant intervention from adults. In a study we conducted in Chicago on the transition to ninth grade, we found that the most striking difference students noticed in high school compared to eighth grade was that they were "free" to go to class or get their work done—nobody made them do it, and they were allowed to simply fall behind in their courses (Rosenkranz et al. 2014). Other researchers have noticed the same pattern (Farrington et al. 2012). Whether they face problems with health, family crises, or peer conflicts, the impersonal nature of high school makes it relatively easy to disengage when these other issues become important.

Although most students show declining grades, attendance, and pass rates when they enter high school, the pattern is not universal and varies considerably depending on the particular high school or middle-grade school students enter. Schools with strong teacher–student relationships tend to have greater student engagement, reduced absences, better pass rates, higher GPAs, and better graduation rates (Allensworth and Easton 2007; Kahne et al. 2006; Pittman and Haughwout 1987; Rosenkranz et al. 2014; Wasley et al. 2000). The relationships students have with teachers and other adults at their high school provide motivation to come to school and support for academic learning and persistence (Akey 2006; Croninger and Lee 2001; Lee and Burkam 2003; Roderick 2003). Punitive practices around discipline can worsen attendance and effectiveness of discipline, and undermine student relationships with school staff. Schools that make frequent use of suspensions have more negative school climates and less student trust of teachers than do schools serving similar students that use fewer punitive measures (Steinberg et al. 2011).

In response to growing awareness of the challenges of the ninth-grade transition and the need to build stronger relationships between students and school staff, educators have made a number of attempts to redesign schools so that their structure makes it easier to provide personalized support for students. Several of these models have shown substantial success using structures such as student advisories and small learning communities to increase teachers' contact with and responsibility for smaller groups of students (Galassi et al. 1997; Herlihy and Quint 2006; Van Ryzin 2010). For example, the Talent Development High School (TDHS) model houses freshmen in a separate "Ninth Grade Success Academy," which facilitates relationship building between students and teachers and provides support to handle a challenging curriculum. A rigorous evaluation of this model showed that it produced higher attendance, course passage, and promotion rates (Kemple et al. 2005). A number of districts have attempted to replace large, anonymous high schools with smaller schools specifically designed to promote stronger relationships between students and faculty. Such initiatives in Chicago and in New York produced improvements in students' reports of academic and personal support, better attendance, and higher graduation rates (Bloom and Unterman 2013; Kahne et al. 2006; Sporte and de la Torre 2010).

Other successful efforts have used adult advocates to provide academic, personal, and social support to students, helping them to address whatever their barriers are to succeeding in school. Two programs that have been successful at improving course pass rates, attendance, and progress toward graduation assign students to mentors who monitor their attendance, behavior, and grades and intervene as soon as problems are identified (Dynarski et al. 2008). In one of these, the Achievement for Latinos Through Academic Success (ALAS) program, adults worked with high-risk Latino middle-grade students to build trusting relationships, attend to their individual needs, and monitor and assist student progress (Larson and Rumberger 1995). With the other program, Check and Connect, adult advocates closely monitored the academic performance of at-risk middle-grade students, provided support, developed conflict resolution skills, and found recreational and service opportunities (Lehr et al. 2004; Sinclair, Christenson and Thurlow 2005).

Schools with high dropout rates need strategies for reaching all of their students, not just those at high risk, by systematically changing the way they support students through the transition to high school. Many schools across the country are now using early warning indicator systems with "real time" data on student performance to make it easy for existing school staff to identify students in need of support and provide them help before it is too late (Dynarski et al. 2008; Neild et al. 2007). There are a number of technological challenges involved in collecting the data and making it available to local practitioners in a timely manner and easy-to-use format, but a number of schools, districts, and states across the country have successfully done so (Bruce et al. 2011). Once these data are available, schools can develop their own local solutions to supporting students, based on each student's level and type of risk. New York City recently engaged in a set of strategies to combat absenteeism across all grade levels, using early warning flags to identify students for intervention, monitor their progress, connect them to mentors, and link community resources to schools. They were successful at improving attendance, and as students' school attendance improved, so did their academic achievement (Balfanz and Byrnes 2013). In Chicago, early warning indicator reports have transformed the ways practitioners support students, with incredible payoff for students' persistence and achievement in school.

17.2 Early Warning Systems Have Successfully Improved Ninth-Grade Achievement in Chicago, and More Students Are Graduating

Fifteen years ago, efforts to reduce high school dropout rates in Chicago seemed to be going nowhere. When school practitioners discussed the problem, conversations tended to focus on students with extremely difficult problems—those returning from incarceration or teens who were pregnant and parenting. Yet, these groups of students were only a very small percentage of school dropouts. Dropout prevention programs at that time were targeted at students who failed half or more of their classes or those who had already dropped out of school and showed very low success rates. The first step in changing practices was to show that it was not just the students with extremely difficult circumstances who were at risk for dropping out. Research came out showing that large numbers of students who seemed to be doing fine in the eighth grade often failed classes when they got to high school (Roderick 2003). Further research showed that even students with just one or two semester course failures in ninth grade were actually at high risk of eventually not graduating, and many of these students entered high school with strong academic skills as measured on tests (Allensworth and Easton 2005). Because these students were not very far behind in ninth grade, especially compared to students failing half of their classes, and many had good test scores, they had rarely been seen as in need of intervention. The new evidence indicated that these students were, in fact, exhibiting warning signals years in advance of leaving school, that the warning signals came from students' attendance and grades rather than their test scores, and that the ninth-grade year was a critical point for intervention.

The school district responded to the research by starting to hold schools accountable for their ninth-grade "on-track" to graduation rates. The on-track metric was a simple indicator of whether students were making basic progress in their ninth-grade year—failing no more than one semester of a core course and accumulating sufficient credits to move on to the tenth grade. However, schools did not yet have strategies for improving ninth-grade failure rates. The on-track rate reports came out at the end of the school year, after students had finished ninth grade, and provided little information about how schools could change their practices to improve ninth-grade achievement.

Then, another study was released, which showed that schools could use data that was available early in the ninth-grade year to identify students' risk of eventual dropout; specifically, information such as attendance and first-quarter grades was highly predictive of graduation 4 years later (Allensworth and Easton 2007). The district responded by developing a system of "hot" data reports for high schools that allowed them to quickly identify which students needed what kinds of support (Ali et al. 2010). In the first year, a few schools started to use the data reports and saw improvements in their ninth-grade pass rates; others tried strategies that were not successful. In the second year, more schools figured out successful strategies for using the data reports. By the third year, more schools showed improvements. Successful strategies spread from school to school, facilitated in some cases by the Network for College Success, an external partner that worked with school leadership teams to help them use their data reports. Successful practices also spread when school staff and administrators took jobs in different schools. Schools did not use standardized approaches to supporting students in ninth grade; instead, they figured out individualized strategies for using the data reports to address the particular needs in their school (Roderick et al. 2014).

Chicago Public Schools' Department of Graduation Pathways developed three types of data reports intended to provide tools that would enable school staff to develop systems for providing support to the students who needed it and keep students from falling through the cracks. One tool was designed to identify incoming high school students who would likely need support, based on their middle-grade academic performance. Another was designed for early intervention—to identify students who showed signs of failure or withdrawal during the ninth-grade year, which enabled staff to reach out early enough to prevent students from failing. The third was designed for recovery—to get students back on track after they failed (Ali et al. 2010).

The first data tool, the "Freshmen Watchlist," alerted high school personnel to which of their incoming ninth graders were at risk of failure so that they could reach out to them over the summer before high school. Some schools used summer programs to establish relationships with students and give them an opportunity to begin earning high school credit before the school year began. One school, for example, invited incoming ninth graders to participate in summer school and activities such as cheerleading and basketball, as an introduction to high school. This allowed incoming students to get to know older students, while school staff working as "on-track coordinators" were able to establish positive relationships with incoming students before the school year started. These preexisting relationships then made it easier for the on-track coordinators to reach out to students during the school year if their attendance slipped, in a way that was seen as positive and supportive rather than punitive.

After the first quarter of the academic year, school leaders received the second data report, called the "Freshmen Success Report," which was similar to the Freshman Watchlist but based on students' ninth-grade performance. This report listed each student by name, flagging those students who had high absences, low course grades (Ds), or course failures during the quarter. The report also showed all students' grades in each of their core courses. Updated monthly for the remainder of the year, the Freshmen Success Report allowed immediate intervention with students whose attendance was lagging. Counselors could easily identify which students were failing or close to failing their classes throughout the year and could develop targeted intervention strategies based on how many courses a student was failing as well as his or her attendance and test scores. Using the reports, teachers could get together and talk about specific students, examining which classes students were struggling in, across the teacher teams. They could then develop coherent messages and plans for working with a particular student across multiple classes and could share information about how to reach students who might be succeeding in some classes and failing in others.

After each semester ended, the district put out a "Credit Recovery" report showing how many and which students needed to make up failed credits, across all grades. Although school-building educators could have produced such information by digging through their files to see who had failed each semester and who had not yet made up the credits, the reports streamlined identification of who needed to make up credits, and which credits needed to be recovered, across all students in the school. School administrators need this information to know which types of classes should be offered and scheduled. A comprehensive list of who needs to make up which credits also helps counselors reach out to all students who need a particular credit to make sure that every student is working to recover needed credits.

This system of data tools allowed school staff to systematically target students for intervention. Having a system that identified students in need of intervention and showed why they were at risk made it much less likely for students to fall through the cracks. In schools where teacher teams met to discuss the success reports, teachers had to confront questions about why students were failing their classes and make plans to reach out to those students. In schools where a counselor or an on-track coordinator was designated to monitor success and recovery reports, students with poor attendance and grades no longer went unnoticed. The counselor could reach out to students, their parents, and their teachers to find out what was happening and put together a plan for the student. The reports moved the problem of course failure from in the level of individual classrooms to something that was a shared responsibility among teachers and school staff.

These reports also changed the nature of relationships between struggling students and school staff as teachers began to see it as their responsibility to reach out to students who were falling behind and find out what they needed to succeed (Allensworth 2013).[1] Reaching out helped teachers to realize that their students were not failing because they did not care about passing, but because they had barriers that interfered with their success in the class. Rather than seeing their job responsibility as strictly teaching math or English—focusing on the content of the course—they reinterpreted their job as assisting students to succeed in their math class or their English class—focusing on the student as a learner. Teachers' different mindset carried over to all students, not just those who were failing, and they began

---

[1] For an example of one successful high school and how its staff has dramatically increased student progress to graduation, see the featured segment on Hancock High School at http://chicagotonight. wttw.com/2013/11/21/american-graduate-special.

reaching out when any student's performance slipped to find out what was happening. When schools started working on improving on-track rates, grades increased at both ends of the spectrum: fewer students failed and more students received As and Bs (Roderick et al. 2014).

Data tools based on individual students are useful for developing intervention strategies and reaching those students who need help. Ultimately, however, schools need to identify structural issues that are leading to low performance among large groups of students if they are to make substantial progress in getting more students on track to graduate. To this end, high schools also received data reports that showed patterns in ninth-grade performance data over time, which could be used to determine whether particular groups of students were struggling and which types of students had responded to previous efforts. They also received reports showing students' responses to surveys about issues such as school safety and teacher support—elements of climate that had been shown to be related to student attendance and engagement in school (see Chap. 12). Using data reports to inform practice is often a struggle for school personnel. However, a number of Chicago high schools were working with the Network for College Success, which brought researchers and school leadership teams together to look at these data reports, analyze the patterns for school improvement planning, and share successful strategies for working with different groups of students. Looking at data from other schools helped school leaders gain insight into how to strengthen their own schools and provided a strong community for sharing practices. In the end, the schools that were part of the Network for College Success showed some of the most dramatic improvements in student performance in the district, and members of those school leadership teams became leaders in changing practices districtwide.

Student progress in high school and graduation rates have improved considerably in Chicago since the district began issuing these individual student data reports in 2008–2009. In the years prior to the 2008–2009 school year, less than 60% of freshmen passed enough classes in their ninth-grade year to be on track to graduate. Then, during the 2008–2009 school year, the percentage of students with sufficient credits to be on track to graduate increased substantially, to 64%. In the following year, on-track-to-graduate rates rose again, to 69%, and in the following year to 73%, and then to 85% among students who entered high school in the 2012–2013 school year. Graduation rates among seniors who had entered high school in 2008–2009 were the highest ever, at 65.4%. The success is continuing in later cohorts as more students are making it to higher grades than ever before.

At the same time, students seem to be learning more while in school. More students than ever are making it to the end of the 11th grade to take the American College Testing (ACT), and test scores have not declined despite more students taking the test. In fact, 11th-grade ACT scores have increased, even though the test scores of students entering the ninth grade have been flat (Luppescu et al. 2011). Paying attention to student attendance and effort in their courses seems to pay off not only in preventing failure but also in getting students to learn more in school.

17.2.1 Schools Serving Highly Disadvantaged Communities Have a Particularly Acute Need for Strong Organization and Systems to Monitor and Support Students

Problems with attendance and poor course performance are not a result simply of students not wanting to come to school but result from a combination of factors pushing and pulling students away from strong engagement in their courses (Rumberger 2004). Most of the "dropout factory" schools in the country serve impoverished communities. Poverty undermines student performance in many ways. It makes school attendance difficult through housing instability, family stress, family health problems, and transportation challenges. Students miss school and fail to complete assignments not only when they are sick but also because they may be taking care of a sick family member or may lack bus fare or clean clothes to wear to school. Crime in students' residential neighborhoods can bring gang problems into schools, make students afraid of other students, raise concerns about being caught up in fights or violence at or around the school, and lead to psychological trauma from witnessing violence, all of which inhibit school engagement (Steinberg et al. 2011). Some schools serve a large concentration of students who have undergone extraordinarily adverse events, with a quarter or more of the students having histories of abuse or neglect and homelessness (Bryk et al. 2010). Student attendance and achievement are particularly difficult to improve in schools where so many students and their families are struggling with extremely stressful and draining problems. When faced with such serious issues, school demands seem a lower priority. A day of class missed here, an assignment there, can seem insignificant until too many missed classes and assignments build up and students become stuck too far behind to catch up.

For schools with small-to-moderate dropout rates, it may be sufficient to have systems in place for monitoring students and plans for how regular school staff can support those who struggle or to have mentoring programs to support the students who are most in need. The more students living in deep poverty, or with a history of low achievement, a school serves, the greater the need for systems and resources to sufficiently address problems with high school dropout. Schools do not all face the same degree of difficulty, or the same problems, in providing services to students. Once schools, districts, and states start keeping data on student performance and monitoring early warning indicators, it is possible to assess the needs of the students in each school and develop plans for addressing them. Some schools will have a greater need for mentors, social workers, and health and mental health care providers than others to address the problems that students face. At many schools, staff may realize they need to collaborate with health-care providers, safety and law enforcement officers, or transportation providers to address the problems that are most prevalent in their particular community.

17.2.2   Systems for Monitoring and Support Make It Possible for Practitioners to Support Students

When high school dropout is viewed as a problem rooted in the struggles of individual children, it is an impossible problem to solve. When viewed as a problem of the design of schools as systems, it becomes solvable—if time and resources available for intervention are commensurate with the level of need across schools. Multiple systems for monitoring and intervention together potentially could dramatically reduce dropout and increase rates of high school graduation.

Systems in the elementary and middle grades, to increase attendance among students with chronic absenteeism, for instance, could provide early intervention to the students at greatest risk. Students and their families face different barriers to getting to school every day, and if they have not figured out how to do so by the middle grades, they will continue to struggle with attendance in high school. These struggles are likely to become more pronounced as students get older and have more responsibility for getting themselves to school. Often, school staff do not even realize they have a substantial problem with chronic absenteeism until they start to track absences (Balfanz and Byrnes 2012). Early warning systems in the middle grades that flag students based on attendance, grades, and behaviors could be used to provide support to students before they arrive in high school and begin to fail classes.

The transition to high school makes students vulnerable to failure, even if they did not show signs of academic failure in the middle grades. Ninth-grade monitoring systems can identify students who are starting to disengage from school before they fail classes. These systems are the most critical component for improving graduation rates as they affect the largest number of students and can lead to substantial improvements without substantial cost. Besides having strong systems for monitoring students, schools can prevent students from struggling in the first place by working to create a safe, orderly environment and structuring the school in ways that encourage the development of supportive relationships between students and keep them from missing their classes. There are many ways schools can address systematic problems with low attendance or failure, or poor levels of trust between students or teachers, once they start to recognize such patterns in their data. For example, one school in Chicago noticed high absence rates in the first period of the day so they programmed students to have only electives first period; another had a problem with ninth graders skipping their last class in order to leave with upperclassmen, so they scheduled ninth-grade classes to have a different bell schedule at the end of the day. Another school wanted to emphasize the importance of attendance among teachers and parents, so they required teachers to call home every time a student missed class to make sure the student knew the course assignments and to encourage attendance (Rosenkranz et al. 2014). There is increasing recognition that school disciplinary practices, which exclude students from instruction (e.g., suspension), can lead students to fall behind in school. Schools can minimize the use of exclusionary disciplinary practices by using alternatives such as restorative justice or Saturday school in place of suspension (Losen and Gillespie 2012).

Some issues that interfere with students' performance in school can be addressed directly by teachers in the building. Other issues stem from stresses outside of school, such as a child's physical or mental illness, illness in the family, or problems resulting from severe poverty. Community partnerships and coordination of services across sectors, including health, transportation, housing, and public safety, could give school personnel greater access to resources to immediately help students when family and personal issues interfere in school. Once school staff start identifying the issues their students are facing, they can figure out the partnerships that are most needed for the population they serve. Some students face specific and difficult barriers to graduation, such as involvement with the criminal justice system, pregnancy/parenting, or beginning high school very old for grade. Schools can be prepared with systems in place for students who have critical specific needs.

Finally, recovery systems can help to get students who have failed classes back on track to graduate before they accumulate too many failures to catch up and to find alternative pathways for students who cannot graduate with their peers. Often, this is where efforts to combat high school dropout start, with students who already have dropped out or are about to do so. But it is easier to get students back on track to graduation if they have not failed many courses. It is easier to find an alternative pathway to graduation for students who already have a fair number of credits toward graduation. It is easier to dedicate intensive resources to a few students who have fallen off track than to thousands of students who are unlikely to make it. The more districts reframe the dropout problem from a recovery problem to a prevention problem, the closer it is to being solved.

References

Akey, T. M. (2006). *School context, student attitudes and behavior, and academic achievement: An exploratory analysis.* New York: MDRC.

Alexander, K. L., Entwisle, D. R., & Dauber, S. L. (2003). *On the success of failure: A reassessment of the effects of retention in the primary grades.* Cambridge: Cambridge University Press.

Ali, K., Basley, J., Flores, Q., Goud, L., Jackson, M. K., Jones, I., & Thomas, R. (2010). *Freshmen on-track: A guide to help you keep your freshmen on-track to graduate.* Chicago: Chicago Public Schools, Department of Graduation Pathways. http://www.chooseyourfuture.org/sites/default/files/fot-freshmen-on-track-handbook.pdf.

Allensworth, E. M. (2013). The use of ninth-grade early warning indicators to improve Chicago schools. *Journal of Education for Students Placed at Risk, 18*(1), 68–83. doi:10.1080/10824669.2013.745181.

Allensworth, E. M., & Easton, J. Q. (2005). *The on-track indicator as a predictor of high school graduation.* Chicago: University of Chicago Consortium on Chicago School Research.

Allensworth, E. M., & Easton, J. Q. (2007). *What matters for staying on-track and graduating in Chicago public high schools: A close look at course grades, failures, and attendance in the freshman year.* Chicago: University of Chicago. Consortium on Chicago School Research.

Allensworth, E. M., Gwynne, J., Moore, P., & de la Torre, M. (2014). *Looking forward to high school and college: Middle school indicators of readiness in Chicago public schools.* Chicago: University of Chicago Consortium on Chicago School Research.

Balfanz, R., & Byrnes, V. (2012). *The importance of being in school: A report on absenteeism in the nation's public schools*. Baltimore: Johns Hopkins University Center for Social Organization of Schools.

Balfanz, R., & Byrnes, V. (2013). *Meeting the challenge of combating chronic absenteeism: Impact of the New York City Mayor's interagency task force on chronic absenteeism and school attendance and its implications for other cities*. Baltimore: Everyone Graduates Center at Johns Hopkins University.

Balfanz, R., & Legters, N. (2004). *Locating the dropout crisis: Which high schools produce the nation's dropouts? Where are they located? Who attends them?* Baltimore: Center for Research on the Education of Students Placed At Risk.

Balfanz, R., Herzog, L., & MacIver, D. J. (2007). Preventing student disengagement and keeping students on the graduation path in urban middle-grades schools: Early identification and effective interventions. *Educational Psychologist, 42*(4), 223–235. doi:10.1080/00461520701621079.

Balfanz, R., Bridgeland, J. M., Bruce, M., & Fox, J. H. (2012). *Building a grad nation report: Progress and challenge in ending the high school dropout epidemic*. Washington, DC: America's Promise Alliance, Civic Enterprises, and Everyone Graduates Center at Johns Hopkins University. http://www.americaspromise.org/Our-Work/Grad-Nation/Building-a-Grad-Nation.aspx.

Belfield, C., & Levin, H. (Eds.). (2007). *The price we pay: Economic and social consequences of inadequate education*. Washington, DC: Brookings Institution.

Benner, A. D., & Graham, S. (2009). The transition to high school as a developmental process among multiethnic urban youth. *Child Development, 80*(2), 356–376. doi:10.1111/j.1467-8624.2009.01265x.

Bloom, H., & Unterman, R. (2013). *Sustained progress: New findings about the effectiveness and operation of small public high schools of choice in New York City*. New York: MDRC.

Bruce, M., Bridgeland, J., Fox, J. H., & Balfanz, R. (2011). *On-track for success: The use of early warning indicator and intervention systems to build a grad nation*. Baltimore: Civic Enterprises and the Everyone Graduates Center at Johns Hopkins University.

Bryk, A. S., Sebring, P. B., Allensworth, E. M., Luppescu, S., & Easton, J. Q. (2010). *Organizing schools for improvement: Lessons from Chicago*. Chicago: University of Chicago Press.

Centers for Disease Control and Prevention. (2008). *National Health Interview Survey, 2007*. Atlanta: Centers for Disease Control and Prevention.

Crockett, L. J., Petersen, A., Graber, J., Schulenberg, J. E., & Ebata, A. (1989). School transitions and adjustment during early adolescence. *Journal of Early Adolescence, 9*(3), 181–210.

Croninger, R. B., & Lee, V. E. (2001). Social capital and dropping out of high school: Benefits to at-risk students of teachers' support and guidance. *Teachers College Record, 103*(4), 548–581.

Currie, J. (2009). Healthy, wealthy, and wise: Socioeconomic status, poor health in childhood, and human capital development. *Journal of Economic Literature, 47*(1), 87–122. doi:10.1257/jel.47.1.87.

Cutler, D. M., & Lleras-Muney, A. (2006). *Education and health: Evaluating theories and evidence (NBER Working Paper No. 12352)*. Cambridge: National Bureau of Economic Research.

Day, J., & Newburger, E. (2002). *The big payoff: Educational attainment and synthetic estimates of work-life earnings (Report P23-210)*. Washington, DC: U.S. Census Bureau.

Dynarski, M., Clarke, L., Cobb, B., Finn, J., Rumberger, R., & Smink, J. (2008). *Dropout prevention: A practice guide* (NCEE 2008–4025). Washington, DC: National Center for Education Evaluation and Regional Assistance, Institute of Education Sciences, U.S. Department of Education. http://ies.ed.gov/ncee/wwc.

Eccles, J. S., Lord, S., & Midgley, C. (1991). What are we doing to early adolescents? The impact of educational contexts on early adolescents. *American Journal of Education, 99*(4), 521–542. doi:10.1086/443996.

Emanuel, R., & Byrd-Bennett, B. (2013, December 13). An education worthy of Chicago's children: Mayor and schools chief challenge outdated perceptions of CPS. *Chicago Tribune*. http://articles.chicagotribune.com/2013-12-13/opinion/ct-emanuel-byrd-bennett-cps-education-perception-s-20131213_1_cps-schools-chicago-public-schools-mayor-and-schools-chief.

Farrington, C. A., Roderick, M., Allensworth, E. M., Nagaoka, J., Seneca Keyes, T., Johnson, D. W., & Beechum, N. O. (2012). *Teaching adolescents to become learners: The role of noncognitive factors in shaping school performance.* Chicago: University of Chicago Consortium on Chicago School Research.

Feldlaufer, H., Midgley, C., & Eccles, J. (1988). Student, teacher, and observer perceptions of the classroom environment before and after the transition to junior high school. *Journal of Early Adolescence, 8*(2), 133–156.

Felner, R. D., Ginter, M., & Primavera, J. (1982). Primary prevention during school transitions: Social support and environmental structure. *American Journal of Community Psychology, 10*(3), 277–290.

Finn, J. D. (1989). Withdrawing from school. *Review of Educational Research, 59*(2), 117–142.

Galassi, J. P., Gulledge, S. A., & Cox, N. D. (1997). Middle school advisories: Retrospect and prospect. *Review of Educational Research, 67*(3), 301–338. doi:10.3102/00346543067003301.

Gleason, P., & Dynarski, M. (2002). Do we know whom to serve? Issues in using risk factors to identify dropouts. *Journal of Education for Students Placed at Risk, 7*(1), 25–41. doi:10.1207/S15327671ESPR0701_3.

Gwynne, J., Lesnick, J., Hart, H. M., & Allensworth, E. M. (2009). *What matters for staying on-track and graduating in Chicago public schools: A focus on students with disabilities.* Chicago: University of Chicago Consortium on Chicago School Research.

Harlow, C. W. (2003). *Education and correctional populations (Bureau of Justice Statistics Special Report, NCJ 195670).* Washington, DC: U.S. Department of Justice. http://www.policyalmanac.org/crime/archive/education_prisons.pdf.

Heckman, J. J., & LaFontaine, P. A. (2007). *The American high school graduation rate: Trends and levels (NBER Working Paper No. 13670).* Cambridge: National Bureau of Economic Research. http://www.nber.org/papers/w13670.

Herlihy, C. M., & Quint, J. (2006). *Emerging evidence on improving high school student achievement and graduation rates: The effects of four popular improvement programs.* Washington, DC: National High School Center.

Kahne, J. E., Sporte, S., de la Torre, M., & Easton, J. Q. (2006). *Small schools on a larger scale: The first three years of the Chicago High School Redesign Initiative.* Chicago: University of Chicago Consortium on Chicago School Research.

Kaplan, D. S., Peck, B. M., & Kaplan, H. B. (1995). Decomposing the academic failure—dropout relationship: A longitudinal analysis. *Journal of Educational Research, 90*(6), 331–343.

Kemple, J. J., Herlihy, C. M., & Smith, T. J. (2005). *Making progress toward graduation: Evidence from the Talent Development High School Model.* New York: MDRC.

Larson, K. A., & Rumberger, R. W. (1995). ALAS: Achievement for Latinos through academic success. In H. Thornton (Ed.), *Staying in school: A technical report of the dropout prevention projects for junior high school students with learning and emotional disabilities (pp. A-1–A-71).* Minneapolis: University of Minnesota, Institute on Community Integration. http://raiseinspiredkids.com/files/alas_program/ALASFinalReportPart 1.pdf.

Lee, V. E., & Burkam, D. T. (2003). Dropping out of high school: The role of school organization and structure. *American Educational Research Journal, 40*(2), 353–393. doi:10.3102/00028312040002353.

Lee, V. E., Bryk, A. S., & Smith, J. B. (1993). The organization of effective secondary schools. *Review of Research in Education, 19,* 171–267.

Lehr, C. A., Sinclair, M. F., & Christenson, S. L. (2004). Addressing student engagement and truancy prevention during the elementary school years: A replication study of the check & connect model. *Journal of Education for Students Placed at Risk, 9*(3), 279–301. doi:10.1207/s15327671espr0903_4.

Losen, D. J., & Gillespie, J. (2012). *Opportunities suspended: The disparate impact of disciplinary exclusion from school.* Los Angeles: Civil Rights Project.

Luppescu, S., Allensworth, E. M., Moore, P., de la Torre, M., Murphy, J., & Jagesic, S. (2011). *Trends in Chicago's schools across three eras of reform.* Chicago: University of Chicago Consortium on Chicago School Research.

Manlove, J. (1998). The influence of high school dropout and school disengagement on the risk of school-age pregnancy. *Journal of Research on Adolescence, 8*(2), 187–220. doi:10.1207/s15327795jra0802_2.

McLanahan, S. (2009). Fragile families and the reproduction of poverty. *Annals of the American Academy of Political and Social Science, 621,* 111–131. doi:10.1177/0002716208324862.

Murnane, R. J. (2013). U.S. high school graduation rates: Patterns and explanations. *Journal of Economic Literature, 51*(2), 370–422. doi:10.1257/jel.51.2.370.

Neild, R. C. (2009). Falling off track during the transition to high school: What we know and what can be done. *Future of Children, 19*(1), 53–76.

Neild, R. C., & Balfanz, R. (2006). *Unfulfilled promise: The dimensions and characteristics of Philadelphia's dropout crisis, 2000–2005.* Philadelphia: Philadelphia Youth Transitions Collaborative.

Neild, R. C., Balfanz, R., & Herzog, L. (2007). An early warning system. *Educational Leadership, 65*(2), 28–33.

Pittman, R. B., & Haughwout, P. (1987). Influence of high school size on dropout rate. *Educational Evaluation & Policy Analysis, 9*(4), 337–343.

Pleis, J. R., & Lucas, J. W. (2009). *Summary health statistics for U.S. adults: National Health Interview Survey, 2007* (Vital and Health Statistics, series 10, no. 240). http://www.cdc.gov/nchs/data/series/sr_10/sr10_240.pdf.

Reyes, O., Gillock, K., & Kobus, K. (1994). A longitudinal study of school adjustment in urban, minority adolescents: Effects of a high school transition program. *American Journal of Community Psychology, 22*(3), 341–369.

Roderick, M. (1993). *The path to dropping out: Evidence for intervention.* Westport: Greenwood Publishing Group.

Roderick, M. (2003). What's happening to the boys? Early high school experiences and school outcomes among African American male adolescents in Chicago. *Urban Education, 33*(5), 538–607. doi:10.1177/0042085903256221.

Roderick, M., & Camburn, E. (1996). Academic difficulty during the high school transition. In P. B. Sebring, A. S. Bryk, M. Roderick & E. Camburn (Eds.), *Charting reform in Chicago: The students speak.* Chicago: University of Chicago Consortium on Chicago School Research.

Roderick, M., & Camburn, E. (1999). Risk and recovery from course failure in the early years of high school. *American Educational Research Journal, 36*(2), 303–343. doi:10.3102/00028312036002303.

Roderick, M., Kelley-Kemple, T., Johnson, D. W., & Beechum, N. (2014). *Preventable failure: Improvements in long-term outcomes when high schools focused on the ninth grade year.* Chicago: University of Chicago Consortium on Chicago School Research.

Rosenkranz, T., de la Torre, M., Stevens, W. D., & Allensworth, E. M. (2014). *Free to fail: Why grades drop when students enter high school and what adults can do about it.* Chicago: University of Chicago Consortium on Chicago School Research.

Rumberger, R. (2004). Why students drop out of school. In G. Orfield (Ed.), *Dropouts in America* (pp. 131–156). Cambridge: Harvard Education Press.

Rumberger, R. W., & Larson, K. A. (1998). Student mobility and the increased risk of high school dropout. *American Journal of Education, 107*(1), 1–35. doi:10.1086/444201.

Schulenberg, J. E., Asp, C. E., & Petersen, A. C. (1984). School from the young adolescent's perspective: A descriptive report. *Journal of Early Adolescence, 4*(2), 107–130.

Seidman, E., LaRue, A., Aber, L. J., Mitchell, C., & Feinman, J. (1994). The impact of school transitions in early adolescence on the self-system and perceived social context of poor urban youth. *Child Development, 65*(2), 507–522. doi:10.2307/1131399.

Seidman, E., Aber, J. L., LaRue, A., & French, S. E. (1996). The impact of the transition to high school on the self-system and perceived social context of poor urban youth. *American Journal of Community Psychology, 24*(4), 489–515. doi:10.1007/BF02506794.

Simmons, R. G., & Blyth, D. A. (1987). *Moving into adolescence: The impact of pubertal change and school context.* Beverly Hills: Sage.

Simmons, R. G., Black, A., & Zhou, Y. (1991). African American versus White children and the transition into junior high school. *American Journal of Education, 99*(4), 481–520.

Sinclair, M. F., Christenson, S. L., & Thurlow, M. L. (2005). Promoting school completion of urban secondary youth with emotional or behavioral disabilities. *Exceptional Children, 71*(4), 465–482.

Sporte, S. E., & de la Torre, M. (2010). *Chicago High School Redesign Initiative: Schools, students, and outcomes.* Chicago: University of Chicago Consortium on Chicago School Research.

Steinberg, M., Allensworth, E. M., & Johnson, D. W. (2011). *Student and teacher safety in Chicago schools: The roles of community context and social organization.* Chicago: University of Chicago Consortium on Chicago School Research.

Sum, A., Khatiwada, I., & McLaughlin, J. (2009). *The consequences of dropping out of high school: Joblessness and jailing for high school dropouts and the high cost for taxpayers.* Boston: Center for Labor Market Studies, Northeastern University.

U.S. Department of Education (USDE), National Center for Education Statistics. (2013). *The condition of education.* http://nces.ed.gov/programs/coe/indicator_coi.asp.

U.S. Department of Education (USDE), National Center for Education Statistics. (n.d.). NCES Common Core of Data, Local Education Agency Universe Survey Dropout and Completion School Years 2008–09 and 2004–05. http://nces.ed.gov/ccd/tables/AFGR.asp.

U.S. Department of Labor, Bureau of Labor Statistics. (2013a). *Earnings and unemployment rates by educational attainment.* http://www.bls.gov/emp/ep_chart_001.htm.

U.S. Department of Labor, Bureau of Labor Statistics. (2013b). *Labor force statistics from the current population survey.* http://data.bls.gov/cgi-bin/surveymost.

Van Ryzin, M. (2010). Secondary school advisors as mentors and secondary attachment figures. *Journal of Community Psychology, 38*(2), 131–154. doi:10.1002/jcop.20356.

Warren, J. R., & Halpern-Manners, A. (2007). Is the glass emptying or filling up? Reconciling divergent trends in high school completion and dropout. *Educational Researcher, 36*(6), 335–343. doi:10.3102/0013189X07306580.

Wasley, P., Fine, M., Gladden, M., Holland, N. E., King, S. P., Mosak, E., & Powell, L. C. (2000). *Small schools: Great strides: A study of new small schools in Chicago.* New York: Bank Street College of Education.

Wong, M., Shapiro, M., Boscardin, W., & Ettner, S. (2002). Contribution of major diseases to disparities in mortality. *New England Journal of Medicine, 347*(20), 1585–1592. doi:10.1056/NEJMsa012979.

Index

© Springer Science+Business Media New York 2015
K. Bosworth (ed.), *Prevention Science in School Settings*,
Advances in Prevention Science, DOI 10.1007/978-1-4939-3155-2

Printed in the United States
By Bookmasters